MONOGRAPH
STATISTICS AND APPLIE... .... Y

General Editors

D.R. Cox, V. Isham, N. Keiding,
N. Reid, and H. Tong

1 Stochastic Population Models in Ecology and Epidemiology
M.S. Bartlett (1960)
2 Queues *D.R. Cox and W.L. Smith* (1961)
3 Monte Carlo Methods *J.M. Hammersley and D.C. Handscomb* (1964)
4 The Statistical Analysis of Series of Events *D.R. Cox and P.A.W. Lewis* (1966)
5 Population Genetics *W.J. Ewens* (1969)
6 Probability, Statistics and Time *M.S. Bartlett* (1975)
7 Statistical Inference *S.D. Silvey* (1975)
8 The Analysis of Contingency Tables *B.S. Everitt* (1977)
9 Multivariate Analysis in Behavioural Research *A.E. Maxwell* (1977)
10 Stochastic Abundance Models *S. Engen* (1978)
11 Some Basic Theory for Statistical Inference *E.J.G. Pitman* (1979)
12 Point Processes *D.R. Cox and V. Isham* (1980)
13 Identification of Outliers *D.M. Hawkins* (1980)
14 Optimal Design *S.D. Silvey* (1980)
15 Finite Mixture Distributions *B.S. Everitt and D.J. Hand* (1981)
16 Classification *A.D. Gordon* (1981)
17 Distribution-free Statistical Methods, 2nd edition *J.S. Maritz* (1995)
18 Residuals and Influence in Regression *R.D. Cook and S. Weisberg* (1982)
19 Applications of Queueing Theory, 2nd edition *G.F. Newell* (1982)
20 Risk Theory, 3rd edition *R.E. Beard, T. Pentikainen and E. Pesonen* (1984)
21 Analysis of Survival Data *D.R. Cox and D. Oakes* (1984)
22 An Introduction to Latent Variable Models *B.S. Everitt* (1984)
23 Bandit Problems *D.A. Berry and B. Fristedt* (1985)
24 Stochastic Modelling and Control *M.H.A. Davis and R. Vinter* (1985)
25 The Statistical Analysis of Compositional Data *J. Aitchison* (1986)
26 Density Estimation for Statistics and Data Analysis *B.W. Silverman* (1986)
27 Regression Analysis with Applications *G.B. Wetherill* (1986)

28 Sequential Methods in Statistics, 3rd edition
   G.B. Wetherill and K.D. Glazebrook (1986)
29 Tensor Methods in Statistics *P. McCullagh* (1987)
30 Transformation and Weighting in Regression *R.J. Carroll and
   D. Ruppert* (1988)
31 Asymptotic Techniques for Use in Statistics *O.E. Barndorff-Nielsen
   and D.R. Cox* (1989)
32 Analysis of Binary Data, 2nd edition *D.R. Cox and E.J. Snell* (1989)
33 Analysis of Infectious Disease Data *N.G. Becker* (1989)
34 Design and Analysis of Cross-over Trials *B. Jones and
   M.G. Kenward* (1989)
35 Empirical Bayes Methods, 2nd edition *J.S. Maritz and T. Lwin* (1989)
36 Symmetric Multivariate and Related Distributions *K.-T. Fang
   S. Kotz and K.W. Ng* (1990)
37 Generalized Linear Models, 2nd edition *P. McCullagh and
   J.A. Nelder* (1989)
38 Cyclic and Computer Generated Designs, 2nd edition
   J.A. John and E.R. Williams (1995)
39 Analog Estimation Methods in Econometrics *C.F. Manski* (1988)
40 Subset Selection in Regression *A.J. Miller* (1990)
41 Analysis of Repeated Measures *M.J. Crowder and D.J. Hand* (1990)
42 Statistical Reasoning with Imprecise Probabilities *P. Walley* (1991)
43 Generalized Additive Models *T.J. Hastie and R.J. Tibshirani* (1990)
44 Inspection Errors for Attributes in Quality Control
   N.L. Johnson, S. Kotz and X. Wu (1991)
45 The Analysis of Contingency Tables, 2nd edition *B.S. Everitt* (1992)
46 The Analysis of Quantal Response Data *B.J.T. Morgan* (1993)
47 Longitudinal Data with Serial Correlation: A State-space Approach
   R.H. Jones (1993)
48 Differential Geometry and Statistics *M.K. Murray
   and J.W. Rice* (1993)
49 Markov Models and Optimization *M.H.A. Davis* (1993)
50 Networks and Chaos – Statistical and Probabilistic Aspects
   *O.E. Barndorff-Nielsen,
   J.L. Jensen and W.S. Kendall* (1993)
51 Number-theoretic Methods in Statistics *K.-T. Fang
   and Y. Wang* (1994)
52 Inference and Asymptotics *O.E. Barndorff-Nielsen
   and D.R. Cox* (1994)
53 Practical Risk Theory for Actuaries *C.D. Daykin, T. Pentikäinen
   and M. Pesonen* (1994)

54 Biplots *J.C. Gower and D.J. Hand* (1996)
55 Predictive Inference: An Introduction *S. Geisser* (1993)
56 Model-Free Curve Estimation *M.E. Tarter and M.D. Lock* (1993)
57 An Introduction to the Bootstrap *B. Efron and R.J. Tibshirani* (1993)
58 Nonparametric Regression and Generalized Linear Models
   P.J. Green and B.W. Silverman (1994)
59 Multidimensional Scaling *T.F. Cox and M.A.A. Cox* (1994)
60 Kernel Smoothing *M.P. Wand and M.C. Jones* (1995)
61 Statistics for Long Memory Processes *J. Beran* (1995)
62 Nonlinear Models for Repeated Measurement Data *M. Davidian
   and D.M. Giltinan* (1995)
63 Measurement Error in Nonlinear Models *R.J. Carroll, D. Ruppert
   and L.A. Stefanski* (1995)
64 Analyzing and Modeling Rank Data *J.I. Marden* (1995)
65 Time Series Models – In econometrics, finance and other fields
   D.R Cox, D.V. Hinkley and O.E. Barndorff-Nielsen (1996)
66 Local Polynomial Modeling and Its Applications *J. Fan and
   I. Gijbels* (1996)
67 Multivariate Dependencies – Models, analysis and interpretation
   D.R. Cox and N. Wermuth (1996)
68 Statistical Inference – Based on the likelihood *A. Azzalini* (1996)
69 Bayes and Empirical Bayes Methods for Data Analysis
   B.P. Carlin and T.A. Louis (1996)
70 Hidden Markov and Other Models for Discrete-valued Time Series
   I.L. MacDonald and W. Zucchini (1997)
71 Statistical Evidence – A likelihood paradigm *R.M. Royall* (1997)
72 Analysis of Incomplete Multivariate Data *J.L. Schafer* (1997)

(Full details concerning this series are available from the Publishers).

Analysis of Incomplete Multivariate Data

J. L. Schafer
Department of Statistics
The Pennsylvania State University
USA

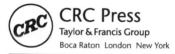

CRC Press
Taylor & Francis Group
Boca Raton London New York

CRC Press is an imprint of the
Taylor & Francis Group, an **informa** business

A CHAPMAN & HALL BOOK

Originally published by Chapman & Hall
First edition 1997

Published 1999 by CRC Press
Taylor & Francis Group
6000 Broken Sound Parkway NW, Suite 300
Boca Raton, FL 33487-2742

First issued in paperback 2022

ISBN 13: 978-1-03-247799-2 (pbk)
ISBN 13: 978-0-412-04061-0 (hbk)

DOI : 10.1201/9780367803025

**Visit the Taylor & Francis Web site at
http://www.taylorandfrancis.com**

**and the CRC Press Web site at
http://www.crcpress.com**

Library of Congress Cataloging-in-Publication Data

Catalog record is available from the Library of Congress.

Contents

Preface   xiii

1 Introduction   1
  1.1 Purpose   1
  1.2 Background   2
    1.2.1 The EM algorithm   3
    1.2.2 Markov chain Monte Carlo   3
  1.3 Why analysis by simulation?   4
  1.4 Looking ahead   6
    1.4.1 Scope of the rest of this book   6
    1.4.2 Knowledge assumed on the part of the reader   7
    1.4.3 Software and computational details   7
  1.5 Bibliographic notes   8

2 Assumptions   9
  2.1 The complete-data model   9
  2.2 Ignorability   10
    2.2.1 Missing at random   10
    2.2.2 Distinctness of parameters   11
  2.3 The observed-data likelihood and posterior   11
    2.3.1 Observed-data likelihood   11
    2.3.2 Examples   13
    2.3.3 Observed-data posterior   17
  2.4 Examining the ignorability assumption   20
    2.4.1 Examples where ignorability is known to hold   20
    2.4.2 Examples where ignorability is not known to hold   22
    2.4.3 Ignorability is relative   23
  2.5 General ignorable procedures   23
    2.5.1 A simulated example   24

2.5.2   Departures from ignorability   26
2.5.3   Notes on nonignorable alternatives   28
2.6   The role of the complete-data model   29
2.6.1   Departures from the data model   29
2.6.2   Inference treating certain variables as fixed   31

3   EM and data augmentation   37
3.1   Introduction   37
3.2   The EM algorithm   37
3.2.1   Definition   37
3.2.2   Examples   41
3.2.3   EM for posterior modes   46
3.2.4   Restrictions on the parameter space   46
3.2.5   The ECM algorithm   49
3.3   Properties of EM   51
3.3.1   Stationary values   51
3.3.2   Rate of convergence   55
3.3.3   Example   59
3.3.4   Further comments on convergence   61
3.4   Markov chain Monte Carlo   68
3.4.1   Gibbs sampling   69
3.4.2   Data augmentation   70
3.4.3   Examples of data augmentation   73
3.4.4   The Metropolis-Hastings algorithm   78
3.4.5   Generalizations and hybrid algorithms   79
3.5   Properties of Markov chain Monte Carlo   80
3.5.1   The meaning of convergence   80
3.5.2   Examples of nonconvergence   80
3.5.3   Rates of convergence   83

4   Inference by data augmentation   89
4.1   Introduction   89
4.2   Parameter simulation   90
4.2.1   Dependent samples   90
4.2.2   Summarizing a dependent sample   93
4.2.3   Rao-Blackwellized estimates   98
4.3   Multiple imputation   104
4.3.1   Bayesianly proper multiple imputations   105
4.3.2   Inference for a scalar quantity   107
4.3.3   Inference for multidimensional estimands   112
4.4   Assessing convergence   118
4.4.1   Monitoring convergence in a single chain   119

	4.4.2	Monitoring convergence with parallel chains	126
	4.4.3	Choosing scalar functions of the parameter	128
	4.4.4	Convergence of posterior summaries	131
4.5	Practical guidelines		134
	4.5.1	Choosing a method of inference	135
	4.5.2	Implementing a parameter-simulation experiment	136
	4.5.3	Generating multiple imputations	138
	4.5.4	Choosing an imputation model	139
	4.5.5	Further comments on imputation modeling	143

5 Methods for normal data   **147**

5.1	Introduction		147
5.2	Relevant properties of the complete-data model		148
	5.2.1	Basic notation	148
	5.2.2	Bayesian inference under a conjugate prior	150
	5.2.3	Choosing the prior hyperparameters	154
	5.2.4	Alternative parameterizations and sweep	157
5.3	The EM algorithm		163
	5.3.1	Preliminary manipulations	163
	5.3.2	The E-step	164
	5.3.3	Implementation of the algorithm	166
	5.3.4	EM for posterior modes	170
	5.3.5	Calculating the observed-data loglikelihood	173
	5.3.6	Example: serum-cholesterol levels of heart-attack patients	175
	5.3.7	Example: changes in heart rate due to marijuana use	178
5.4	Data augmentation		181
	5.4.1	The I-step	181
	5.4.2	The P-step	183
	5.4.3	Example: cholesterol levels of heart-attack patients	185
	5.4.4	Example: changes in heart rate due to marijuana use	189

6 More on the normal model   **193**

6.1	Introduction		193
6.2	Multiple imputation: example 1		193
	6.2.1	Cholesterol levels of heart-attack patients	193
	6.2.2	Generating the imputations	194
	6.2.3	Complete-data point and variance estimates	194

6.2.4   Combining the estimates   197
6.2.5   Alternative choices for the number of impu-
        tations   197
6.3   Multiple imputation: example 2   200
6.3.1   Predicting achievement in foreign language
        study   200
6.3.2   Applying the normal model   202
6.3.3   Exploring the observed-data likelihood and
        posterior   204
6.3.4   Overcoming the problem of inestimability   206
6.3.5   Analysis by multiple imputation   208
6.4   A simulation study   211
6.4.1   Simulation procedures   212
6.4.2   Complete-data inferences   214
6.4.3   Results   216
6.5   Fast algorithms based on factored likelihoods 218
6.5.1   Monotone missingness patterns   218
6.5.2   Computing alternative parameterizations   220
6.5.3   Noniterative inference for monotone data   223
6.5.4   Monotone data augmentation   226
6.5.5   Implementation of the algorithm   229
6.5.6   Uses and extensions   234
6.5.7   Example   236

7   Methods for categorical data   **239**
7.1   Introduction   239
7.2   The multinomial model and Dirichlet prior   240
7.2.1   The multinomial distribution   240
7.2.2   Collapsing and partitioning the multinomial 243
7.2.3   The Dirichlet distribution   247
7.2.4   Bayesian inference   250
7.2.5   Choosing the prior hyperparameters   251
7.2.6   Collapsing and partitioning the Dirichlet   255
7.3   Basic algorithms for the saturated model   257
7.3.1   Characterizing an incomplete categorical
        dataset   257
7.3.2   The EM algorithm   260
7.3.3   Data augmentation   264
7.3.4   Example: victimization status from the
        National Crime Survey   267
7.3.5   Example: Protective Services Project for
        Older Persons   272

7.4   Fast algorithms for near-monotone patterns   275
       7.4.1   Factoring the likelihood and prior density   275
       7.4.2   Monotone data augmentation   279
       7.4.3   Example: driver injury and seatbelt use   282

8 Loglinear models   289
   8.1   Introduction   289
   8.2   Overview of loglinear models   289
          8.2.1   Definition   289
          8.2.2   Eliminating associations   292
          8.2.3   Sufficient statistics   294
          8.2.4   Model interpretation   295
   8.3   Likelihood-based inference with complete data   297
          8.3.1   Maximum-likelihood estimation   297
          8.3.2   Iterative proportional fitting   298
          8.3.3   Hypothesis testing and goodness of fit   302
          8.3.4   Example: misclassification of seatbelt use
                  and injury   303
   8.4   Bayesian inference with complete data   305
          8.4.1   Prior distributions for loglinear models 305
          8.4.2   Inference using posterior modes   307
          8.4.3   Inference by Bayesian IPF   308
          8.4.4   Why Bayesian IPF works   312
          8.4.5   Example: misclassification of seatbelt use
                  and injury   318
   8.5   Loglinear modeling with incomplete data   320
          8.5.1   ML estimates and posterior modes   320
          8.5.2   Goodness-of-fit statistics   322
          8.5.3   Data augmentation and Bayesian IPF   324
   8.6   Examples   325
          8.6.1   Protective Services Project for Older Persons 325
          8.6.2   Driver injury and seatbelt use   328

9 Methods for mixed data   333
   9.1   Introduction   333
   9.2   The general location model   334
          9.2.1   Definition   334
          9.2.2   Complete-data likelihood   336
          9.2.3   Example   338
          9.2.4   Complete-data Bayesian inference   339
   9.3   Restricted models   341
          9.3.1   Reducing the number of parameters   341

9.3.2   Likelihood inference for restricted models   344
9.3.3   Bayesian inference   346
9.4   Algorithms for incomplete mixed data   348
9.4.1   Predictive distributions   348
9.4.2   EM for the unrestricted model   352
9.4.3   Data augmentation   355
9.4.4   Algorithms for restricted models   357
9.5   Data examples   359
9.5.1   St. Louis Risk Research Project   359
9.5.2   Foreign Language Attitude Scale   367
9.5.3   National Health and Nutrition Examination
        Survey   372

10 Further topics   379
10.1 Introduction   379
10.2 Extensions of the normal model   379
10.2.1 Restricted covariance structures   379
10.2.2 Heavy-tailed distributions   380
10.2.3 Interactions   380
10.2.4 Semicontinuous variables   381
10.3 Random-effects models   382
10.4 Models for complex survey data   383
10.5 Nonignorable methods   384
10.6 Mixture models and latent variables   384
10.7 Coarsened data and outlier models   385
10.8 Diagnostics   386

Appendices
A   Data examples   387
B   Storage of categorical data   395
C   Software   399

References   401

Index   415

Preface

The last quarter of a century has seen enormous developments in general statistical methods for incomplete data. The EM algorithm and its extensions, multiple imputation and Markov chain Monte Carlo provide a set of flexible and reliable tools for inference in large classes of missing-data problems. Yet, in practical terms, these developments have had surprisingly little impact on the way most data analysts handle missing values on a routine basis. My hope is that this book will help to bridge the gap between theory and practice, making a multipurpose kit of missing-data tools accessible to anyone who may need them.

This book is intended for applied statisticians, graduate students and methodologically-oriented researchers in search of practical tools to handle missing data. The focus is applied rather than theoretical, but technical details have been included where necessary to help readers thoroughly understand the statistical properties of these methods and the behavior of the accompanying algorithms.

The methods presented here rely on three fully parametric models for multivariate data: the unrestricted multivariate normal distribution, loglinear models for cross-classified categorical data and the general location model for mixed continuous and categorical variables. In addition, the missing data are assumed to be missing at random, in the sense defined by Rubin (1976). My reviewers have correctly pointed out that many other vitally important topics could (and perhaps should) have been addressed: non-normal models such as the contaminated normal and multivariate-t; repeated measures and restricted covariance structures; censored and coarsened data; models for nonignorable nonresponse; latent variables; and hierarchical or random-effects models. Imputation for complex surveys and censuses, a topic in which I am deeply interested, deserves much more attention than it received. For better or worse, I decided to limit the material to a few important subjects, but to treat these subjects thoroughly and illustrate them with non-trivial data examples. This book would not have been possible without the generous support and encouragement of many friends, colleagues and agencies. Don Rubin, whose countless contributions to the area of missing data provided a springboard for this work, was the first to suggest publishing it as a book. The initial round of software development was sponsored by Frank Sulloway, whose wonderfully incomplete dataset provided the first and most colorful application of these methods. Additional support was provided by the Bureau of the Census, the United States Department of Agriculture and the National Center for Health Statistics. Many helpful comments and suggestions were given by John Barnard, Rose Brunner, Andrew Gelman, Bonnie Ghosh, Xiao-Li Meng, Susan Murphy, Maren Olsen, Fritz Scheuren, Stef van Buuren, Recai Yucel and Alan Zaslavsky, and the editorial and production staff at Chapman & Hall. Data on the Foreign Language Attitude Scale were contributed by Mark Raymond. My parents, Chester and Dolores Schafer, created a loving and stable childhood environment, and my wife Sharon did not fail to encourage and inspire. Prayer support was provided by Dr. Samuel C. Lee and members of University Bible Fellowship.

Finally, I must acknowledge my debt to the late Clifford C. Clogg, to whom this book is dedicated. Cliff's steady encouragement and careful review greatly improved the quality of the book, especially the first five chapters. His warmth, love for learning, hard work and faith continue to inspire the many who were close to him. Personally and professionally, it is most gratifying to know that Cliff regarded this book as 'good stuff'.

Joseph L. Schafer
University Park, Pennsylvania
October 1996

CHAPTER 1

Introduction

1.1 Purpose

This book presents methods of statistical inference from multivariate datasets with missing values where missingness may occur on any or all of the variables. Such datasets arise frequently in statistical practice, but the tools for effectively dealing with them are not readily available to data analysts. It is our goal to provide these tools, along with the knowledge of how to use them.

When faced with missing values, practitioners frequently resort to ad hoc methods of *case deletion* or *imputation* to force the incomplete dataset into a rectangular complete-data format. Many statistical software packages, for example, automatically omit from a linear regression analysis any case that has a missing value for any variable. Imputation is a generic term for filling in missing data with plausible values. In a multivariate dataset, each missing value may be replaced by the observed mean for that variable, or, in a slightly less naive approach, by some sort of predicted value from a regression model. Almost invariably, after the dataset has been altered by one of these methods no additional provision for missing data is made in the subsequent analysis. The research usually proceeds as if the omitted cases had never really been observed, or as if the imputed values were real data.

When the incomplete cases comprise only a small fraction of all cases (say, five percent or less) then case deletion may be a perfectly reasonable solution to the missing-data problem. In multivariate settings where missing values occur on more than one variable, however, the incomplete cases are often a substantial portion of the entire dataset. If so, deleting them may be inefficient, causing large amounts of information to be discarded. Moreover, omitting them from the analysis will tend to introduce bias, to the extent that the incompletely observed cases differ systematically from the completely observed ones. The completely observed cases that remain will be unrepresentative of the population for which the inference is usually intended: the population of *all* cases, rather than the population of cases with no missing data.

Ad hoc methods of imputation are no less problematic. Imputing averages on a variable-by-variable basis preserves the observed sample means, but it distorts the covariance structure, biasing estimated variances and covariances toward zero. Imputing predicted values from regression models, on the other hand, tends to inflate observed correlations, biasing them away from zero. When the pattern of missingness is complex, devising an ad hoc imputation scheme that preserves important aspects of the joint distribution of the variables can be a daunting task. Moreover, even if the joint distribution of all variables could be adequately preserved, it may be a serious mistake to treat the imputed data as if they were real. Standard errors, p-values and other measures of uncertainty calculated by standard complete-data methods could be misleading, because they fail to reflect any uncertainty due to missing data.

This book presents a unified approach to the analysis of incomplete multivariate data. We will consider datasets for which the variables are continuous, categorical, or both. This approach allows one to analyze the data by virtually any technique that would be appropriate if the data were complete. This is accomplished not by simply modifying the data in an ad hoc fashion to make them appear complete, but by principled methods that account for the missing values, and the uncertainty they introduce, at each step of the analysis in a formal way. These methods tend to be computationally intensive, requiring more computer time than ad hoc alternatives. However, they do not require a heavy investment of analyst time, and can be applied to a wide variety of problems more or less routinely without special efforts to develop new technology unique to each problem. This book is written from an applied perspective, attempting to bring together theory, computational methods, data examples and practical advice in a single source.

1.2 Background

The methods presented here have their origins in two distinct bodies of statistical literature. The first concerns likelihood-based inference with incomplete data and, in particular, the EM algorithm. The second concerns techniques of Markov chain Monte Carlo: Gibbs sampling, data augmentation, the Metropolis-Hastings algorithm, and related methods.

1.2.1 The EM algorithm

The EM algorithm is a general technique for finding maximum-likelihood estimates for parametric models when the data are not fully observed. Although special cases of EM appear far back in the statistical literature, it was not until Dempster, Laird and Rubin (1977) coined the term *EM* and established its fundamental properties that the generality and usefulness of this algorithm were realized. EM spawned a revolution in the analysis of incomplete data, making it possible to compute efficient parameter estimates, and thus obviating the need for ad hoc methods like case deletion, in wide classes of statistical problems.

The influence of EM has been far reaching, not merely as a computational technique, but as a paradigm for approaching difficult statistical problems. There are many statistical problems which, at first glance, may not appear to involve missing data, but which can be reformulated as missing-data problems: mixture models, hierarchical or random effects models, experiments with unbalanced data and many more. In the last fifteen years, a surprisingly large number of applications for EM have been found in a wide variety of fields. Unfortunately, major producers of statistical software have been rather slow to incorporate general-purpose EM algorithms for incomplete data into their products. One notable exception is BMDP, which has EM algorithms for the multivariate normal model and for unbalanced repeated measures with structured covariance matrices (BMDP Statistical Software, Inc., 1992).

1.2.2 Markov chain Monte Carlo

Markov chain Monte Carlo is a body of methods for generating pseudorandom draws from probability distributions via Markov chains. A Markov chain is a sequence of random variables in which the distribution of each element depends on the value of the previous one. As we proceed along the sequence, provided that certain regularity conditions are met, the distributions of the elements stabilize to a common distribution known as the *stationary distribution*. In Markov chain Monte Carlo, one constructs a Markov chain whose stationary distribution is a distribution of interest. By repeatedly simulating steps of the chain, one is able eventually to simulate draws from the distribution of interest.

The two most popular methods of Markov chain Monte Carlo are Gibbs sampling and the Metropolis-Hastings algorithm. In Gibbs sampling (Geman and Geman, 1984; Gelfand and Smith, 1990), one draws from the conditional distribution of each component of a multivariate random variable given the other components in a cyclic fashion. In Metropolis-Hastings (Metropolis *et al.*, 1953; Hastings, 1970), one draws from a probability distribution intended to approximate the distribution actually of interest, and then accepts or rejects the drawn value with a specified probability. Many variations of these are possible, for example, hybrid algorithms that perform steps of Metropolis-Hastings within iterations of Gibbs. These methods are related to more traditional Monte Carlo methods such as importance sampling (e.g. Kleijnan, 1974) and rejection sampling (e.g. Kennedy and Gentle, 1980).

As with EM, specific applications of Markov chain Monte Carlo have been in use for many years, notably in areas of statistical mechanics and image reconstruction. In the past decade, however, many new uses for these methods have been discovered and implemented that are of special interest to statisticians. In particular, Markov chain Monte Carlo has spawned a revolution of its own in the area of applied Bayesian inference.

In Bayesian inference, information about unknown parameters is expressed in the form of posterior probability distribution. Even with relatively simple probability models, the posterior distribution is often intractable: important summaries such as moments, marginal densities and quantiles are not readily available in closed form. Practitioners have typically resorted to asymptotic approximation, numerical integration and importance sampling to elicit meaningful summaries of intractable posteriors. Through Markov chain Monte Carlo, however, it is now possible in many cases to simulate the entire joint posterior distribution of the unknown quantities, and thereby obtain simulation-based estimates of virtually any features of the posterior that are of interest.

1.3 Why analysis by simulation?

Simulation of posterior distributions enjoys many advantages over more traditional methods of parametric inference. Some of these are listed below.

1. In complex problems it may be easier to implement than other methods, both conceptually and computationally.

2. It may be the only method currently feasible when the unknown parameter is of high dimension.

3. It does not rely on asymptotic approximations. The algorithms converge stochastically to posterior distributions that are exact, regardless of sample size.

In an era when computing environments are becoming increasingly powerful and less expensive, simulation promises to be one of the mainstays of applied parametric modeling and data analysis in the years ahead.

Simulation is especially attractive at the present time as a general approach to the analysis of incomplete multivariate data. There are at least two major reasons for this. First, simulation by Markov chain Monte Carlo is a natural companion and complement to the current tools for handling missing data, and, in particular, the EM algorithm. Markov chain Monte Carlo can be applied to precisely the same types of problems as EM, and, computationally speaking, its implementation is often remarkably similar to that of EM. Whereas EM provides only point estimates of the unknown parameters, however, Markov chain Monte Carlo provides random draws from their joint posterior distribution. A point estimate, even if it is efficient, is not especially useful unless there is also some measure of uncertainty associated with it. With Markov chain Monte Carlo, Bayesian analogues of the standard tools of frequentist inference (standard errors, confidence intervals and p-values) are now readily simulated, providing these measures of uncertainty.

A second reason why simulation is a natural choice for missing-data problems is that it facilitates inference by *multiple imputation*. Multiple imputation (Rubin, 1987) is a technique in which each missing value is replaced by $m > 1$ simulated values. The m sets of imputations reflect uncertainty about the true values of the missing data. After the multiple imputations are created, m plausible versions of the complete data exist, each of which are analyzed by standard complete-data methods. The results of the m analyses are then combined to produce a single inferential statement (e.g. a confidence interval or a p-value) that includes uncertainty due to missing data.

Until now, the task of generating multiple imputations has been problematic except in some simple cases, such as univariate examples and datasets with only one variable subject to nonresponse. No straightforward, general-purpose algorithms have been available for generating proper multiple imputations in a multivariate setting. Using techniques of Markov chain Monte Carlo, however, it is now possible to do this quite easily.

Like other methods of inference, simulation based on Markov chains has certain disadvantages. Carrying out a simulation for a large dataset or a complicated model may require access to a fast computer with substantial memory. Monitoring the convergence of Markov chain Monte Carlo algorithms can be difficult. Moreover, the use of the Bayesian paradigm and the introduction of prior distributions for unknown parameters, even if the impact on conclusions is minimal, may be regarded by some as artificial or undesirably subjective. In the chapters ahead, we will try to address these issues carefully and thoughtfully as they arise.

1.4 Looking ahead

This book presents iterative algorithms for simulating multiple imputations of missing values in incomplete datasets under some important classes of multivariate models. The same algorithms may also be used to draw values of parameters from their posterior distributions. The algorithms are described in detail, focusing on practical issues of computation. The computational efficiency and low data-storage requirements of the algorithms make them suitable even for datasets that are quite large, and they have been applied routinely to datasets with over 10 000 observations and 30 variables. The use of these algorithms is demonstrated on a variety of real data examples, with accompanying discussion on issues of practical importance to data analysts.

Because of their good performance, we believe that these algorithms will find widespread use in a variety of applications. We expect that they will become standard supplements to the current tools of missing-data analysis. Perhaps the most important aspect of this work is that now, for the first time, multiple imputation and parameter simulation are made available to nonspecialists who know the importance of adjusting for missing data in their inference, but who lack the resources or special expertise needed to develop and implement these techniques on their own.

1.4.1 Scope of the rest of this book

Chapter 2 presents the key assumptions that will be made throughout this book, the parametric data model and the assumption of ignorable missingness, and discusses their relevance in various applied settings. Chapter 3 presents necessary background material on EM and Markov chain Monte Carlo. Chapter 4 discusses in practical terms the various methods of conducting inference by simulation. The remaining chapters describe algorithms for specific multivariate models and illustrate their use in a variety of examples. Chapters 5-6 discuss methods for the multivariate normal distribution; Chapters 7-8, models for cross-classified categorical data; and Chapter 9, multivariate models for datasets with both continuous and categorical variables.

Chapters 3 and 4 serve as a reference for the subsequent chapters. Readers interested primarily in applications may find it helpful to initially skim through Chapters 3 and 4 and then return to them as necessary while working through Chapters 5-9.

1.4.2 Knowledge assumed on the part of the reader

We assume that the reader is familiar with basic concepts of probability theory, inference based on the likelihood function, and multivariate distributions, especially the multivariate normal and the multinomial. Matrix notation will be used throughout. We assume that the reader is also comfortable with the basic concepts of Bayesian inference, although not necessarily having experience with applying Bayesian techniques in real examples. Some knowledge of standard categorical-data techniques, especially loglinear models, is also helpful but not absolutely necessary.

1.4.3 Software and computational details

The algorithms described in this book have been implemented by the author for general use as functions in the statistical language S (Becker, Chambers, and Wilks, 1988), using subroutines written in Fortran-77. The programs are available to anyone free of charge, and information on them is provided in Appendix C.

As you read this book, especially the later chapters, you may be surprised at the unusual amount of attention devoted to computational issues. Enough detail has been provided to enable a dedicated reader to reinvent the crucial portions of computer programs, if he or she chooses to do so. These details were provided for the following reasons:

1. to encourage others to implement the algorithms in other computer languages or software packages, if they are better served by these environments;

2. to encourage others to improve upon these algorithms, if they discover ways to make them more efficient; and

3. to foster development of similar algorithms for more general classes of models, perhaps using these routines as building blocks for larger and more complex programs.

1.5 Bibliographic notes

A general overview of techniques for missing data, with discussion of various ad hoc approaches as well as the EM algorithm, is given by Little and Rubin (1987). The original article on EM by Dempster, Laird, and Rubin (1977) with discussion, now almost twenty years old, still provides a helpful introduction to EM; its simple examples anticipate many of the major types of EM algorithms in use today. For a comprehensive bibliographic review of EM, see Meng and Pedlow (1992).

Excellent overviews of Markov chain Monte Carlo methods, including data augmentation, Gibbs, sampling, and the Metropolis-Hastings algorithm, appear in books by Tanner (1993) and Gilks, Richardson, and Spiegelhalter (1996). Tanner's book also contains an entire chapter on EM.

A classic introduction to Bayesian inference is given by Box and Tiao (1992), and Gelman *et al.* (1995) discuss practical Bayesian data analysis from a modern perspective.

Good reference material on cross-classified categorical data and loglinear models is given by Bishop, Fienberg and Holland (1975) and Agresti (1990).

CHAPTER 2

Assumptions

2.1 The complete-data model

We will consider rectangular datasets whose rows can be modeled as independent, identically distributed (iid) draws from some multivariate probability distribution. A schematic representation of such a dataset is shown in Figure 2.1. The n rows represent observational units and the p columns represent variables recorded for those units. Missing values, denoted by question marks, may occur in any pattern.

Let Y denote the $n \times p$ matrix of complete data, which is not fully observed, and let y_i denote the ith row of Y, $i = 1, \ldots, n$. By the iid assumption, the probability density or probability function

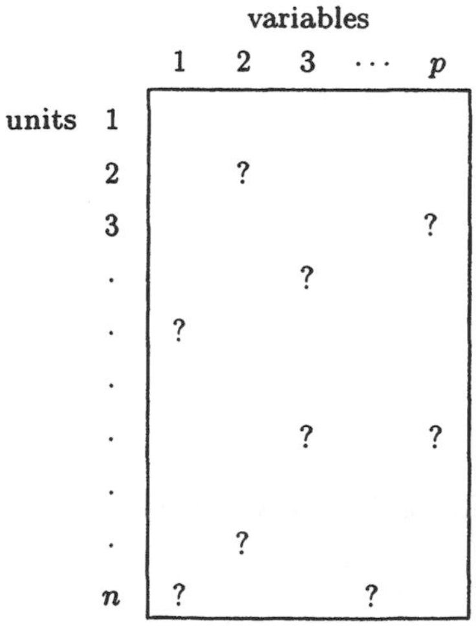

Figure 2.1. *Multivariate dataset with missing values.*

of the complete data may be written

$$P(Y \,|\, \theta) = \prod_{i=1}^{n} f(y_i \,|\, \theta), \qquad (2.1)$$

where f is the density or probability function for a single row, and θ is a vector of unknown parameters. We will consider three classes of distributions f:

1. the multivariate normal distribution;

2. the multinomial model for cross-classified categorical data, including loglinear models; and

3. a class of models for mixed normal and categorical data (Krzanowski, 1980, 1982; Little and Schluchter, 1985).

On occasion, the two crucial modeling assumptions above, that the rows are iid, and that the we have correctly specified (up to the unknown θ) the full joint distribution of all p variables, will not be needed in their entirety and may be partially relaxed. We will sometimes be able to accommodate situations like regression, in which we seek to model the conditional distribution of one or more response variables given some predictor variables without specifying any probability model for the predictors. A discussion of this point will be given in Section 2.6. For now, we turn our attention to the mechanism of missingness.

2.2 Ignorability

2.2.1 Missing at random

Denote the observed part of Y by Y_{obs}, and the missing part by Y_{mis}, so that $Y = (Y_{obs}, Y_{mis})$. Throughout this book, we will assume that the missing data are *missing at random* (MAR) in the sense defined by Rubin (1976).

A precise definition for MAR will be given momentarily, but first we describe it in an informal way: the probability that an observation is missing may depend on Y_{obs} but not on Y_{mis}. Another useful heuristic definition of MAR is the following. Let U and V be any two variables or non-overlapping groups of variables. Suppose that we restrict attention to units for which U is observed and equal to a specific value, say u. MAR means that among these units, the distribution of V is, apart from ordinary sampling variability, the same among the cases for which V is observed as it is among the cases for which V is missing.

Despite its name, then, MAR does not suggest that the missing data values are a simple random sample of all data values. The latter condition is known as *missing completely at random* (MCAR). MCAR is only a special case of MAR. MAR is less restrictive than MCAR because it requires only that the missing values behave like a random sample of all values within subclasses defined by observed data. In other words, MAR allows the probability that a datum is missing to depend on the datum itself, but only indirectly through quantities that are observed.

More formally, Rubin (1976) defines MAR in terms of a probability model for the missingness. Let R be an $n \times p$ matrix of indicator variables whose elements are zero or one depending on whether the corresponding elements of Y are missing or observed. We would not in general expect the distribution of R to be unrelated to Y, so we posit a probability model for R, $P(R|Y, \xi)$, which depends on Y as well as some unknown parameters ξ. The MAR assumption is that this distribution does not depend on Y_{mis},

$$P(R|Y_{obs}, Y_{mis}, \xi) = P(R|Y_{obs}, \xi). \tag{2.2}$$

2.2.2 Distinctness of parameters

To proceed further, we also need to assume that the parameters θ of the data model and the parameters ξ of the missingness mechanism are *distinct*. From a frequentist perspective, this means that the joint parameter space of (θ, ξ) must be the Cartesian cross-product of the individual parameter spaces for θ and ξ. From a Bayesian perspective, this means that any joint prior distribution applied to (θ, ξ) must factor into independent marginal priors for θ and ξ. In many situations this is intuitively reasonable, as knowing θ will provide little information about ξ and vice-versa. If both MAR and distinctness hold, then the missing-data mechanism is said to be *ignorable* (Little and Rubin, 1987; Rubin, 1987).

2.3 The observed-data likelihood and posterior

2.3.1 Observed-data likelihood

Following arguments given by Rubin (1976) and Little and Rubin (1987), it can be shown that under ignorability, we do not need to consider the model for R nor the nuisance parameters ξ when making likelihood-based or Bayesian inferences about θ.

Because the 'observed data' truly consist not only of Y_{obs} but also of R, the probability distribution of the observed data is actually given by

$$P(R, Y_{obs} | \theta, \xi) = \int P(R, Y | \theta, \xi) \, dY_{mis}$$

$$= \int P(R | Y, \xi) P(Y | \theta) \, dY_{mis}, \qquad (2.3)$$

where the integral is understood to mean summation for distributions that are discrete. Under the MAR assumption, (2.3) becomes

$$P(R, Y_{obs} | \theta, \xi) = P(R | Y_{obs}, \xi) \int P(Y | \theta) \, dY_{mis}$$

$$= P(R | Y_{obs}, \xi) P(Y_{obs} | \theta). \qquad (2.4)$$

The likelihood of the observed data under MAR can thus be factored into two pieces, one pertaining to the parameter of interest θ and the other pertaining to the nuisance parameter ξ. When the two parameters are distinct, then likelihood-based inferences about θ will be unaffected by ξ or $P(R | Y_{obs}, \xi)$. Maximum-likelihood estimation of θ, likelihood-ratio tests concerning θ, and so on can then be performed without regard for the missing-data mechanism; that is, the missing-data mechanism may be safely ignored.

The factor in (2.4) pertaining to θ (or, more precisely, any function proportional to this factor) is referred to by Little and Rubin (1987) as the likelihood ignoring the missing-data mechanism,

$$L(\theta | Y_{obs}) \propto P(Y_{obs} | \theta). \qquad (2.5)$$

For brevity, we will refer to (2.5) as the *observed-data likelihood*, although that name should, strictly speaking, be reserved for the complete function (2.4). Because we assume ignorability throughout, however, there is never a need to work with the complete function (2.4), and thus there will be no ambiguity.

Notice that at first glance, the factorization (2.4) seems to contain no implicit assumptions about the missingness mechanism. The joint distribution of any two random variables, say Z_1 and Z_2, can always be written as the marginal distribution of Z_1 multiplied by the conditional distribution of Z_2 given Z_1. A subtle but important difference exists between this basic rule of probability and the factorization (2.4), however, and the distinction lies in the definition of θ. In our framework, θ refers to the parameters of the model for the complete data $Y = (Y_{obs}, Y_{mis})$, not the parameters for the distribution of Y_{obs} alone. We assume that the ultimate goal of the analysis is to draw inferences about the parameters of the complete-data model, not the parameters governing the marginal distribution of Y_{obs}. If θ were re-defined to pertain only to Y_{obs}, then assumptions like MAR would not be necessary. This approach has some major conceptual difficulties, however, and may lead to results that are very hard to interpret, so we will not consider it further. For an interesting discussion related to this point, see the exchange between Efron (1994) and Rubin (1994).

2.3.2 Examples

Example 1: *Incomplete univariate data.* Suppose that a single variable is observed for units $1, 2, \ldots, n_1 < n$ and missing for units $n_1 + 1, \ldots, n$. Let $Y = (y_1, y_2, \ldots, y_n)$ denote the complete data and $R = (r_1, r_2, \ldots, r_n)$ the response indicators, where $r_i = 1$ if y_i is observed and $r_i = 0$ if y_i is missing. If the distribution of R does not depend on Y then the missingness mechanism is MAR. In fact, in this case it is MCAR. One such mechanism is simple Bernoulli selection in which each unit is observed with probability ξ independently of all other units,

$$P(R|Y,\xi) = \prod_{i=1}^{n} \xi^{r_i} (1 - \xi)^{1-r_i}.$$

Another MAR mechanism arises when the responding units are a simple random sample of all units,

$$P(R|Y,\xi) = \begin{cases} \binom{n}{n_1}^{-1} & \text{if } \sum_{i=1}^{n} r_i = n_1, \\ 0 & \text{otherwise.} \end{cases}$$

The latter regards n_1 as fixed whereas the former regards n_1 as random. Under either of these mechanisms or any other mechanism that is MAR, it is appropriate to base inferences about parameters of the distribution of Y on the observed-data likelihood. This likelihood may be written

$$L(\theta|Y_{obs}) = \int P(Y|\theta)\, dY_{mis}$$

$$= \int \cdots \int \prod_{i=1}^{n_1} P(y_i|\theta) \prod_{i=n_1+1}^{n} P(y_i|\theta)\, dy_{n_1+1} \cdots dy_n.$$

The first product in the integrand does not involve Y_{mis} and can be brought out of the integral, and the second product integrates

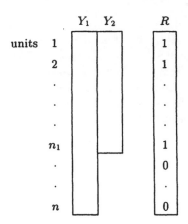

Figure 2.2. *Bivariate data with one variable subject to nonresponse.*

to one, yielding

$$L(\theta \mid Y_{obs}) = \prod_{i=1}^{n_1} P(y_i \mid \theta),$$

which is simply a complete-data likelihood based on the reduced sample $(y_1, \ldots, y_{n_1})$.

Example 2: Bivariate data with one variable subject to nonresponse. Consider a dataset with variables Y_1 and Y_2 as shown in Figure 2.2, where Y_1 is observed for units $1, 2, \ldots, n$ but Y_2 is observed only for units $1, 2, \ldots, n_1 < n$. The missing data will be MAR if the probability that Y_2 is missing does not depend on Y_2, although it may possibly depend on Y_1. Let y_{i1} and y_{i2} denote the values of Y_1 and Y_2, respectively, for unit i. The observed-data likelihood may be written

$$\int \prod_{i=1}^{n_1} P(y_{i1}, y_{i2} \mid \theta) \prod_{i=n_1+1}^{n} P(y_{i1} \mid \theta) \prod_{i=n_1+1}^{n} P(y_{i2} \mid y_{i1}, \theta) \, dY_{mis}.$$

The first two products in the integrand do not involve Y_{mis} and the last product integrates to one, hence

$$L(\theta \mid Y_{obs}) = \prod_{i=1}^{n_1} P(y_{i1}, y_{i2} \mid \theta) \prod_{i=n_1+1}^{n} P(y_{i1} \mid \theta) \quad (2.6)$$

$$= \prod_{i=1}^{n} P(y_{i1} \mid \theta) \prod_{i=1}^{n_1} P(y_{i2} \mid y_{i1}, \theta). \quad (2.7)$$

For example, suppose that Y_1 and Y_2 have a bivariate normal distribution with parameter

$$\theta = (\mu_1, \sigma_{11}, \mu_2, \sigma_{22}, \sigma_{12}),$$

where $\mu_i = E(Y_i \mid \theta)$ and $\sigma_{ij} = \text{Cov}(Y_i, Y_j \mid \theta)$, $i, j = 1, 2$. The observed-data likelihood may be written as in (2.6),

$$L(\theta \mid Y_{obs}) \;\propto\; |\Sigma|^{-n_1/2} \exp\left\{ -\tfrac{1}{2} \sum_{i=1}^{n_1} (y_i - \mu)^T \Sigma^{-1} (y_i - \mu) \right\}$$

$$\times \sigma_{11}^{-(n-n_1)/2} \exp\left\{ -\frac{1}{2\sigma_{11}} \sum_{i=n_1+1}^{n} (y_{i1} - \mu_1)^2 \right\}, \quad (2.8)$$

where $y_i = (y_{i1}, y_{i2})^T$, $\mu = (\mu_1, \mu_2)^T$ and Σ is the 2×2 matrix with elements σ_{ij}. Alternatively, the parameter of the bivariate normal distribution may be expressed as

$$\phi = (\mu_1, \sigma_{11}, \beta_0, \beta_1, \sigma_{22 \cdot 1}),$$

where $\beta_1 = \sigma_{12}/\sigma_{11}$, $\beta_0 = \mu_2 - \beta_1 \mu_1$ and $\sigma_{22 \cdot 1} = \sigma_{22} - \sigma_{12}^2/\sigma_{11}$, so that $E(Y_2 \mid Y_1, \phi) = \beta_0 + \beta_1 Y_1$ and $V(Y_2 \mid Y_1, \phi) = \sigma_{22 \cdot 1}$. The transformation $\phi = \phi(\theta)$ is one-to-one. Following (2.7), the observed-data likelihood may be written in terms of ϕ as

$$L(\phi \mid Y_{obs}) \;\propto\; \sigma_{11}^{-n/2} \exp\left\{ -\frac{1}{2\sigma_{11}} \sum_{i=1}^{n} (y_{i1} - \mu_1)^2 \right\} \quad (2.9)$$

$$\times \sigma_{22 \cdot 1}^{-n_1/2} \exp\left\{ -\frac{1}{2\sigma_{22 \cdot 1}} \sum_{i=1}^{n_1} (y_{i2} - \beta_0 - \beta_1 y_{i1})^2 \right\},$$

an expression first given by Anderson (1957).

Expressions (2.8) and (2.9) are equivalent, but the latter has a convenient interpretation as the product of two complete-data likelihood functions: the univariate normal likelihood for Y_1 based on units $1, 2, \ldots, n$, and the likelihood for the normal linear regression of Y_2 on Y_1 based on units $1, 2, \ldots, n_1$. Because the parameters $\phi_1 = (\mu_1, \sigma_{11})$ and $\phi_2 = (\beta_0, \beta_1, \sigma_{22 \cdot 1})$ corresponding to these two factors are distinct, inferences about them may proceed independently. For example, maximum-likelihood estimates may be obtained by independently maximizing the likelihoods for ϕ_1 and ϕ_2, each of which corresponds to a straightforward complete-data problem. Expression (2.8) also appears to be the product of two complete-data likelihoods, but the parameters in the two factors are not distinct because μ_1 and σ_{11} appear in both.

Example 3: *Multivariate normal data with arbitrary patterns of missing values.* Now consider a p-variate normal data matrix with missing values on any or all variables as in Figure 2.1. It is convenient to group the rows of the matrix according to their missingness patterns. A missingness pattern is a unique combination of response statuses (observed or missing) for $Y_1, Y_2, \ldots, Y_p$. With p variables there are 2^p possible missingness patterns. It is usually the case, especially when p is large, that not all possible patterns are represented in the sample. Index the unique missingness patterns that actually appear in the sample by s, where $s = 1, 2, \ldots, S$, and let $\mathcal{I}(s)$ denote the subset of the rows $i = 1, 2, \ldots, n$ that exhibit pattern s. A generalization of the arguments leading to (2.6) and (2.8) allows us to write the observed-data likelihood as

$$\prod_{s=1}^{S} \prod_{i \in \mathcal{I}(s)} |\Sigma_s^*|^{-1/2} \exp\left\{ -\tfrac{1}{2} (y_i^* - \mu_s^*)^T \Sigma_s^{*-1} (y_i^* - \mu_s^*) \right\}, \quad (2.10)$$

where y_i^* denotes the observed part of row i of the data matrix, and μ_s^* and Σ_s^* denote the subvector of the mean vector μ and the square submatrix of the covariance matrix Σ, respectively, that pertain to the variables that are observed in pattern s. Notice that if any rows of the data matrix are completely missing, then those rows drop out of the observed-data likelihood; under the ignorability assumption, these rows contribute nothing to the inference and may be ignored.

Despite the concise appearance of (2.10), this likelihood tends to be a complicated function of the individual means μ_i and covariances σ_{ij}, $i, j = 1, 2, \ldots, p$. Except in special cases, there is no way to express this likelihood as in (2.7) and (2.9), the product of simple complete-data likelihoods whose parameters are distinct (Rubin, 1974). Moreover, the first two derivatives of (2.10) or its logarithm with respect to the individual μ_i and σ_{ij} tend to be very complicated as well, making (2.10) awkward to maximize by gradient methods such as Newton-Raphson. A much more convenient method for maximizing this likelihood is provided by the EM algorithm (Beale and Little, 1975; Dempster, Laird, and Rubin, 1977), to be introduced in Chapter 3.

The complicated nature of (2.10) is typical of the observed-data likelihood functions one encounters with incomplete multivariate data. Except in special cases, meaningful summaries of these functions (e.g. modes) are not available in closed form, nor are they readily computable from classical numerical methods; we typically need to resort to special iterative techniques like EM.

2.3.3 Observed-data posterior

Definition

In the Bayesian framework all inferences are based on a posterior probability distribution for the unknown parameters that conditions on the quantities that are observed. Returning to the notation of Section 2.3.1, the unknown parameters are (θ, ξ) and the observed quantities are Y_{obs} and R. By Bayes's Theorem, the posterior distribution may be written as

$$P(\theta, \xi \,|\, Y_{obs}, R) = k^{-1} P(R, Y_{obs} \,|\, \theta, \xi)\, \pi(\theta, \xi), \qquad (2.11)$$

where $\pi(\cdot)$ denotes a prior distribution applied to (θ, ξ) and k is the normalizing constant

$$k = \int \int P(R, Y_{obs} \,|\, \theta\xi)\, \pi(\theta, \xi)\, d\theta\, d\xi.$$

Under the assumption of MAR, we may substitute (2.4) into (2.11) to obtain

$$P(\theta, \xi \,|\, Y_{obs}, R) \propto P(R \,|\, Y_{obs}, \xi)\, P(Y_{obs} \,|\, \theta)\, \pi(\theta, \xi).$$

Bayesian inferences about θ alone are based on the marginal posterior obtained by integrating this function over the nuisance parameter ξ. When θ and ξ are distinct according to the definition in Section 2.2.2, the prior distribution factors as

$$\pi(\theta, \xi) = \pi_\theta(\theta)\, \pi_\xi(\xi).$$

Hence the marginal posterior for θ is, under ignorability,

$$
\begin{aligned}
P(\theta \,|\, Y_{obs}, R) &= \int P(\theta, \xi \,|\, Y_{obs}, R)\, d\xi \\
&\propto P(Y_{obs} \,|\, \theta)\, \pi_\theta(\theta) \int P(R \,|\, Y_{obs}, \xi)\, \pi_\xi(\xi)\, d\xi \\
&\propto L(\theta \,|\, Y_{obs})\, \pi_\theta(\theta), \qquad (2.12)
\end{aligned}
$$

where the proportionality is up to a multiplicative factor that does not involve θ. Note that R does not appear on the right-hand side of (2.12) and therefore $P(\theta \,|\, Y_{obs}, R) = P(\theta \,|\, Y_{obs})$. We have thus shown that under ignorability all information about θ is summarized in the posterior that ignores the missing-data mechanism,

$$P(\theta \,|\, Y_{obs}) \propto L(\theta \,|\, Y_{obs})\, \pi_\theta(\theta). \qquad (2.13)$$

We shall refer to (2.13) as the *observed-data posterior*.

In most practical applications one would not be interested in the function (2.13) itself but in meaningful summaries of it: posterior moments, marginal posterior densities and quantiles of univariate components of θ, etc. Note that these summaries are typically integrals of the density (2.13) or functions involving it over the parameter space. In many commonly used probability models with complete data, computation of these integrals can be simplified by choosing a prior distribution for θ within a natural conjugate class (e.g. Box and Tiao, 1992). With incomplete data, however, the usual natural conjugate priors no longer lead to posteriors that are recognizable or easy to summarize.

A bivariate normal example

Let us return to Example 2 of Section 2.3.2 in which Y_1 is observed for all units but Y_2 is missing for some. Assuming that the complete data are bivariate normal with parameter $\theta = (\mu, \Sigma)$, the observed-data likelihood is given by (2.8). In the absence of strong prior beliefs about θ, a prior 'distribution' commonly used with complete data is

$$\pi_\theta(\theta) \propto |\Sigma|^{-3/2}, \qquad (2.14)$$

which can be derived by applying the invariance principle of Jeffreys to μ and Σ (e.g. Box and Tiao, 1992). The prior (2.14) is said to be *improper* because it is not a true probability density function; its integral over the parameter space is not finite. With complete data this prior leads to a posterior distribution for θ that is the product of an inverted-Wishart distribution for Σ and a normal distribution for μ given Σ. The properties of this normal-inverted Wishart distribution are well known, and summaries (marginal densities, moments, etc.) are readily available in closed form. When some values of Y_2 are missing, however, the posterior under (2.14) is no longer normal-inverted Wishart.

One way to characterize this posterior is to express it in terms of the alternative parameterization $\phi = (\mu_1, \sigma_{11}, \beta_0, \beta_1, \sigma_{22\cdot1})$, where $\beta_1 = \sigma_{12}/\sigma_{11}$, $\beta_0 = \mu_2 - \beta_1\mu_1$ and $\sigma_{22\cdot1} = \sigma_{22} - \sigma_{12}^2/\sigma_{11}$. As shown in (2.9), the likelihood for ϕ factors neatly into a complete-data likelihood for $\phi_1 = (\mu, \sigma_{11})$ based on all the sample units and a complete-data likelihood for $\phi_2 = (\beta_0, \beta_1, \sigma_{22\cdot1})$ based on the units for which Y_2 is observed. Moreover, the prior distribution (2.14) also factors into independent priors for ϕ_1 and ϕ_2. To see this, note that $\phi = \phi(\theta)$ is a one-to-one transformation, and the density for ϕ implied by (2.14) can thus be written as

$$\pi_\phi(\phi) = \pi_\theta(\phi^{-1}(\phi)) \, \|J\|^{-1},$$

where $\theta = \phi^{-1}(\phi)$ denotes the transformation from ϕ back to θ, and $\|J\|$ denotes the absolute value of the determinant of the Jacobian (first-derivative) matrix for the transformation from θ to ϕ. Notice that $|\Sigma| = \sigma_{11}\sigma_{22} - \sigma_{12}^2 = \sigma_{11}\sigma_{22\cdot1}$. Moreover, it will be shown in Section 5.2.4 that $\|J\| = \sigma_{11}^{-1}$, and thus

$$\pi_\phi(\phi) = \sigma_{11}^{-1/2}\sigma_{22\cdot1}^{-3/2}. \tag{2.15}$$

Combining (2.15) with the likelihood (2.9), the observed-data posterior can be written as

$$P(\phi|Y_{obs}) = P(\phi_1|Y_{obs})\, P(\phi_2|Y_{obs}), \tag{2.16}$$

where

$$P(\phi_1|Y_{obs}) \propto \sigma_{11}^{-(n+1)/2}\exp\left\{-\frac{1}{2\sigma_{11}}\sum_{i=1}^{n}(y_{i1} - \mu_1)^2\right\}$$

and

$$P(\phi_2|Y_{obs}) \propto \sigma_{22\cdot1}^{-(n_1+3)/2}\exp\left\{-\frac{1}{2\sigma_{22\cdot1}}\sum_{i=1}^{n_1}(y_{i2} - \beta_0 - \beta_1 y_{i1})^2\right\}.$$

After some manipulation, it can be shown that $P(\phi_1|Y_{obs})$ is the product of a normal and a scaled-inverted chisquare density,

$$\mu_1 \mid \sigma_{11}, Y_{obs} \sim N(\bar{y}_1, n^{-1}\sigma_{11}),$$
$$\sigma_{11} \mid Y_{obs} \sim (n-1)S_{11}\,\chi_{n-2}^{-2}, \tag{2.17}$$

where $\bar{y}_1$ and S_{11} are the usual sample mean and variance of Y_1 based on all n units and χ_{n-2}^{-2} denotes an inverted chisquare variate (i.e. the reciprocal of a chisquare variate) with $n-2$ degrees of freedom. Moreover, $P(\phi_2|Y_{obs})$ can be shown to be the product of a bivariate normal and an inverted chisquare,

$$\beta \mid \sigma_{22\cdot1}, Y_{obs} \sim N(\hat{\beta}, \sigma_{22\cdot1}(X^TX)^{-1}),$$
$$\sigma_{22\cdot1} \mid Y_{obs} \sim \hat{\varepsilon}^T\hat{\varepsilon}\,\chi_{n_1-1}^{-2}, \tag{2.18}$$

where $\beta = (\beta_0, \beta_1)^T$,

$$X = \begin{bmatrix} 1 & y_{11} \\ 1 & y_{21} \\ \vdots & \vdots \\ 1 & y_{n_1,1} \end{bmatrix}, \quad y = \begin{bmatrix} y_{12} \\ y_{22} \\ \vdots \\ y_{n_1,2} \end{bmatrix},$$

$\hat{\beta} = (X^T X)^{-1} X^T y$ and $\hat{\varepsilon} = y - X\hat{\beta}$. Details of the calculations lead-ing to these posteriors may be found in standard texts on Bayesian analysis and will be reviewed in Chapters 5–6.

In the above example, a particular factorization of the observed-data likelihood enabled us to express the posterior in a tractable form. This will not always be the case. One cannot always factor the observed-data likelihood into complete-data likelihoods whose parameters are distinct. The techniques of Markov chain Monte Carlo to be introduced in Chapter 3 will free us from many of the constraints of mathematical tractability, allowing us to create random draws from the observed-data posterior whether or not it can be written in a tractable form.

2.4 Examining the ignorability assumption

The statistician unaccustomed to missing-data problems might be led to believe that the observed-data likelihood is *always* the rele-vant likelihood function for θ whenever data are not fully observed; it is, after all, simply the marginal distribution of Y_{obs}, the observed part of Y. But as we have seen, the 'observed data' consist of both Y_{obs} and R, and one needs the special condition of ignorability to make the observed value of R noninformative with respect to θ. Therefore it is crucial for the data analyst to understand the im-plications of the ignorability assumption, particularly MAR, and assess its appropriateness in any given problem.

2.4.1 Examples where ignorability is known to hold

On occasion, the MAR condition is known to hold exactly. Some examples of this are given below.

Double sampling. In sample surveys that employ double sampling (e.g. Cochran, 1977), some characteristics, say $Y_1, Y_2, \ldots, Y_k$, are recorded for all units in the sample, and then additional charac-teristics $Y_{k+1}, \ldots, Y_p$ are recorded for a subsample of the original sample. If this subsample is selected by a mechanism that depends on $Y_1, Y_2, \ldots, Y_k$ alone, even in a systematic or deterministic way, then the missing values of $Y_{k+1}, \ldots, Y_p$ for those units not included in the subsample are MAR.

Sampling for nonresponse followup. In censuses and large sur-veys, initial attempts to collect data may fail for a substantial proportion of units. In a mail-based household survey, for example, some residents will inevitably fail to mail back their forms. In many cases, more intensive data-collection efforts (e.g. personal interviews) would be successful, but attempting to follow up every nonresponding unit may be economically infeasible. If the intensive followup effort is applied to a random sample of nonresponding units, then the missing data for the remaining nonrespondents is MAR. A famous early discussion of this method is given by Hansen and Hurwitz (1946).

Randomized experiments with unequal numbers of cases per treatment group. In many designed experiments, the researcher strives to assign an equal number of cases or subjects to each treatment, because data that are balanced in this fashion are typically easier to analyze than data that are unbalanced. Moreover, principles of efficiency often support the use of balanced designs. Sometimes balance is not feasible, however, and the data are unbalanced by design. The analysis of unbalanced data can often be simplified by imagining a number of additional cases which, if they were included in the experiment under the appropriate treatment groups, would result in a balanced experiment. Because the hypothetical missing data within each treatment group were missing with probability one, they are MAR.

Medical screening with multiple tests, where not all tests are administered to all subjects. In many medical studies, an inexpensive or easily administered test is given to a large number of subjects, and for purposes of calibration a second, more expensive, and more reliable test is administered to a subsample. The calibrating sample may be chosen completely at random, on the basis of subject-specific covariates, or even on the basis of the outcome of the first test. As long as all the information used to choose the subsample is recorded and regarded as part of the observed data Y_{obs}, then the missing data will be MAR.

Matrix sampling for questionnaire or test items. In matrix sampling (e.g. Thayer, 1983) a test or questionnaire is divided into sections, and groups of sections are administered to subjects in a randomized fashion. The resulting data matrix will have rectangular patches of missing data corresponding to sections of the test or questionnaire that were not administered to subject groups. If all the variables used in the sampling plan are included in Y_{obs}, then the missing data will be MAR.

In most of the above examples, the missing data may be said to be *missing by design*, because it was never the intention of the investigator to record all potential variables for all subjects. When missing data are missing by design, they tend also to be MAR.

2.4.2 Examples where ignorability is not known to hold

In many other missing-data contexts, however, it is not known whether or not the MAR condition is satisfied. Examples include:

1. Sample surveys where some sampled individuals are not at home, unwilling to be interviewed, or do not otherwise provide useful responses to some or all of the questionnaire items. Notice, however, that if followup data can later be obtained for a probability sample of nonrespondents, the missing data can be converted to MAR.

2. Planned experiments where, for reasons unforeseen or unintended by the investigator, one or more outcomes of interest cannot be recorded: culture dishes break, production runs fail, subjects drop out of the study, etc.

3. Observational studies in which data of economic, historic or other scientific interest are collected for analysis, but for reasons beyond the control of the investigator some of the variables desired are simply not available for some cases.

Sometimes the fact that a numerical observation is not recorded is more like a response than a missing value. In a laboratory experiment, for example, an animal may die for reasons related to the treatment that was applied to it. If so, then the hypothetical missing data, the measurements that could not be recorded because the animal died, are counterfactual and poorly defined. In such instances, careful thought should be given to whether it is sensible to analyze such data by missing-data methods.

When data are missing for reasons beyond the investigator's control, one can never be certain whether MAR holds. The MAR hypothesis in such datasets cannot be formally tested unless the missing values, or at least a sample of them, are available from an external source. When such an external source is unavailable, deciding whether or not MAR is plausible will necessarily involve some guesswork, and will require careful consideration of conditions specific to the problem at hand.

2.4.3 Ignorability is relative

One final point that must be made is that MAR and ignorability are relative, defined with respect to a particular set of observed data Y_{obs}. In many situations, the status of the missing data (whether or not they are MAR) may change if the definition of Y_{obs} is changed. For example, consider a sample survey that involves probability sampling for nonresponse followup. Let Y_{mis} refer to the data for nonrespondents not included in the followup effort. If Y_{obs} is the data for nonrespondents who were included in the followup effort, then the missing data are MAR. If the definition of Y_{obs} is expanded to include the original respondents, however, and no information (e.g. dummy indicator) is retained to distinguish them from the nonrespondents who were subsequently followed up, then the missing data are no longer MAR.

In other situations, a nonresponse mechanism may not be exactly known to the analyst, but covariates are available that could plausibly explain or predict the missingness to a great extent. The plausibility of MAR would then depend on whether these covariates are included in the analysis. Further discussion of this point is given by Graham et al. (1994) with regard to attrition in a longitudinal study of adolescent drug use.

2.5 General ignorable procedures

Virtually all of the missing-data procedures used in statistical practice, both ad hoc approaches and principled ones, rely at least implicitly on an assumption of ignorability. Often the assumptions made are even stronger. For example, the case-deletion method used by many statistical packages (omitting all incomplete cases from the analysis) may introduce bias into inferences about θ unless the missing data are MCAR. Even if MCAR holds, case deletion may still be grossly inefficient.

We shall call a missing-data procedure a *general ignorable procedure* if it is based upon either an observed-data likelihood or an observed-data posterior. The EM algorithm, for example, will be seen to be a general ignorable procedure because it maximizes the observed-data likelihood. Omitting all incomplete cases from an analysis, however, is not a general ignorable procedure because it leads to a different likelihood or posterior, one based only on the complete cases. All of the methods developed in this book are general ignorable procedures.

A common feature of ad hoc missing-data treatments like case deletion is that they tend to discard information from certain units and/or variables in order to make the estimation problem more tractable. General ignorable procedures by nature, however, do not discard such information because the observed-data likelihood or posterior conditions fully on Y_{obs}. From standpoints of efficiency and bias, full conditioning on Y_{obs} is advantageous because it leads to inferences that are proper under any missing-data mechanism that is ignorable, whereas procedures that are not fully conditional may perform well in some but not all ignorable scenarios. This point can be illustrated with a simple hypothetical example.

2.5.1 A simulated example

Consider again the bivariate data described in Example 2 of Section 2.3.2, in which Y_1 is always observed but Y_2 is sometimes missing. Under a bivariate normal data model with ignorable missingness, we may easily find the value $\hat{\phi}$ that maximizes the observed-data likelihood function $L(\phi \mid Y_{obs})$ in (2.9) and then apply the inverse transformation $\hat{\theta} = \phi^{-1}(\hat{\phi})$ to find the maximum-likelihood (ML) estimate for θ. Straightforward calculation shows that the ML estimate of μ_2 is $\hat{\mu}_2 = \hat{\beta}_0 + \hat{\beta}_1 \hat{\mu}_1$, where $\hat{\beta}_0$ and $\hat{\beta}_1$ are least-squares estimates from the regression of Y_2 on Y_1 based on units $1, 2, \ldots, n_1$ and $\hat{\mu}_1$ is the average value of Y_1 among units $1, 2, \ldots, n$ (Anderson, 1957). Alternatively, one may compute $\hat{\mu}_2$ by first imputing regression-based predictions for the missing values of Y_2, i.e. letting $y_{i2} = \hat{\beta}_0 + \hat{\beta}_1 y_{i1}$ for $i = n_1 + 1, \ldots, n$, and then computing the average of Y_2 among units $1, 2, \ldots, n$ in the imputed dataset.

Estimating μ_2 by $\hat{\mu}_2$ is a general ignorable procedure because $\hat{\mu}_2$ is obtained by maximizing the observed-data likelihood $L(\phi \mid Y_{obs})$. Another plausible estimate is the complete-case (CC) estimate $\bar{\mu}_2 = n_1^{-1} \sum_{i=1}^{n_1} y_{i2}$, the average of Y_2 among the completely observed cases. Estimating μ_2 by $\bar{\mu}_2$ may certainly be regarded as an ignorable procedure because it is consistent with the belief that the missing data are MCAR, a special case of MAR. It is not, however, a general ignorable procedure because it does not condition fully on Y_{obs}; in particular, it discards the observed values of Y_1 for units $n_1 + 1, \ldots, n$. Consequently, the ML estimate tends to be more efficient than the CC estimate, and it exhibits better performance over a variety of missingness mechanisms.

We can easily compare the performance of the ML and CC estimates by simulation. As shown in Figure 2.2, let us define

Table 2.1. *Simulated means (standard deviations) of the CC and ML estimates under three MAR mechanisms*

Missingness mechanism	$\rho = 0$		$\rho = 0.5$		$\rho = 0.9$	
	CC	ML	CC	ML	CC	ML
Constant	.00	.00	.00	.00	.00	.00
$a_1 = 0.5$	(.14)	(.15)	(.14)	(.13)	(.14)	(.11)
Probit selection (Y_1)	.00	.00	.28	.00	.51	.00
$a_2 = 0,\ b_2 = 1$	(.14)	(.18)	(.14)	(.16)	(.12)	(.12)
Interval selection (Y_1)	.00	.00	.14	.00	.25	.00
$a_3 = -0.385,\ b_3 = 1.036$	(.14)	(.18)	(.13)	(.17)	(.08)	(.12)

$R = (r_1, \ldots, r_n)$ to be a vector of response indicators where $r_i = 1$ if Y_2 is observed and $r_i = 0$ if Y_2 is missing for unit i, $i = 1, 2, \ldots, n$. In particular, consider the class of ignorable mechanisms in which $P(r_i = 1 \mid Y) = g(y_{i1})$ independently for units $i = 1, 2, \ldots, n$, where g is some function that maps the real line into the unit interval $[0, 1]$. Three possible choices for g are

constant $g_1(y_{i1}) = a_1,\ 0 \leq a_1 \leq 1$,

probit selection $g_2(y_{i1}) = \Phi(a_2 + b_2 y_{i1})$,

interval selection $g_3(y_{i1}) = 1$ if $a_3 \leq y_{i1} \leq b_3$, else 0,

where $\Phi(\cdot)$ denotes the standard normal cumulative distribution function. The constant function g_1 is MCAR, whereas g_2 and g_3 are MAR but not MCAR. A simulation was conducted in which samples of size $n = 100$ were drawn from bivariate normal populations with $\mu_1 = \mu_2 = 0$, $\sigma_{11} = \sigma_{22} = 1$ and $\sigma_{12} = \rho = 0$, 0.5 and 0.9, respectively. Random patterns of missingness were imposed on each sample according to g_1 with $a_1 = 0.5$, g_2 with $a_2 = 0$, $b_2 = 1$ and g_3 with $a_3 = \Phi^{-1}(0.35) = -0.385$, $b_3 = \Phi^{-1}(0.85) = 1.036$. These constants were chosen to yield an expected response rate n_1/n of 50% under each mechanism, a level higher than is found in most typical applications.

The means and standard deviations of the CC and ML estimates over 5000 repetitions are shown in Table 2.1. Under the non-MCAR mechanisms, the CC estimate is biased whenever $\rho \neq 0$. Except under the unrealistic condition that $n_1/n \to 1$, this bias does not vanish as $n \to \infty$, causing $\bar{\mu}_2$ to be inconsistent. The ML estimate, however, is unbiased and consistent under the three mechanisms used here, as well as under essentially all other ignorable mechanisms. From considerations of bias and consistency, the ML estimate has a clear advantage over the CC estimate.

In fairness, one should note that it is possible to construct a missingness mechanism for which the ML estimate would be less biased than the CC estimate. Such a mechanism would be neither MAR nor MCAR, but a peculiar nonignorable mechanism in which Y_1 and Y_2 would have correlations of opposite sign among the respondent and nonrespondent groups. Such mechanisms, although mathematically possible, are somewhat atypical and should not be expected to occur often in practice with real data. Further discussion of this point in an applied setting is given by Schafer (1992).

Under the more restrictive condition of MCAR, both the ML and CC estimates are unbiased, but ML still has an advantage over CC for $\rho = 0.5$ and $\rho = 0.9$ because its variance is lower. This reduction in variance occurs because Y_1 becomes an increasingly valuable predictor of the missing values of Y_2 as ρ increases. The only situations in Table 2.1 for which CC appears to dominate ML are when Y_1 and Y_2 are unrelated ($\rho = 0$), in which case $\hat{\mu}_2$ has more variability than $\bar{\mu}_2$. Here CC enjoys an advantage because it correctly assumes that the correlation between Y_1 and Y_2 is zero, whereas ML uses an estimated regression line whose slope $\hat{\beta}_1$ randomly varies about zero. This advantage of CC over ML would be much less dramatic if the average missingness rate were lower. Moreover, the benefit of CC's lower variance in this special situation tends to be outweighed by the protection against bias afforded by ML when $\rho \neq 0$ and the mechanism is not MCAR.

2.5.2 Departures from ignorability

The above example illustrates the advantages of general ignorable procedures when missing data are MAR. Even when the missing data are not precisely MAR, however, general ignorable procedures still tend to be better than ad hoc procedures such as case deletion for the following reason: general ignorable procedures remove all of the nonresponse bias explainable by Y_{obs}, whereas ad hoc procedures may not.

To demonstrate this point, let us modify the example of Section 2.5.1 to include a mechanism that is not MAR. Suppose that propensity to respond for Y_2 is no longer a function of Y_1 but is now directly related to Y_2. We will assume that $P(r_i = 1 \,|\, Y) = g(y_{i2})$ independently for $i = 1, 2, \ldots, n$. A simulation was conducted using probit selection, $g(y_{i2}) = \Phi(a_2 + b_2 y_{i2})$ with $a_2 = 0$, $b_2 = 1$ and all

Table 2.2. *Simulated means (standard deviations) of $\bar{\mu}_2$ and $\hat{\mu}_2$ under a non-MAR mechanism*

Missingness mechanism	$\rho = 0$		$\rho = 0.5$		$\rho = 0.9$	
	CC	ML	CC	ML	CC	ML
Probit selection (Y_2)	.56	.56	.56	.46	.56	.14
$a_2 = 0$, $b_2 = 1$	(.12)	(.12)	(.12)	(.12)	(.12)	(.11)

other parameters as before. Results shown in Table 2.2 show that the CC estimate $\bar{\mu}_2$ and the general ignorable ML estimate $\hat{\mu}_2$ are equally biased when $\rho = 0$ but that ML becomes substantially less biased for larger values of ρ. By making use of Y_1 to predict missing values of Y_2, the ML procedure removes the nonresponse bias in the observed values of Y_2 attributable to Y_1. In this example nonresponse is related to Y_2 rather than Y_1, but as ρ increases Y_1 becomes an increasingly useful proxy for Y_2.

Limited practical experience with real data also suggests that general ignorable procedures may tend to perform well even when the ignorability assumption is suspect, especially in multivariate settings. In surveys containing questions about income, for example, nonresponse rates on income-related questions tend to be high, and both experience and common sense suggest that the probability of response is likely to be related to level of income. In a study of missing-data methods for an income question in the Current Population Survey, Greenlees *et al.* (1982) established definite relationships between response and income itself. Upon further investigation, David *et al.* (1986) found little evidence of bias in ignorable procedures that imputed missing values of income on the basis of other demographic and questionnaire items that were observed. This evidence came from knowledge of the missing values obtained from an external source, the actual wages and salary reported to the Internal Revenue Service on the individuals' tax returns. David *et al.* (1986) also concluded that further improvements in the missing-data procedures would probably come from better modeling of the multivariate structure of the data, not from nonignorable modeling.

The crucial assumption made by ignorable methods is not that the propensity to respond is completely unrelated to the missing data, but that this relationship can be explained by data that are observed. Whether ignorability is plausible in a particular setting is therefore closely related to the richness of the observed data Y_{obs} and the complexity of the data model $P(Y \mid \theta)$. If Y_{obs} contains a lot of information relevant for predicting Y_{mis}, and if the data model is sufficiently complex to make use of this information, then we should expect the residual dependence of R upon Y_{mis} after conditioning on Y_{obs} to be relatively minor. Thus in multivariate datasets where both the observed data and the complete-data model are rich, general ignorable procedures may tend to perform well in practice. Even if they do not perform well, they still may provide an important and useful baseline for assessing and comparing any available alternatives.

2.5.3 Notes on nonignorable alternatives

Various approaches to incomplete data that do not assume ignorability have also appeared in the literature. A detailed review of nonignorable methods is beyond the scope of this text, but we note that these nonignorable methods tend to have a common approach. They generally involve joint probability modeling of both the data $P(Y \mid \theta)$ and the missingness mechanism $P(R \mid Y, \xi)$ and joint estimation of θ and ξ from Y_{obs} and R. These joint models for Y and R typically involve more parameters than can be estimated from Y_{obs} and R alone. In order to make them identifiable, one must either (a) impose a priori restrictions on the joint parameter space for θ and ξ, or (b) impose an informative Bayesian prior distribution on (θ, ξ).

For continuous data, one group of nonignorable methods is based on models known in the econometric literature as stochastic censoring or selection models (Heckman, 1976; Amemiya, 1984). For categorical data, nonignorable contingency-table approaches are described by Fay (1986); Baker and Laird (1988); Rubin, Schafer and Schenker (1988); Winship and Mare (1989); and Park and Brown (1994). A review of some nonignorable methods is given by Little and Rubin (1987, chap. 11). Glynn, Laird and Rubin (1993) describe nonignorable modeling based on followup data. Approaches to nonignorable modeling for longitudinal data are discussed by Conaway (1992, 1994); Diggle and Kenward (1994); and Baker (1994). Little (1993) discusses in general terms a class of nonignorable models called pattern-mixture models, in which the joint distribution of Y and R is specified in terms of the marginal distribution of R and the conditional distribution of Y given R.

2.6 The role of the complete-data model

Having discussed at length the assumption of ignorability, we now return to the role of the model for the complete data presented in Section 2.1. A good model should be plausible and have sufficient flexibility to preserve the subtle features of the data at hand, but in realistic settings one must also consider issues of convenience and mathematical tractability. The classes of models considered in this book, the multivariate normal for continuous data, loglinear models for cross-classified categorical data and the class of models for mixed continuous and categorical data, are general-purpose multivariate models that are both mathematically tractable and appropriate in many but not all situations. With categorical and mixed data, the analyst has considerable freedom to tailor a model to the particular dataset; two-way, three-way or higher associations between variables may be included if they are thought to be important. The multivariate normal model for continuous data is less flexible, however, because it fits only pairwise associations. Sometimes the normality assumption may be made more plausible by applying suitable transformations to one or more variables (Box and Cox, 1964; Emerson, 1991).

2.6.1 Departures from the data model

When making inferences about a parameter θ, the assumed parametric form of the model and the iid assumption often play a crucial role. If these assumptions are seriously violated, then even under ignorability the likelihood (2.5) may be a poor summary of the data's evidence about θ. Indeed, if the data model does not hold, the interpretation of θ itself may be ambiguous. Selection of a data model should proceed with care, and diagnostics for assessing goodness of fit should be used whenever possible. Of course, in all analyses of real (not simulated) data a probability model is only an approximation to reality, and some departures from modeling assumptions are inevitable. In practice one must judge whether these departures are of a magnitude and nature that seriously impairs the quality of the inference about θ, or whether they are of only minor importance and may be safely ignored.

Complex sample surveys

The assumption (2.1) that the rows of the data matrix are independent and identically distributed (iid) can be problematic, especially when the rows do not correspond to observational units that are *exchangeable* (i.e. like a simple random sample). This assumption is commonly violated in large-scale surveys, which typically employ complex probability sampling methods. Sample surveys often have special features (unequal probabilities of selection, stratification, clustering, etc.) that cause the units to be non-exchangeable.

In some cases, it may be possible to apply the models of this book to survey data in a way that preserves the integrity of the complex design. Stratification and the general issue of design variables are discussed in Section 2.6.2 below. Data with clusters, naturally occurring groups of observations that are potentially intercorrelated, should not in general be handled by iid models. If the clusters are few and large, it may be feasible to fit separate models for each cluster that treat the units within clusters as exchangeable. Another possibility is to add a cluster identifier to the model as an additional categorical variable, and posit some simple associations between this variable and the other variables in the dataset; an example of this approach is described in Section 9.5.3.

When the number of clusters is large, and there are relatively few observations per cluster, the data are more appropriately described by hierarchical probability models with an explicit multilevel error structure. These models, sometimes called random-effects or mixed models, have been extensively applied in the univariate setting with continuous responses (Laird and Ware, 1982; Searle *et al.*, 1992). Recent advances in computational methods have allowed extensions to discrete (Zeger and Karim, 1991) and multivariate continuous (Everson and Morris, 1996) response models. Application to problems of missing data in surveys, however, will typically require hierarchical models for multivariate categorical responses. A proper treatment of these models is well beyond the scope of this book. For a detailed example of such a model in the context of the U.S. Decennial Census, see Schafer (1995). More discussion of missing-data problems in complex surveys will appear in Sections 4.3 and 4.5.

The role of imputation

It may be possible to mitigate some of the effects of model failure through multiple imputation (Section 4.3). Inference by multiple imputation proceeds in two stages. First, m simulated versions of the missing data are created under a data model. Second, the m versions of the complete data are then analyzed by complete-data statistical techniques, and the results are combined to produce one overall inference. Sometimes the complete-data statistical analyses of the second stage will involve different models than the one used to produce the multiple imputations in the first stage. When analyzing data from a sample survey, for example, one may impute the missing data on the basis of an elaborate multivariate model, but then proceed to analyze the data using classical nonparametric survey methods in which inferences are based entirely on the randomization used to draw the sample (e.g. Cochran, 1977). Even if the model used for imputation is somewhat restrictive or unrealistic, it will effectively be applied not to the entire dataset but only to its missing part. Multiple imputation thus has a natural advantage over some other methods of inference in that it may tend to be more robust to departures from the complete-data model, especially when the amounts of missing information are not large. Hence, even though the classes of models examined in this book may not realistically describe many of the multivariate datasets one encounters in the real world, we suspect that they will still prove useful in a wide variety of data analyses if applied within the framework of multiple imputation. The role of modeling assumptions in multiple imputation will be revisited in Section 4.5.4.

2.6.2 Inference treating certain variables as fixed

Sometimes the only relevant analysis of a multivariate dataset involves modeling the conditional distribution of certain variables given others. In regression analysis, for example, the goal is to model one or more response variables given one or more predictors. When analyzing data from surveys, it is common practice to estimate means, proportions, etc. not for the population as a whole but within subdomains (strata or poststrata) that are considerably smaller. The individual subdomain estimates are then combined, using population proportions derived from an external source (e.g. a census), to yield estimates for larger domains. The relative sizes of the subdomains in the population are assumed to be known and are not estimated from the sample. Similarly, with data from planned experiments, the relevant analysis is usually a comparison of mean responses across two or more treatment groups; the manner in which experimental units are allocated to treatments is determined by the experimenter and does not need to be modeled.

In discussing situations like these, we will refer to variables in a generic sense as either *response* variables or *design* variables, with the latter being those that the statistical analysis ultimately regards as fixed. Predictors in regression analyses, variables defining strata or poststrata in sample surveys and indicators of treatment groups in planned experiments are all examples of design variables. When a dataset contains one or more design variables, the iid assumption (2.1) is typically violated, as design variables are often under direct control of the investigator and are thus not random in the same sense as the response variables are random. It is usually not desirable to impose any probability model at all on the design variables, but to model only the conditional distribution of the response variables given the design variables.

Datasets with design variables can be accommodated in our framework with just a few additional assumptions. Suppose that each row y_i of the complete-data matrix can be partitioned into two parts, a vector u_i of design variables and a vector v_i of response variables. Furthermore, suppose that the density of y_i can be factored as

$$f(y_i \mid \theta) = f_u(u_i \mid \alpha) \, f_{v\mid u}(v_i \mid u_i, \beta), \qquad (2.19)$$

where α and β are distinct parameters. Finally, suppose that the design variables are completely observed for all units. Under these assumptions, we can write the complete-data matrix as

$$Y = (Y_{obs}, Y_{mis}) = (U, V_{obs}, V_{mis}),$$

where U denotes the design variables, V_{obs} the observed response variables, and V_{mis} the missing response variables, so that $Y_{obs} = (U, V_{obs})$ and $Y_{mis} = V_{mis}$. The probability distribution of the observed quantities may then be written as

$$\int P(R \mid U, V_{obs}, V_{mis}, \xi) \, P(U \mid \alpha) \, P(V_{obs}, V_{mis} \mid U, \beta) \, dV_{mis}, \quad (2.20)$$

where ξ is a set of parameters governing the response mechanism. Under ignorability, this response mechanism does not depend on V_{mis},

$$P(R \mid U, V_{obs}, V_{mis}, \xi) = P(R \mid U, V_{obs}, \xi).$$

Thus the first two factors in the integrand of (2.20) do not involve V_{mis}, so (2.20) becomes

$$P(R, Y_{obs} \mid \theta, \xi) = P(R \mid U, V_{obs}, \xi) \, P(U \mid \alpha) \, P(V_{obs} \mid U, \beta). \quad (2.21)$$

The factorization in (2.21) implies that inferences about β, the parameters of the conditional distribution of V given U, may be based on the conditional observed-data likelihood function

$$L(\beta\,|\,U, V_{mis}) \propto P(V_{obs}\,|\,U, \beta), \qquad (2.22)$$

or on the observed-data posterior

$$P(\beta\,|\,U, V_{mis}) \propto L(\beta\,|\,U, V_{mis})\,\pi_\beta(\beta), \qquad (2.23)$$

where π_β is a prior distribution applied to β independently of any prior on α or ξ. Notice that (2.22) and (2.23) are the same for all α and even for all $P(U\,|\,\alpha)$. In other words, we will obtain a correct inference about β even if the marginal model for the design variables is misspecified.

To summarize, when design variables are present we can often apply a joint probability model such as (2.1) to the complete data Y, even a model in which the distribution of the design variables is misspecified. We will obtain correct inferences about the parameters of interest provided that (a) the design variables U are observed for all units in the sample, and (b) the joint density of (U, V) factors into densities for U and for $V\,|\,U$, with the parameters of the two densities being distinct. Assumption (b) will be a characteristic of some, but not all, of the multivariate models used in this book. Assumption (a) often does hold in practice; it would be somewhat unusual, for example, for stratification variables in a sample survey or treatment indicators in a planned experiment to be missing. In regression analysis with incomplete predictors, the factorization in (2.21) will not precisely hold, but it may still be approximately true provided that the amount of information missing on the predictors is not large.

Example: a comparison of two sample means

The experimental data in Table 2.3 reported by Snedecor and Cochran (1989, Table 6.9.1) show the weight gains of two groups of female rats, one fed a low-protein diet and the other fed a high-protein diet. The low-protein group has 7 rats and the high-protein group has 12. Snedecor and Cochran perform a classical analysis assuming that the observations are independent and normally distributed and the within-group variances are equal. A pooled estimate of the common variance is

$$\frac{6(425) + 11(457)}{17} = 445.7$$

Table 2.3. *Weight gains in grams of two groups of female rats (28-84 days old) under two diets*

Low protein	70	118	101	85	107	132
	94					
	mean = 101		variance = 425			
High protein	134	146	104	119	124	161
	107	83	113	129	97	123
	mean = 120		variance = 457			

Source: Snedecor and Cochran (1989, Table 6.9.1)

on 17 degrees of freedom, and a 95% confidence interval for the difference in mean weight gain between the two groups is

$$(120 - 101) \pm t_{17,.975} \sqrt{445.7 \left(\frac{1}{7} + \frac{1}{12} \right)}, \qquad (2.24)$$

where $t_{\nu,p}$ denotes the pth quantile of the t distribution with ν degrees of freedom. The interval (2.24) extends from -2.2 to 40.2, barely covering zero, so the difference in means is almost significant at the 0.05 level.

Let us now regard Table 2.3 as incomplete data from a balanced experiment; that is, we now suppose that the low-protein group had 12 potential observations, 5 of which are missing. This supposition is for illustrative purposes only, because the analysis of variance for an experiment with a single factor is no more difficult when the data are unbalanced than when they are balanced. The complete data could then be regarded as a 24×2 matrix in which the first variable Y_1 is a treatment indicator (0=low protein, 1=high protein) and the second variable Y_2 is weight gain.

Suppose that we modeled the joint distribution of Y_1 and Y_2 as bivariate normal. The implied marginal normal distribution of the design variable Y_1 would be clearly erroneous. But note the conditional distribution of Y_2 given Y_1 implied by this model, a normal linear regression with constant variance, is precisely the same model that underlies the classical analysis and the confidence interval (2.24). Because Y_1 is coded as 0 or 1, the slope of this regression is identical to the difference in mean weight gain between the two groups. Likelihood-based or Bayesian inferences about the regression slope would yield essentially the same result as the classical interval (2.24), perhaps with minor differences depending on how the observed-data likelihood is summarized or on what prior distribution is chosen.

One possible advantage of using the bivariate normal model here is that a general ignorable procedure devised for incomplete multivariate normal data could be applied to this dataset and the resulting inference about the regression slope would still be valid, provided, of course, that the conditional normal model for Y_2 given Y_1 was correct. When design variables are present it will often be convenient to apply model-fitting and simulation algorithms devised for iid probability models like the multivariate normal, even though parts of the model pertaining to the design variables may be incorrect, because developing a more specialized algorithm then becomes unnecessary.

This example also raises an unrelated but important issue regarding unbalanced experimental data. Classical methods of analysis such as the t-interval in (2.24), and other methods for unbalanced data arising from more complicated designs (e.g. Dodge, 1985), almost invariably contain an implicit assumption that the mechanism causing the imbalance is ignorable. If the data are unbalanced not by design but by accident, e.g. if responses for one or more units could not be recorded because of mishaps or other unforeseen occurrences, then these methods should not be applied without first considering the plausibility of MAR.

CHAPTER 3

EM and data augmentation

3.1 Introduction

Assuming that the complete-data model and ignorability assumptions are correct, all relevant statistical information about the parameters is contained in the observed-data likelihood $L(\theta \mid Y_{obs})$ or observed-data posterior $P(\theta \mid Y_{obs})$. Except in special cases, however, these tend to be complicated functions of θ, and extracting meaningful summaries such as parameter estimates and standard errors requires special computational tools. EM and data augmentation provide those tools. The key ideas behind EM and data augmentation are the same: to solve a difficult incomplete-data problem by repeatedly solving tractable complete-data problems. As a result, the two methods share many features in common, and their implementation in specific examples is often remarkably similar. In this chapter, EM and data augmentation are introduced together to highlight the similarities between them.

3.2 The EM algorithm

3.2.1 Definition

EM capitalizes on the interdependence between missing data Y_{mis} and parameters θ. The fact that Y_{mis} contains information relevant to estimating θ, and θ in turn helps us to find likely values of Y_{mis}, suggests the following scheme for estimating θ in the presence of Y_{obs} alone: 'Fill in' the missing data Y_{mis} based on an initial estimate of θ, re-estimate θ based on Y_{obs} and the filled-in Y_{mis} and iterate until the estimates converge. This idea is so intuitively appealing that specific applications of it have appeared in the statistical literature as far back as 1926 (Little and Rubin, 1987; Meng and Pedlow, 1992). Dempster, Laird and Rubin (1977) formalized the meaning of filling in the missing data at each step and presented the algorithm in its full generality, naming it Expectation-Maximization or EM.

In any incomplete-data problem, the distribution of the complete data Y can be factored as

$$P(Y|\theta) = P(Y_{obs}|\theta)\, P(Y_{mis}|Y_{obs},\theta). \tag{3.1}$$

Viewing each term in (3.1) as a function of θ, it follows that

$$l(\theta|Y) = l(\theta|Y_{obs}) + \log P(Y_{mis}|Y_{obs},\theta) + c \tag{3.2}$$

where $l(\theta|Y) = \log P(Y|\theta)$ denotes the complete-data loglikelihood, $l(\theta|Y_{obs}) = \log L(\theta|Y_{obs})$ the observed-data loglikelihood, and c an arbitrary constant. The term $P(Y_{mis}|Y_{obs},\theta)$, which we shall call the *predictive distribution of the missing data given* θ, plays a central role in EM because it captures the interdependence between Y_{mis} and θ. When viewed as a probability distribution it summarizes knowledge about Y_{mis} for any assumed value of θ, and when viewed as a function of θ it conveys the evidence about θ contained in Y_{mis} beyond that already provided by Y_{obs}.

Because Y_{mis} is unknown we cannot calculate the second term on the right-hand side of (3.2), so instead we take the average of (3.2) over the predictive distribution $P(Y_{mis}|Y_{obs},\theta^{(t)})$, where $\theta^{(t)}$ is a preliminary estimate of the unknown parameter. This averaging yields

$$Q(\theta|\theta^{(t)}) = l(\theta|Y_{obs}) + H(\theta|\theta^{(t)}) + c, \tag{3.3}$$

where

$$Q(\theta|\theta^{(t)}) = \int l(\theta|Y)\, P(Y_{mis}|Y_{obs},\theta^{(t)})\, dY_{mis}$$

and

$$H(\theta|\theta^{(t)}) = \int \log P(Y_{mis}|Y_{obs},\theta)\, P(Y_{mis}|Y_{obs},\theta^{(t)})\, dY_{mis}.$$

A central result of Dempster, Laird, and Rubin (1977) is that if we let $\theta^{(t+1)}$ be the value of θ that maximizes $Q(\theta|\theta^{(t)})$, then $\theta^{(t+1)}$ is a better estimate than $\theta^{(t)}$ in the sense that its observed-data loglikelihood is at least as high as that of $\theta^{(t)}$,

$$l(\theta^{(t+1)}|Y_{obs}) \geq l(\theta^{(t)}|Y_{obs}). \tag{3.4}$$

This can be seen by writing

$$\begin{aligned} l(\theta^{(t+1)}|Y_{obs}) - l(\theta^{(t)}|Y_{obs}) &= Q(\theta^{(t+1)}|\theta^{(t)}) - Q(\theta^{(t)}|\theta^{(t)}) \\ &\quad + H(\theta^{(t)}|\theta^{(t)}) - H(\theta^{(t+1)}|\theta^{(t)}). \end{aligned}$$

The quantity $Q(\theta^{(t+1)}|\theta^{(t)}) - Q(\theta^{(t)}|\theta^{(t)})$ is non-negative because $\theta^{(t+1)}$ has been chosen to satisfy

$$Q(\theta^{(t+1)}|\theta^{(t)}) \geq Q(\theta|\theta^{(t)}) \text{ for all } \theta. \tag{3.5}$$

The remainder $H(\theta^{(t)}|\theta^{(t)}) - H(\theta^{(t+1)}|\theta^{(t)})$, which can be written

$$\int \log \left[\frac{P(Y_{mis}|Y_{obs},\theta^{(t)})}{P(Y_{mis}|Y_{obs},\theta^{(t+1)})} \right] P(Y_{mis}|Y_{obs},\theta^{(:)}) \, dY_{mis},$$

is easily shown to be non-negative by Jensen's inequality and the convexity of the function $x \log x$.

It is convenient to think of one iteration of EM, defined by (3.5), as consisting of two distinct steps:

1. the Expectation or E-step, in which the function $Q(\theta|\theta^{(t)})$ is calculated by averaging the complete-data loglikelihood $l(\theta|Y)$ over $P(Y_{mis}|Y_{obs},\theta^{(t)})$; and

2. the Maximization or M-step, in which $\theta^{(t+1)}$ is found by maximizing $Q(\theta|\theta^{(t)})$.

Alternately performing the E- and M-steps beginning with a starting value $\theta^{(0)}$ defines a sequence of iterates $\{\theta^{(t)}: t = 0, 1, 2, \ldots\}$. Dempster, Laird, and Rubin (1977) and Wu (1983) provide conditions under which this sequence converges reliably to a stationary point of the observed-data loglikelihood. In well-behaved problems this stationary point is a global maximum and EM yields the unique maximum-likelihood estimate (MLE) of θ, the maximizer of $l(\theta|Y_{obs})$. Not all problems are well-behaved, however, and sometimes EM does not converge to a unique global maximum; these situations are taken up in Section 3.3.1 below.

EM for regular exponential families

The E-step of EM clarifies the intuitive idea of filling in the missing data under an assumed value of θ. In some problems (e.g. incomplete data that are purely categorical), we shall see that the E-step actually does correspond to filling in the missing data in the sense that it replaces Y_{mis} with its average or expected value $E(Y_{mis}|Y_{obs},\theta)$ under the assumption $\theta = \theta^{(t)}$. In other problems, however, it does not. In particular, when the complete-data probability model falls in a *regular exponential family*, the complete-data loglikelihood based on n iid (possibly multivariate) observations $Y = (y_1, y_2, \ldots, y_n)$ may be written

$$l(\theta|Y) = \eta(\theta)^T T(Y) + ng(\theta) + c, \tag{3.6}$$

where
$$\eta(\theta) = (\eta_1(\theta), \eta_2(\theta), \ldots, \eta_s(\theta))^T$$
is the canonical form of the parameter θ,
$$T(Y) = (T_1(Y), T_2(Y), \ldots, T_s(Y))^T$$
is an s-dimensional vector of complete-data sufficient statistics and c is a constant term that does not involve θ. Moreover, each of the sufficient statistics has an additive form,

$$T_j(Y) = \sum_{i=1}^{n} h_j(y_i)$$

for some function h_j. Because $l(\theta \mid Y)$ is a linear function of the sufficient statistics, the E-step replaces $T_j(Y)$ by $E(T_j(Y) \mid Y_{obs}, \theta^{(t)})$ for $j = 1, 2, \ldots, s$; in other words, the E-step fills in not the missing elements of Y per se, but rather the missing portions of the complete-data sufficient statistics. In our regular exponential-family models, the expectations $E(T_j(Y) \mid Y_{obs}, \theta^{(t)})$ will be available in closed form and thus the E-step will be computationally straightforward.

In many cases the M-step will also be straightforward; $Q(\theta \mid \theta^{(t)})$ will have the same functional form as a complete-data loglikelihood, so finding $\theta^{(t+1)}$ will be computationally no different from finding the MLE in the complete-data case. For regular exponential families, the complete-data MLE can be found as the solution to the moment equations

$$E(T(Y) \mid \theta) = t, \tag{3.7}$$

where t is the realized value of the vector $T(Y)$ and the expectation is taken with respect to $P(Y \mid \theta)$ (e.g. Cox and Hinkley, 1974). If these equations can be solved for an arbitrary t, then they can just as easily be solved when t is replaced by the output of an E-step. In many of the models appearing in this book, the moment equations can be solved for θ algebraically, and thus the M-step will be available in closed form. When an algebraic solution is not available, one can still maximize the loglikelihood numerically for any given t using standard complete-data iterative techniques such as Newton-Raphson. In the latter situation, implementation of EM would require undesirable nested iterations because each M-step would itself be iterative. When this arises, however, we are often able to streamline the computation by applying a generalization of EM known as ECM, to be discussed in Section 3.2.5.

3.2.2 Examples

Example 1: *Incomplete univariate normal data.* Suppose that $Y = (y_1, y_2, \ldots, y_n)$ represents n iid observations from a univariate normal distribution with mean μ and variance ψ, so that $\theta = (\mu, \psi)$ is the unknown parameter. The reader may easily verify that the complete-data loglikelihood $l(\theta|Y)$ can be written in exponential-family form (3.6) with sufficient statistics

$$T(Y) = (T_1, T_2)^T = \left(\sum_{i=1}^n y_i, \sum_{i=1}^n y_i^2 \right)^T.$$

Letting t_1 and t_2 denote the realized values of T_1 and T_2 respectively, the moment equations

$$
\begin{aligned}
E(T_1) &= n\mu = t_1, \\
E(T_2) &= n\psi + n\mu^2 = t_2
\end{aligned}
$$

lead immediately to the well-known MLEs $\hat{\mu} = \bar{y} = n^{-1} \sum_{i=1}^n y_i$ and $\hat{\psi} = n^{-1} \sum_{i=1}^n y_i^2 - (\bar{y})^2$.

Now suppose that only the first n_1 components of the data vector Y are observed, and the remaining $n_0 = n - n_1$ components are missing at random (which, in this simple example, is equivalent to MCAR). It follows from Example 1, Section 2.3.2 that the observed-data likelihood $L(\theta \mid Y_{obs})$ is just a complete-data likelihood based only on $Y_{obs} = (y_1, y_2, \ldots, y_{n_1})$, and the observed-data MLEs for μ and ψ are thus $\bar{y}_{obs} = n_1^{-1} \sum_{i=1}^{n_1} y_i$ and $n_1^{-1} \sum_{i=1}^{n_1} y_i^2 - (\bar{y}_{obs})^2$, respectively. In this trivial example the observed-data MLEs exist in closed form, but one could also compute them using the EM algorithm. Because of the iid structure the predictive distribution of the missing data given θ does not depend on the observed data, and

$$P(Y_{mis}|Y_{obs}, \theta) = P(Y_{mis}|\theta) = \prod_{i=n_1+1}^{n} P(y_i|\theta). \qquad (3.8)$$

The E-step replaces T_1 and T_2 by their expected values under $P(Y_{mis}|Y_{obs}, \theta)$,

$$
\begin{aligned}
E(T_1|Y_{obs}, \theta) &= E\left[\sum_{i=1}^{n_1} y_i + \sum_{i=n_1+1}^{n} y_i \right] \\
&= \sum_{i=1}^{n_1} y_i + n_0 \mu, \\
E(T_2|Y_{obs}, \theta) &= E\left[\sum_{i=1}^{n_1} y_i^2 + \sum_{i=n_1+1}^{n} y_i^2 \right] \\
&= \sum_{i=1}^{n_1} y_i^2 + n_0(\psi + \mu^2).
\end{aligned}
$$

Inserting these expected sufficient statistics into the expressions for the complete-data MLEs yields a single iteration of EM,

$$\mu^{(t+1)} = n^{-1}\left[\sum_{i=1}^{n_1} y_i + n_0\mu^{(t)}\right], \qquad (3.9)$$

$$\psi^{(t+1)} = n^{-1}\left[\sum_{i=1}^{n_1} y_i^2 + n_0\psi^{(t)} + n_0(\mu^{(t)})^2\right] \qquad (3.10)$$
$$-n^{-2}\left[\sum_{i=1}^{n_1} y_i + n_0\mu^{(t)}\right]^2.$$

In this simple example, the fixed-point equations $\mu^{(t+1)} = \mu^{(t)}$ and $\psi^{(t+1)} = \psi^{(t)}$ can be solved explicitly to show that the iterations converge to the correct observed-data MLEs (Little and Rubin, 1987).

The behavior of this EM algorithm in a small numerical example is displayed in Table 3.1. A sample of $n_1 = 10$ observations is shown with mean $\hat{\mu} = 48.1$ and sample (maximum-likelihood) variance $\hat{\psi} = 59.4$. Arbitrarily choosing the number of missing observations to be $n_0 = 3$ and the starting values to be $\mu^{(0)} = 30$, $\psi^{(0)} = 70$, the algorithm converges to within four decimal places of the MLEs by the 11th iteration. It is apparent from (3.9)–(3.10) that convergence can be accelerated by taking n_0 to be small, and with $n_0 = 0$ the MLE is achieved after just one iteration regardless of the starting values. We shall see in Section 3.3.3 that the rate of convergence in this example is determined by $n_0/(n_0 + n_1)$, the proportion of observations that are missing. More generally, the convergence rate of EM is governed by the fractions of information about components of θ missing due to nonresponse.

Example 2: Two binary variables with missing data on both. Suppose that Y_1 and Y_2 are two potentially related dichotomous variables, each taking values 1 or 2. If the n units in a sample are iid, the complete data may, without loss of information, be reduced to an array of counts $x = (x_{11}, x_{12}, x_{21}, x_{22})$ having a multinomial distribution, where x_{ij} is the number of sample units having $Y_1 = i$ and $Y_2 = j$. Let $\theta = (\theta_{11}, \theta_{12}, \theta_{21}, \theta_{22})$, where θ_{ij} is the probability that a unit has $Y_1 = i$ and $Y_2 = j$. We will use the notation $x \sim M(n, \theta)$ to indicate that x has a multinomial distribution with index n and parameter θ. Because the complete-data loglikelihood is linear in the cell counts x_{ij},

$$l(\theta \,|\, x) = x_{11}\log\theta_{11} + x_{12}\log\theta_{12} + x_{21}\log\theta_{21} + x_{22}\log\theta_{22},$$

the counts are the sufficient statistics and the MLEs are found by equating each x_{ij} with its expectation $n\theta_{ij}$; hence the complete-data MLEs are simply the sample proportions $\hat{\theta}_{ij} = x_{ij}/n$ for $i, j = 1, 2$.

Table 3.1. *Example of EM for incomplete univariate normal data with* $n_1 = 10$ *values observed and* $n_0 = 3$ *values missing*

<table>
<tr><td colspan="2">(a) Observed data</td><td colspan="3">(b) Iterations of EM</td></tr>
<tr><td>50.1</td><td>49.6</td><td>t</td><td>$\mu^{(t)}$</td><td>$\psi^{(t)}$</td></tr>
<tr><td>39.8</td><td>48.7</td><td></td><td></td><td></td></tr>
<tr><td>46.4</td><td>49.7</td><td>0</td><td>30.0000</td><td>70.0000</td></tr>
<tr><td>31.2</td><td>53.4</td><td>1</td><td>43.9231</td><td>120.0218</td></tr>
<tr><td>50.0</td><td>62.1</td><td>2</td><td>47.1361</td><td>76.5067</td></tr>
<tr><td></td><td></td><td>3</td><td>47.8776</td><td>63.5326</td></tr>
<tr><td colspan="2">$\hat{\mu} = 48.1$</td><td>4</td><td>48.0487</td><td>60.3825</td></tr>
<tr><td colspan="2">$\hat{\psi} = 59.4$</td><td>5</td><td>48.0882</td><td>59.6472</td></tr>
<tr><td></td><td></td><td>6</td><td>48.0973</td><td>59.4771</td></tr>
<tr><td></td><td></td><td>7</td><td>48.0994</td><td>59.4378</td></tr>
<tr><td></td><td></td><td>8</td><td>48.0999</td><td>59.4287</td></tr>
<tr><td></td><td></td><td>9</td><td>48.1000</td><td>59.4266</td></tr>
<tr><td></td><td></td><td>10</td><td>48.1000</td><td>59.4261</td></tr>
<tr><td></td><td></td><td>11</td><td>48.1000</td><td>59.4260</td></tr>
<tr><td></td><td></td><td>∞</td><td>48.1000</td><td>59.4260</td></tr>
</table>

If missing values occur on both Y_1 and Y_2, we can partition the sample into three parts denoted by A, B and C, respectively, where A includes units having both variables observed, B includes those having only Y_1 observed and C includes those having only Y_2 observed. (Any units that have neither Y_1 nor Y_2 observed contribute nothing to the observed-data likelihood and may be excluded from the analysis under ignorability.) Each complete-data count x_{ij} can then be expressed as the sum of contributions from each of the three sample parts, $x_{ij} = x_{ij}^A + x_{ij}^B + x_{ij}^C$. Although x_{ij}^A is observed, x_{ij}^B and x_{ij}^C are not; for sample parts B and C, we observe only the marginal totals $x_{i+}^B = x_{i1}^B + x_{i2}^B$ and $x_{+j}^C = x_{1j}^C + x_{2j}^C$, respectively. The observed data $Y_{obs} = \{x_{ij}^A, x_{i+}^B, x_{+j}^C : i, j = 1, 2\}$ can be displayed as in Table 3.2, with a 2×2 table cross-classifying the units in A by Y_1 and Y_2, a 2×1 table classifying the units in B by Y_1 alone, and a 1×2 table classifying the units in C by Y_2 alone.

A convenient feature of the multinomial distribution is that if we regard the sum of any set of components of x as fixed, the conditional distribution of those components becomes another multinomial and is independent of the remaining components (e.g. Agresti, 1990). For example, the conditional distribution of (x_{11}, x_{12}) given

Table 3.2. *Classification of sample units by two incompletely observed binary variables*

(a) Both variables observed			(b) Y_2 missing	(c) Y_1 missing	
	$Y_2 = 1$	$Y_2 = 2$		$Y_2 = 1$	$Y_2 = 2$
$Y_1 = 1$	x_{11}^A	x_{12}^A	x_{1+}^A	$Y_1 = 1$	x_{1+}^B	x_{+1}^C	x_{+2}^C
$Y_1 = 2$	x_{21}^A	x_{22}^A	x_{2+}^A	$Y_1 = 2$	x_{2+}^B		
	x_{+1}^A	x_{+2}^A				

$x_{1+} = x_{11} + x_{12}$ is multinomial with parameter $(\theta_{11}/\theta_{1+}, \theta_{12}/\theta_{1+})$ where $\theta_{1+} = \theta_{11} + \theta_{12}$; furthermore, (x_{11}, x_{12}) is conditionally independent of (x_{21}, x_{22}). Applying this property within parts B and C of the sample, the predictive distribution of the missing data given θ and the observed data becomes a set of independent multinomials or a *product multinomial*,

$$(x_{i1}^B, x_{i2}^B) \mid Y_{obs}, \theta \sim M(x_{i+}^B, (\theta_{i1}/\theta_{i+}, \theta_{i2}/\theta_{i+})), \quad i = 1, 2,$$
$$(x_{1j}^C, x_{2j}^C) \mid Y_{obs}, \theta \sim M(x_{+j}^C, (\theta_{1j}/\theta_{+j}, \theta_{2j}/\theta_{+j})), \quad j = 1, 2.$$

The E-step of EM replaces the unknown counts x_{ij}^B and x_{ij}^C in x_{ij} by their conditional expectations under an assumed value for θ,

$$
\begin{aligned}
E(x_{ij} \mid Y_{obs}, \theta) &= E(x_{ij}^A + x_{ij}^B + x_{ij}^C \mid Y_{obs}, \theta) \\
&= x_{ij}^A + x_{i+}^B \theta_{ij}/\theta_{i+} + x_{+j}^C \theta_{ij}/\theta_{+j}.
\end{aligned}
$$

The M-step then estimates θ_{ij} by $E(x_{ij} \mid Y_{obs}, \theta)/n$. Combining the two steps yields a single iteration of EM,

$$\theta_{ij}^{(t+1)} = n^{-1} \left[x_{ij}^A + x_{i+}^B \left(\frac{\theta_{ij}^{(t)}}{\theta_{i+}^{(t)}} \right) + x_{+j}^C \left(\frac{\theta_{ij}^{(t)}}{\theta_{+j}^{(t)}} \right) \right],$$

$i, j = 1, 2$, an expression first given by Chen and Fienberg (1974).

The data in Table 3.3, previously analyzed by Kadane (1985), were obtained through the National Crime Survey conducted by the U.S. Bureau of the Census. Housing unit occupants were interviewed to determine whether they had been victimized by crime in the preceding six-month period. Six months later the units were visited again to determine whether the occupants had been victimized in the intervening months. Discarding the 115 households that

Table 3.3. *EM algorithm applied to victimization status of households on two occasions*

(a) Victimization status from the National Crime Survey

	Second visit		
First visit	Crime-free	Victims	Nonrespondents
Crime-free	392	55	33
Victims	76	38	9
Nonrespondents	31	7	115

Source: Kadane (1985, Table 1)

(b) Iterations of EM

t	$\theta_{11}^{(t)}$	$\theta_{12}^{(t)}$	$\theta_{21}^{(t)}$	$\theta_{22}^{(t)}$
0	.2500	.2500	.2500	.2500
1	.6615	.1170	.1498	.0718
2	.6947	.1003	.1370	.0680
3	.6969	.0988	.1359	.0684
4	.6971	.0987	.1358	.0684
5	.6971	.0986	.1358	.0685
∞	.6971	.0986	.1358	.0685

did not respond to the survey at either visit, we are left with a sample of $n = 641$ for which responses are available at one or both occasions. The EM algorithm for this example converges quite rapidly. Starting from a table of uniform probabilities (all $\theta_{ij} = 0.25$), the estimated cell probabilities converge to four decimal places by the fifth iteration as shown in Table 3.3 (b).

One way to summarize the association between two binary variables is by the cross-product or odds ratio

$$\omega = \frac{\theta_{11}\theta_{22}}{\theta_{12}\theta_{21}},$$

with $\omega = 1$ under independence. The ML estimate of the odds ratio is $(\hat{\theta}_{11}\hat{\theta}_{22})/(\hat{\theta}_{12}\hat{\theta}_{21}) = 3.57$. Households that were victimized during the first period appear to be more than 3.5 times as likely, on the odds scale, to have been victimized in the second period than households that were crime-free in the first period. The question of whether this result is statistically significant will be addressed shortly.

3.2.3 EM for posterior modes

The EM algorithm is typically presented as a technique for finding MLEs. As pointed out by Dempster, Laird, and Rubin (1977), however, EM may also be used to compute posterior modes, values of θ for which the observed-data posterior density rather than the observed-data likelihood is highest.

Because the complete-data posterior density under the prior $\pi(\theta)$ is $P(\theta|Y) \propto P(Y|\theta)\,\pi(\theta)$, it follows from (3.2) that

$$\log P(\theta|Y) = l(\theta|Y_{obs}) + \log P(Y_{mis}|Y_{obs}, \theta) + \log \pi(\theta) + c.$$

Averaging this equation over the predictive distribution of Y_{mis} given $\theta = \theta^{(t)}$ gives

$$Q^*(\theta|\theta^{(t)}) = \log P(\theta|Y_{obs}) + H(\theta|\theta^{(t)}) + \log \pi(\theta) + c,$$

where

$$Q^*(\theta|\theta^{(t)}) = Q(\theta|\theta^{(t)}) + \log \pi(\theta^{(t)}),$$

and the functions $Q(\theta|\theta^{(t)})$ and $H(\theta|\theta^{(t)})$ are defined as before. If we choose the next iterate $\theta^{(t+1)}$ to maximize $Q^*(\theta|\theta^{(t)})$, i.e. to satisfy

$$Q^*(\theta^{(t+1)}|\theta^{(t)}) \geq Q^*(\theta|\theta^{(t)}) \text{ for all } \theta, \qquad (3.11)$$

then each iteration will increase $\log P(\theta \mid Y_{obs})$, and in a well-behaved problem the sequence of parameter estimates will converge to the mode of $P(\theta|Y_{obs})$.

It is evident that when the prior $\pi(\theta)$ is chosen to be a constant function over the parameter space, this algorithm reduces to the maximum-likelihood version of EM. If the prior is not constant the M-step will change, requiring maximization of $Q^*(\theta \mid \theta^{(t)})$ rather than $Q(\theta \mid \theta^{(t)})$. The E-step procedure will be the same as in the maximum-likelihood version, however, because the E-step is dependent upon a fixed value of θ and therefore does not involve the prior.

3.2.4 Restrictions on the parameter space

Thus far little has been said about the parameter space or domain of θ. In many problems it will be the natural parameter space, the set of all values of θ for which $P(Y \mid \theta)$ is a valid probability density or probability function. In Example 2 of Section 3.2.2, for instance, we assumed nothing about the multinomial parameter π except the minimal requirements $\pi_{ij} \geq 0$ for $i, j = 1, 2$ and $\pi_{++} = \pi_{11} + \pi_{12} + \pi_{21} + \pi_{22} = 1$. In other situations, however, it is desirable to restrict θ to lie within some smaller set Θ_0, a subset of the natural parameter space which is typically of lower dimension. In the 2×2 contingency table, for example, we could require the cell probabilities to satisfy the condition of row-column independence, $\pi_{ij} = \pi_{i+}\pi_{+j}$ for all i and j. Appropriate choices for Θ_0 generate useful classes of models in a variety of continuous and categorical-data contexts.

It often happens that we want to test a null hypothesis $\theta \in \Theta_0$ versus an alternative $\theta \in \Theta_1$, where Θ_0 is a lower-dimensional subset of Θ_1. If $\hat{\theta}_0$ is the maximizer of $l(\theta \mid Y_{obs})$ over Θ_0 and $\hat{\theta}_1$ the maximizer over Θ_1, then the well known large-sample approximation

$$2\,l(\hat{\theta}_1 \mid Y_{obs}) - 2\,l(\hat{\theta}_0 \mid Y_{obs}) \sim \chi_d^2 \qquad (3.12)$$

under the null hypothesis, where $d = \dim \Theta_1 - \dim \Theta_0$, forms the basis for a *likelihood-ratio test* (e.g. Cox and Hinkley, 1974). If the drop in $2\,l(\theta \mid Y_{obs})$ as we move from $\hat{\theta}_1$ to $\hat{\theta}_0$ is unusually large when compared to the χ_d^2 distribution, then the evidence against the null hypothesis in favor of the alternative is strong. In performing this test one needs to maximize the likelihood twice, once over Θ_0 and once over Θ_1.

Using the EM algorithm to maximize a likelihood or posterior over a restricted parameter space is conceptually no different from applying EM without such restrictions. The form of the E-step will not change, because taking the expectation of a quantity with respect to $P(Y_{mis} \mid Y_{obs}, \theta)$ is computationally the same whether or not $\theta \in \Theta_0$. The M-step, however, will become a constrained maximization of the expected complete-data likelihood or posterior over Θ_0 and hence may require special, often iterative, optimization techniques. To avoid implementing an iterative M-step which would make the EM algorithm doubly iterative, it is often helpful to apply a recent extension of EM known as ECM, described below in Section 3.2.5.

Example: testing hypotheses for an incomplete 2×2 table

Returning to the National Crime Survey data in Table 3.3, we can apply the EM algorithm under the restriction that victimization status on the first occasion is independent of victimization status on the second occasion. The E-step is the same as in the unrestricted case, but the M-step is different. It is well known that with complete data, the ML estimates under independence are

$$\tilde{\theta}_{ij} = \frac{x_{i+}x_{+j}}{n^2} = \frac{(x_{i1} + x_{i2})(x_{1j} + x_{2j})}{n^2} \qquad (3.13)$$

for $i, j = 1, 2$. The M-step of EM uses (3.13) with each count x_{ij} replaced by $E(x_{ij} \,|\, \theta, Y_{obs})$, the output of the E-step. Starting from a uniform table, EM converges after four iterations to the restricted ML estimate

$$\tilde{\theta} = (\tilde{\theta}_{11}, \tilde{\theta}_{12}, \tilde{\theta}_{21}, \tilde{\theta}_{22})$$
$$= (0.6631, 0.1329, 0.1699, 0.0341).$$

Notice that the estimated cross-product ratio $(\tilde{\theta}_{11}\tilde{\theta}_{22})/(\tilde{\theta}_{12}\tilde{\theta}_{21}) = 1.00$ satisfies the independence condition as required.

To test whether row-column independence is plausible, we can perform a likelihood-ratio test. For the households that responded to the survey on both occasions, the loglikelihood contribution has the form of a complete-data multinomial loglikelihood,

$$l_A(\theta \,|\, Y_{obs}) = x_{11}^A \log \theta_{11} + x_{12}^A \log \theta_{12} + x_{21}^A \log \theta_{21} + x_{22}^A \log \theta_{22}.$$

The households that responded to the survey only on the first occasion provide information only about the marginal probabilities $\theta_{1+} = \theta_{11} + \theta_{12}$ and $\theta_{2+} = \theta_{21} + \theta_{22}$; their loglikelihood contribution has the form of a binomial,

$$l_B(\theta \,|\, Y_{obs}) = x_{1+}^B \log (\theta_{11} + \theta_{12}) + x_{2+}^B \log (\theta_{21} + \theta_{22}).$$

Similarly, the households that responded only on the second occasion contribute

$$l_C(\theta \,|\, Y_{obs}) = x_{+1}^C \log (\theta_{11} + \theta_{21}) + x_{+2}^C \log (\theta_{12} + \theta_{22}).$$

The observed-data loglikelihood is the sum of the loglikelihood contributions from each missingness pattern,

$$l(\theta \,|\, Y_{obs}) = l_A(\theta \,|\, Y_{obs}) + l_B(\theta \,|\, Y_{obs}) + l_C(\theta \,|\, Y_{obs}).$$

Plugging in the observed data and the restricted ML estimate $\tilde{\theta}$ yields $l(\tilde{\theta} \,|\, Y_{obs}) = -575.19$, the highest loglikelihood achievable under independence. Plugging in the unrestricted ML estimate $\hat{\theta}$ from Table 3.3 (b) yields $l(\hat{\theta} \,|\, Y_{obs}) = -562.50$. The likelihood-ratio test statistic is thus $2(-562.50 + 575.19) = 25.38$, which is well beyond the plausible range of a χ_1^2 random variate. We therefore conclude, not surprisingly, that victimization status on the two occasions is related.

Perhaps a more interesting and appropriate question for these data is not whether victimization during the two periods seems independent, but whether the victimization rate seems to have changed over time. That is, it may be of interest to test the hypothesis of marginal homogeneity, $\theta_{k+} = \theta_{+k}$, $k = 1, 2$, which for a 2×2 table is equivalent to the hypothesis of off-diagonal symmetry, $\theta_{12} = \theta_{21}$. With complete data, a commonly used procedure for assessing marginal homogeneity/symmetry in a 2×2 table is *McNemar's test*, in which the statistic

$$M = \frac{x_{12} - x_{21}}{\sqrt{x_{12} + x_{21}}}$$

is compared to the standard normal distribution (McNemar, 1947; Agresti, 1990). With incomplete data, we can perform a likelihood-ratio test by maximizing the likelihood subject to $\theta_{12} = \theta_{21}$. Under this restriction, we may collapse the off diagonal cells into a single cell and express the complete-data loglikelihood as that of a trinomial,

$$l(\theta \mid Y) = x_{11} \log \theta_{11} + (x_{12} + x_{21}) \log (2\theta_{12}) + x_{22} \log \theta_{22},$$

with sufficient statistics x_{11}, x_{22} and $(x_{12} + x_{21})$; the moment equations (3.7) lead immediately to the ML estimates $\breve{\theta}_{11} = x_{11}/n$, $\breve{\theta}_{22} = x_{22}/n$, and $\breve{\theta}_{12} = \breve{\theta}_{21} = (x_{12} + x_{21})/(2n)$. Revising the M-step to include the marginal homogeneity/symmetry restriction, EM quickly converges to

$$\breve{\theta} = (0.6970, \ 0.1173, \ 0.1173, \ 0.0685).$$

The loglikelihood at this estimate is $l(\breve{\theta} \mid Y_{obs}) = -564.25$, so the statistic for testing the null hypothesis of marginal homogeneity/symmetry is $2(-562.50 + 564.25) = 3.50$ with a p-value of $P(\chi_1^2 \geq 3.50) = 0.06$. The evidence against marginal homogeneity/symmetry is thus fairly strong. Extensions of this procedure for testing marginal homogeneity in $r \times r$ tables for $r > 2$ are more complicated, because ML estimates do not exist in closed form; the M-step may be carried out using techniques of nonlinear programming, as discussed by Shih (1987).

3.2.5 The ECM algorithm

The ECM or Expectation-Conditional Maximization algorithm is a useful extension of EM for situations where the M-step cannot be carried out without iteration (Meng and Rubin, 1993). ECM replaces a complicated M-step with a sequence of simpler conditional or constrained maximizations known as a CM-step. ECM retains the reliable convergence properties of EM while simplifying, and often reducing, the required computations.

The CM step of ECM is comprised of S conditional maximizations in which the Q function is maximized not over the entire parameter space as in (3.5), but over a smaller set in which a vector-valued function $g_s(\theta)$ is fixed at its previous value for $s = 1, 2, \ldots, S$. The set of functions $G = \{g_s(\theta) : s = 1, \ldots, S\}$ must be pre-selected and must satisfy precise conditions defined by Meng and Rubin (1993). Once G is specified, one iteration of ECM proceeds as follows. Given the current value of the parameter $\theta^{(t)}$, first perform an E-step to obtain $Q(\theta \mid \theta^{(t)})$ as in the EM algorithm. Then find $\theta^{(t+1)}$ by maximizing $Q(\theta \mid \theta^{(t)})$ subject to the constraint

$$g_s(\theta) = g_s(\theta^{(t+(s-1)/S)})$$

for $s = 1, 2, \ldots, S$. The resulting parameter value $\theta^{(t+S/S)} = \theta^{(t+1)}$ becomes the input to the next E-step. Clearly $Q(\theta^{(t+1)} \mid \theta^{(t)})$ must be at least as large as $Q(\theta^{(t)} \mid \theta^{(t)})$, so subsequent iterations will never decrease the observed-data loglikelihood. Moreover, it can be shown that a stationary point of ECM, i.e. a value $\theta^{(t)}$ such that $\theta^{(t+1)} = \theta^{(t)}$, is also a stationary point and typically a maximum of the observed-data loglikelihood.

The basic condition required of the set of constraints G in ECM is that repeated application of the CM-step in the absence of missing data would result in the likelihood being maximized over the whole parameter space. Many, but not all, iterative algorithms used for maximizing likelihoods with complete data can be interpreted as repeated application of a CM-step. One example is the method of cyclic ascent or iterated conditional modes (Besag, 1986), in which θ is partitioned into a set of S subvectors and the likelihood function is successively maximized with respect to each subvector holding the others constant. Another example is iterative proportional fitting of loglinear models for contingency tables (Bishop, Fienberg and Holland, 1975), in which the estimated cell probabilities are proportionately adjusted at each step to match the observed cell proportions on sets of margins determined by the model. These algorithms have often been regarded as less desirable than gradient methods such as Newton-Raphson, because they tend to converge more slowly in complete-data problems. When paired with an E-step and applied to incomplete data, however, they tend to produce computationally stable and reliable ECM algorithms that are guaranteed to increase the likelihood at each step.

Our uses of the ECM algorithm will be confined to loglinear models for categorical data (Chapter 8) and models for mixed continuous and categorical data that employ loglinear constraints (Chapter 9). Other examples of ECM and further references are given by Meng and Rubin (1993).

3.3 Properties of EM

3.3.1 Stationary values

For incomplete-data problems, the most attractive features of EM relative to other optimization techniques are its simplicity and its stability. Rather than maximizing the potentially complicated function $l(\theta \mid Y_{obs})$ directly, we repeatedly maximize the Q function, which is typically much easier and often equivalent to finding MLEs with complete data. Moreover, successive iterations of EM are guaranteed never to decrease $l(\theta \mid Y_{obs})$, which is not generally true of gradient methods like Newton-Raphson. In practice, evaluating $l(\theta \mid Y_{obs})$ at each step to ensure that it is increasing is often helpful for assessing the progress of EM and for detecting and diagnosing programming errors.

As with any optimization technique, however, EM is not guaranteed to always converge to a unique global maximum. In well-behaved problems the function $l(\theta \mid Y_{obs})$ is unimodal and concave over the entire parameter space, in which case EM converges to the unique MLE $\hat{\theta}$ from any starting value. Exceptions occur both in theory and in practice, however, and one needs to be alert to detect these abnormalities when they arise.

Multiple modes

Table 3.4 shows a hypothetical bivariate dataset reported by Murray (1977) with twelve sample units and four missing values for each variable. Under the assumption that the complete data are iid observations of a bivariate normal vector (Y_1, Y_2), one may calculate the observed-data likelihood using (2.10). It is apparent that the likelihood function is symmetric with respect to Y_1 and Y_2, and that the marginal means (μ_1, μ_2) and variances $(\sigma_{11}, \sigma_{22})$ are relatively better estimated than the correlation coefficient $\rho = \sigma_{12}/\sqrt{\sigma_{11}\sigma_{22}}$. Using analytical methods or the EM algorithm for multivariate normal data to be presented in Section 5.3, one may

Table 3.4. *Bivariate dataset with missing values*

1	1	-1	-1	2	2	-2	-2	?	?	?	?
1	-1	1	-1	?	?	?	?	2	2	-2	-2

verify that $l(\theta \mid Y_{obs})$ has two modes, one at $\theta = (\mu_1, \mu_2, \sigma_{11}, \sigma_{22}, \rho)$ $= (0, 0, 2.67, 2.67, 0.5)$ and the other at $\theta = (0, 0, 2.67, 2.67, -0.5)$. EM will converge to the first mode if started with $\rho^{(0)} > 0$ and to the second mode if $\rho^{(0)} < 0$.

The bimodality in this example is due to the symmetry of the data and the unusual pattern of missingness in which the observations with high leverage, i.e. those that would contribute the most information about ρ, have one of the two components missing. In real multivariate datasets where the data are sparse and/or the missingness pattern is unusually pernicious, multiple modes do sometimes occur. Unlike this symmetric example in which the likelihood values at the two modes are equal, there will typically be one major and one or more minor modes, and the mode to which EM converges may change depending on the choice of $\theta^{(0)}$. To detect multiple modes, it is helpful to run EM from a variety of starting values to see whether it always converges to the same answer.

Saddlepoints

A saddlepoint is a value of θ at which the directional derivatives of $l(\theta \mid Y_{obs})$ are zero but which is neither a local maximum nor a local minimum. EM could possibly converge to a saddlepoint, but in practice this is quite rare. Convergence to a saddlepoint requires not only that the saddlepoint exist, but that the successive iterates of θ approach it only from certain directions. The loglikelihood for the data in Table 3.4 has a saddlepoint at $\theta = (0, 0, 2.5, 2.5, 0)$, and EM converges to it if started from $\rho^{(0)} = 0$. However, even a very slight perturbation from $\rho = 0$ will cause EM to leave the saddle and go to one of the two modes. In real data examples convergence to a saddlepoint is rarely encountered, and thus saddlepoints are not a cause for concern.

Likelihood ridges

It may happen that the maximum value of the likelihood function is achieved not at a single value of θ but at a whole continuum of values. This phenomenon occurs when one or more components or functions of θ are inestimable in the sense that they do not appear in the likelihood, and thus $l(\theta \mid Y_{obs})$ is the same for any value of those components; that is, $l(\theta \mid Y_{obs})$ is flat in certain directions. Consider the bivariate dataset shown below.

−2	−1	0	1	2	?	?	?	?	?
?	?	?	?	?	2	1	0	−1	−2

Under the bivariate normal model $l(\theta \mid Y_{mis})$ is the sum of two complete-data loglikelihoods, one pertaining to (μ_1, σ_{11}) and the other pertaining to (μ_2, σ_{22}), and the correlation ρ is inestimable. The maximum value of $l(\theta \mid Y_{mis})$ is achieved for $\hat{\mu}_1 = \hat{\mu}_2 = 0$, $\hat{\sigma}_{11} = \hat{\sigma}_{22} = 2$, and any value of ρ, so the likelihood is said to have a one-dimensional ridge. If EM were applied to this dataset from various starting values, it would converge to different points on the ridge. When the likelihood has a ridge, any value along the ridge is a stationary value of EM. The algorithm does not wander aimlessly on the ridge but stops once the ridge is reached.

When two normal variables are not observed together, the correlation between them will be inestimable and the likelihood will have a ridge. Similar results apply to incomplete datasets with three or more variables. Consider the trivariate case where Y_1 and Y_2 are sometimes observed together, Y_1 and Y_3 are sometimes observed together, but Y_2 and Y_3 are never jointly observed; in this case it can be shown that the partial correlation of Y_2 and Y_3 given Y_1 is inestimable. Estimability of parameters in multivariate normal datasets where not all variables are observed together is discussed by Rubin (1974) and Rubin and Thayer (1978). It should be noted that merely having joint observations of all variables is not sufficient to guarantee uniqueness of the MLE, as in the example below.

−2	−1	1	2	0	0	?	?	?	?
?	?	?	?	0	0	2	1	−1	−2

Here the two joint observations of Y_1 and Y_2 are identical and thus provide no information about ρ.

Boundary estimates

Yet another abnormality is an ML estimate on the boundary of the parameter space. Consider the dataset below for which the ML estimates are $\hat{\mu}_1 = \hat{\mu}_2 = 0$, $\hat{\sigma}_{11} = \hat{\sigma}_{22} = 1.80$, and $\hat{\rho} = -1$.

−2	0	0	2	−1	1	?	?	?	?
?	?	?	?	1	−1	2	0	0	−2

If convergence is assessed by relative changes in the components of $\theta = (\mu_1, \mu_2, \sigma_{11}, \sigma_{22}, \rho)$, then EM will converge reliably in this example. If ρ is examined on some open-ended scale, however (for example, the familiar Fisher's z-transformation

$$z = \tfrac{1}{2} \log \frac{1 + \rho}{1 - \rho}, \tag{3.14}$$

which takes values on the whole real line) then the iterations of EM will appear to diverge as $z \to -\infty$.

General comments on the method of maximum likelihood

It is important to note that the abnormalities described above, multiple modes, saddlepoints, ridges and boundary solutions, are not shortcomings of the EM algorithm but inherent features of $l(\theta \mid Y_{obs})$ that would impact any optimization method. Indeed, when such features exist, EM is often remarkably well-behaved in comparison with other computational methods. With incomplete multivariate data, these abnormalities are typically associated with small samples, high rates of missingness and models that are clearly overparameterized (i.e. having too many parameters) relative to the amount of information in Y_{obs}. In the data of Table 3.4, for example, an unusually large portion of the information in Y about ρ is concentrated in Y_{mis}, and inferences about ρ will be highly sensitive to untestable assumptions about missing data and the missing-data mechanism.

From a theoretical point of view, the desirability of ML estimates stems primarily from their large-sample properties. Under suitable regularity conditions, MLEs are asymptotically unbiased, normal, and efficient with variance determined by the curvature of the loglikelihood near the mode (e.g. Cox and Hinkley, 1974). In large samples the loglikelihood function tends to be unimodal and approximately quadratic. In such cases an MLE and an estimate of its variance provide an excellent summary of the data's information about θ, and large-sample procedures such as asymptotic confidence intervals, likelihood-ratio tests, etc. will tend to be reliable. When this is not the case, however, when the loglikelihood is oddly-shaped with multiple modes, suprema on the boundary, etc., the behavior of large-sample procedures may be seriously impaired and attractiveness of the ML method is greatly diminished.

When abnormalities are found in $l(\theta \,|\, Y_{obs})$, the analyst is faced with several options. One option is to reduce the size of the model by eliminating parameters or imposing restrictions on the parameter space. Another possibility is to introduce additional information about θ through a prior distribution π and base inference on the observed-data posterior $P(\theta \,|\, Y_{obs})$ rather than the observed-data likelihood. A posterior mode will tend to be a better estimate of θ than the MLE when substantial prior knowledge about θ is available. Even when prior knowledge is scarce, however, we will find that adding small amounts of information through π may be a useful technique for ensuring that EM converges to a unique value of θ in the interior of the parameter space. When data are sparse or missing values occur in such a way that one or more components of θ are poorly estimated, a judiciously chosen prior may greatly improve the numerical stability of computations and perhaps even strengthen the estimate of θ from a statistical point of view.

3.3.2 Rate of convergence

Like any algorithm for successive approximation, EM implicitly defines a function that maps the parameter space to itself. Let $\theta = (\theta_1, \theta_2, \ldots, \theta_k)^T$ be the k-dimensional parameter. Denote a single iteration of EM by

$$\theta^{(t+1)} = M(\theta^{(t)}) = (\, M_1(\theta^{(t)}), M_2(\theta^{(t)}), \ldots M_k(\theta^{(t)})\,)^T$$

so that both the E and M-steps are incorporated into the vector function M. Expanding $M(\theta^{(t)})$ in a Taylor series about $\hat{\theta}$ gives a first-order approximation

$$M(\theta^{(t)}) - M(\hat{\theta}) \approx M'(\hat{\theta})(\theta^{(t)} - \hat{\theta}) \qquad (3.15)$$

in the neighborhood of $\hat{\theta}$, where $M'(\theta)$ is the $k \times k$ first-derivative or Jacobian matrix for $M(\theta)$ with typical element $\partial M_i(\theta)/\partial \theta_j$. If $\hat{\theta}$ is a stationary value of EM, then $M(\hat{\theta}) = \hat{\theta}$ and (3.15) becomes

$$(\theta^{(t+1)} - \hat{\theta}) \approx M'(\hat{\theta})(\theta^{(t)} - \hat{\theta}) \qquad (3.16)$$

or $\varepsilon^{(t+1)} = D\varepsilon^{(t)}$, where $\varepsilon^{(t)} \approx \theta^{(t)} - \hat{\theta}$ is the error in approximation at step t and D is shorthand for $M'(\hat{\theta})$. EM's convergence is thus said to be linear, because $\varepsilon^{(t+1)}$ is approximately a linear transformation of $\varepsilon^{(t)}$ near the mode. Newton-Raphson and other superlinear methods have the property that $D = 0$ so the Taylor series approximation in (3.15) is dominated by the smaller second-order term.

The speed at which EM converges in any particular application is determined by the rate matrix D. In the case of a scalar parameter we have $|\varepsilon^{(t+1)}| \approx D|\varepsilon^{(t)}|$ where D is a single number between 0 and 1. The convergence will be rapid when D is near zero and slow when D is near one. The situation for $k \geq 2$ is more complicated, however, and depends on the eigenstructure of D.

Any vector v such that $Dv = \lambda v$ for some constant λ is said to be an *eigenvector* of D, and λ is its associated *eigenvalue*. The eigenvalues must also satisfy the equation $|D - \lambda I| = 0$, and because the determinant of a $k \times k$ matrix is a polynomial of order k this equation has at most k distinct roots. When the roots $\lambda_1, \lambda_2, \ldots, \lambda_k$ are distinct the corresponding eigenvectors $v_1, v_2, \ldots, v_k$ are linearly independent, and any k-dimensional vector can be written as a linear combination of the eigenvectors. In particular, we can write the error vector $\varepsilon^{(t)} = \theta^{(t)} - \hat{\theta}$ as

$$\varepsilon^{(t)} = c_1 v_1 + c_2 v_2 + \cdots c_k v_k.$$

Then the error at the next iteration becomes

$$\begin{aligned} \varepsilon^{(t+1)} &\approx D(c_1 v_1 + c_2 v_2 + \cdots c_k v_k) \\ &\approx c_1 \lambda_1 v_1 + c_2 \lambda_2 v_2 + \cdots + c_k \lambda_k v_k, \end{aligned}$$

and after r iterations,

$$\varepsilon^{(t+r)} \approx c_1 \lambda_1^r v_1 + c_2 \lambda_2^r v_2 + \cdots + c_k \lambda_k^r v_k.$$

In ordinary problems all the eigenvalues will satisfy $0 \leq \lambda_j < 1$ and successive iterations of EM beginning from any $\theta^{(t)}$ in a neighborhood of $\hat{\theta}$ will shrink the error toward zero. If $\hat{\theta}$ is a saddlepoint then one or more eigenvalues could exceed one. If $\varepsilon^{(t)}$ happens to be precisely orthogonal to the eigenvectors corresponding to those eigenvalues, then EM will converge to the saddlepoint. For a randomly chosen $\theta^{(t)}$ in the neighborhood of $\hat{\theta}$, however, this will happen with negligible probability, so in most cases the iterates will diverge from a saddlepoint. One or more eigenvalues equal to one indicates that the likelihood is flat in certain directions and is maximized along a ridge (Dempster, Laird and Rubin, 1977).

The missing information principle

It is well known that in regular problems the large-sample precision of the MLE is determined by the curvature of the loglikelihood function. With complete data, the *Fisher information* is defined to be

$$I^*(\theta|Y) = -\int \left[\frac{\partial^2}{\partial\theta^2} l(\theta|Y)\right] P(Y|\theta) \, dY, \qquad (3.17)$$

where $\partial^2 l(\theta \mid Y)/\partial\theta^2$ is the $k \times k$ matrix with typical element $\partial^2 l(\theta \mid Y)/\partial\theta_i\partial\theta_j$. One estimate of the covariance matrix of $\hat{\theta}$ in large samples is $[I^*(\hat{\theta}|Y)]^{-1}$, the inverse of the Fisher information matrix evaluated at the complete-data MLE. Another, asymptotically equivalent, estimate is the inverse of

$$I(\hat{\theta}|Y) = -\frac{\partial^2}{\partial\theta^2} l(\theta|Y) \Big|_{\theta=\hat{\theta}}, \qquad (3.18)$$

which fixes Y in the loglikelihood function at its realized value rather than averaging over its distribution.

With incomplete data, differentiating (3.2) twice yields

$$-\frac{\partial^2}{\partial\theta^2} l(\theta|Y) = -\frac{\partial^2}{\partial\theta^2} l(\theta|Y_{obs}) - \frac{\partial^2}{\partial\theta^2} \log P(Y_{mis}|Y_{obs},\theta).$$

Taking the expectation of this over $P(Y_{mis} \mid Y_{obs},\theta)$, we obtain a fundamental relationship: the complete information is equal to the observed information plus the missing information. This relationship, called the *missing information principle* by Orchard and Woodbury (1972), was also investigated by Dempster, Laird and Rubin (1977), Louis (1982) and Meng and Rubin (1991a). Assuming sufficient regularity to interchange the order of differentiation and integration, we can write the complete information as

$$I_c(\theta) = -\frac{\partial^2}{\partial\theta^2} Q(\theta|\theta),$$

the observed information as

$$I_o(\theta) = -\frac{\partial^2}{\partial\theta^2} l(\theta|Y_{obs}),$$

and the missing information as

$$I_m(\theta) = -\frac{\partial^2}{\partial\theta^2} H(\theta|\theta),$$

so that

$$I_c(\theta) = I_o(\theta) + I_m(\theta). \qquad (3.19)$$

Note that each quantity in (3.19) is a function of Y_{obs}, although this fact has been suppressed in the notation. Also note that the concept of information used in (3.19) is more consistent with (3.18) than with (3.17), because we have fixed Y_{obs} at its realized value and averaged only over the distribution of the unknown Y_{mis}. A natural large-sample estimate of the covariance matrix with incomplete data is

$$I_o^{-1}(\hat{\theta}) = \left[-\frac{\partial^2}{\partial \theta^2} l(\theta \,|\, Y_{obs}) \right]_{\theta = \hat{\theta}}^{-1}, \qquad (3.20)$$

where $\hat{\theta}$ is now the observed-data MLE, the maximizer of $l(\theta \,|\, Y_{obs})$.

Missing information and convergence

Dempster, Laird and Rubin (1977) established an important connection between these information quantities and $D = M'(\hat{\theta})$, the asymptotic rate matrix of EM. In regular problems where $\theta^{(t+1)}$ is obtained as a solution to $\partial Q(\theta \,|\, \theta^{(t)})/\partial \theta = 0$, they showed that

$$D = I_c^{-1}(\hat{\theta}) \, I_m(\hat{\theta}). \qquad (3.21)$$

In the extreme case where Y_{mis} provides no additional information about θ not already contained in Y_{obs}, then $I_m(\hat{\theta}) = 0$ and (3.21) implies that EM essentially converges in a single iteration. More generally, for a scalar parameter (3.21) implies that D is the ratio of the missing information to the complete information. For brevity we will call this ratio the *fraction of missing information*, although a more precise term would be the fraction of information missing due to nonresponse. If we denote the fraction of missing information in the scalar case by $D = \lambda$, then each iteration approximately multiplies the error by λ,

$$(\theta^{(t+1)} - \hat{\theta}) \approx \lambda \, (\theta^{(t)} - \hat{\theta}), \qquad (3.22)$$

which demonstrates one of the fundamental properties of the EM algorithm: the rate of convergence of EM is determined by the fraction of missing information.

When θ is a vector of length $k > 1$ the 'fraction of missing information' is no longer a number but a matrix; yet a result similar to (3.22) holds for multiparameter problems as well. Suppose we order the eigenvalues of D so that $\lambda_1 \geq \lambda_2 \geq \cdots \geq \lambda_k$, and let $v_1, v_2, \ldots, v_k$ be eigenvectors of D corresponding to these ordered eigenvalues. As before, we can write the error vector as

$$\varepsilon^{(t)} = \theta^{(t)} - \hat{\theta} = c_1 v_1 + c_2 v_2 + \cdots c_k v_k$$

for some $c_1, c_2, \ldots, c_k$, so that after r iterations

$$\varepsilon^{(t+r)} \approx c_1 \lambda_1^r v_1 + c_2 \lambda_2^r v_2 + \cdots + c_k \lambda_k^r v_k.$$

By analogy with (3.22) we may regard $\lambda_1, \lambda_2, \ldots, \lambda_k$ as fractions of missing information corresponding to the particular directions $v_1, v_2, \ldots, v_k$. Moreover, if λ_2 is strictly less than λ_1 we have

$$\varepsilon^{(t+r)} \approx \lambda_1^r (c_1 v_1 + R), \qquad (3.23)$$

where the remainder term

$$R = c_2 \left(\frac{\lambda_2}{\lambda_1}\right)^r v_2 + \cdots + c_k \left(\frac{\lambda_k}{\lambda_1}\right)^r v_k$$

approaches zero at a rate determined by λ_2/λ_1. Thus in the vicinity of the mode,

$$(\theta^{(t+1)} - \hat{\theta}) \approx \lambda_1 (\theta^{(t)} - \hat{\theta}) \qquad (3.24)$$

where λ_1 is the largest eigenvalue of D. If the s largest eigenvalues happen to be equal, then (3.23) becomes

$$\varepsilon^{(t+r)} \approx \lambda_1^r (c_1 v_1 + \cdots + c_s v_s + R)$$

where R approaches zero at a rate determined by λ_{s+1}/λ_1, and (3.24) still holds. In the multiparameter case, we can thus say that *EM's rate of convergence is governed by the largest fraction of missing information*. Exceptions to this rule are possible; for example, if $\varepsilon^{(t)}$ happens to be precisely orthogonal to the eigenvector(s) corresponding to the largest eigenvalue, then convergence will be dominated by the next largest eigenvalue. For most real-data problems, however, this basic result does hold. Further results and discussion on the convergence of EM are given by Meng (1990).

3.3.3 Example

In Example 1 of Section 3.2.2, we derived the EM algorithm for incomplete univariate normal data and applied it to the $n_1 = 10$ observations displayed in Table 3.1 (a) by assuming that an additional $n_0 = 3$ observations were missing. By varying the choice of n_0 we can make the rate of convergence in this example arbitrarily large or small. Figure 3.1 displays the iterations of EM in this two-parameter problem from a variety of starting values under $n_0 = 10$ and $n_0 = 90$, corresponding to missingness rates of 50% and 90%, respectively. For visual clarity the variance ψ is shown on the log scale. With $n_0 = 10$ the convergence is quite rapid, whereas for $n_0 = 90$ it is much slower. Unlike gradient methods EM does not necessarily follow the path of steepest ascent, but often climbs the loglikelihood surface by a more circuitous route.

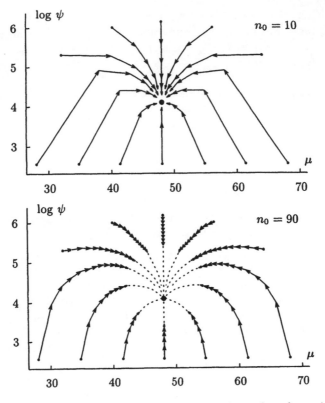

Figure 3.1. *Iterations of EM from various starting values for univariate normal data with $n_0 = 10$ and $n_0 = 90$.*

In simple examples like this one, it is feasible to investigate the convergence properties analytically. The elements of the matrix $M'(\theta^{(t)})$, obtained by differentiating (3.9)–(3.10), are

$$\frac{\partial \mu^{(t+1)}}{\partial \mu^{(t)}} = \frac{n_0}{n},$$

$$\frac{\partial \mu^{(t+1)}}{\partial \psi^{(t)}} = 0,$$

$$\frac{\partial \psi^{(t+1)}}{\partial \mu^{(t)}} = 2\left(\frac{n_0 n_1}{n^2}\right)\left(\mu^{(t)} - \bar{y}_{obs}\right),$$

$$\frac{\partial \psi^{(t+1)}}{\partial \psi^{(t)}} = \frac{n_0}{n},$$

where $\bar{y}_{obs} = n_1^{-1} \sum_{i=1}^{n_1} y_i$ is the observed-data MLE for μ. Evaluating these derivatives at the mode (i.e. taking $\theta^{(t)} = \hat{\theta}$) gives

$$D = M'(\hat{\theta}) = \left[\begin{array}{cc} n_0/n & 0 \\ 0 & n_0/n \end{array} \right].$$

The eigenvalues of this matrix are $\lambda_1 = \lambda_2 = \lambda = n_0/n$. Whenever eigenvalues are repeated, the corresponding eigenvectors are not uniquely defined. In fact, because D is proportional to the identity matrix in this example, any error vector $\varepsilon^{(t)}$ is an eigenvector. Yet the overall convergence rate is still governed by λ, and a single iteration of EM can be expressed as $\varepsilon^{(t+1)} \approx \lambda \varepsilon^{(t)}$.

In this and other univariate examples, the fraction of missing information λ is also the rate of missing observations. In multivariate applications, however, the fractions of missing information corresponding to various components of θ will typically differ from the rates of missing observations, both overall and on a variable-by-variable basis, depending on the pattern of missingness and the observed interrelationships among variables.

3.3.4 Further comments on convergence

Monitoring and detecting convergence

Two basic methods for monitoring the convergence of EM involve (a) successive parameter values $\theta^{(t)}$, and (b) successive values of the observed-data loglikelihood $l(\theta^{(t)} \,|\, Y_{obs})$. In practice both are quite useful. Because each iteration of EM is guaranteed never to decrease the likelihood, evaluating $l(\theta \,|\, Y_{obs})$ at each step is helpful for detecting programming errors as well as for monitoring the progress of EM in specific examples. Convergence is typically judged by examining changes in individual components of $\theta = (\theta_1, \theta_2, \ldots, \theta_k)$ from one iteration to the next. If the changes are all relatively small, for example, if

$$|\theta_j^{(t)} - \theta_j^{(t-1)}| \leq \epsilon |\theta_j^{(t)}|$$

for $j = 1, 2, \ldots, k$ and a suitably small ϵ (say, 0.0001), then we may say that EM has 'converged' by iteration t.

If the elements of θ continue to change for many iterations with very little increase in $l(\theta \,|\, Y_{obs})$, then it should be taken as a sign that the loglikelihood is nearly flat in certain directions and that one or more functions of θ are very poorly estimated. Often in these problems there is little to be gained from additional iterations, because the value of θ to which EM would ultimately converge has loglikelihood only slightly higher than the current value; the observed data do little to distinguish between these values of θ. Slow convergence is also a sign that the fractions of missing information corresponding to certain aspects of θ are close to one, and that most of the information about them is being contributed by $P(Y_{mis} \mid Y_{obs}, \theta)$, the model for the missing data, rather than by Y_{obs}. Because the correctness of $P(Y_{mis} \mid Y_{obs}, \theta)$ rests on both the complete-data model and the ignorability assumption, slow convergence warns us that inferences about certain aspects of θ are highly model-dependent. This does not automatically mean that all inferences about θ are suspect, because in some problems (e.g. when the missing data are missing by design and therefore known to be MAR) the model may be quite trustworthy. In other problems, however, particularly when it is not known whether the data are MAR, slow convergence is a useful warning that the estimate of θ may rest largely on our assumptions about the unknown Y_{mis} rather than on the known Y_{obs}. If so, then a simplification of the model, perhaps by imposing restrictions on the parameter or by eliminating variables with high rates of missingness, may be a sensible strategy.

Asymptotic covariance matrices from EM

One drawback of EM relative to other optimization techniques is that it does not automatically provide standard errors associated with the parameter estimates. The asymptotic covariance matrix $I_o^{-1}(\hat\theta)$ defined in (3.20) is not readily available because implementation of EM does not require calculation of the derivatives of $l(\theta \mid Y_{obs})$, which are often complicated and tedious to derive.

In a comment on the original EM paper, Smith (1977) noted that for a scalar parameter the iterations of EM provide a good estimate of λ. From (3.22) it is apparent that after a large number of iterations λ will be well approximated by $\varepsilon^{(t+1)}/\varepsilon^{(t)}$ or, equivalently, by $\hat\lambda^{(t)} = (\theta^{(t+1)} - \theta^{(t)})/(\theta^{(t)} - \theta^{(t-1)})$, because

$$\hat\lambda^{(t)} = \frac{\theta^{(t+1)} - \theta^{(t)}}{\theta^{(t)} - \theta^{(t-1)}} = \frac{\varepsilon^{(t+1)} - \varepsilon^{(t)}}{\varepsilon^{(t)} - \varepsilon^{(t-1)}} \approx \frac{\lambda\varepsilon^{(t)} - \varepsilon^{(t)}}{\varepsilon^{(t)} - \lambda^{-1}\varepsilon^{(t)}} = \lambda.$$

This estimate of λ may be used to obtain a large-sample standard error for $\hat\theta$, because (3.19) and (3.21) imply that the asymptotic variance of $\hat\theta$ is

$$I_o^{-1}(\hat\theta) = I_c^{-1}(\hat\theta)/(1 - \lambda).$$

For exponential families, $I_c^{-1}(\hat{\theta})$ is the complete-data asymptotic variance calculated from the expected sufficient statistics obtained at the last E-step. In other words, a standard error for $\hat{\theta}$ can be obtained simply by inflating the complete-data standard error by $\sqrt{1 - \lambda}$, where λ is estimated from the steps of EM.

In most real-data applications, of course, θ is multidimensional, and obtaining a covariance matrix for $\hat{\theta}$ is less straightforward. A general numerical procedure for approximating $I_o^{-1}(\hat{\theta})$, given by Meng and Rubin (1991a), is called Supplemented EM or SEM. From (3.19) and (3.21) it can be shown that

$$I_o^{-1}(\hat{\theta}) = I_c^{-1}(\hat{\theta}) + I_c^{-1}(\hat{\theta}) (I - D)^{-1} D. \tag{3.25}$$

Meng and Rubin show how the elements of $D = M'(\hat{\theta})$ can be estimated by repeated runs of a 'forced EM' in which all but one of the individual elements of θ are fixed at their MLEs. The procedure corresponds to numerical differentiation with step sizes determined by EM. For a k dimensional parameter one needs to perform k runs of forced EM, one to estimate each row of D. Using (3.25), the numerical estimate of D is then combined with the complete-data asymptotic covariance matrix $I_c^{-1}(\hat{\theta})$ to produce $I_o^{-1}(\hat{\theta})$. Implementation of SEM thus requires only the code for computing an asymptotic covariance matrix from complete data and the code for the EM algorithm itself.

An asymptotic covariance matrix for $\hat{\theta}$ is typically used in conjunction with the large-sample normal approximation

$$(\hat{\theta} - \theta) \sim N(0, I_o^{-1}(\hat{\theta})), \tag{3.26}$$

which can be justified from either a frequentist or a Bayesian perspective (e.g. Cox and Hinkley, 1974). This approximation is expected to work well when the sample size is sufficiently large that $l(\theta \mid Y_{obs})$ resembles a quadratic function in the vicinity of $\hat{\theta}$. In practice the validity of (3.26) often depends on the scale of the parameter, and transformations may need to be applied to one or more components of θ to make the approximation more accurate. Transformations to improve normality will alter the form of the complete-data covariance matrix $I_c^{-1}(\hat{\theta})$. When $l(\theta \mid Y_{obs})$ has unusual features such as multiple modes, ridges or suprema on a boundary, then the value of an asymptotic covariance matrix is dubious at best, and (3.26) should not be used for making inferential statements about θ.

For many of the multivariate models and data examples in this book, the potentially large number of parameters makes the implementation of SEM computationally prohibitive. In some cases the validity of the normal approximation (3.26) will be suspect as well, even on a carefully chosen scale for θ. For this reason, we will adopt simulation rather than asymptotic approximation as the primary method of inference. In multiparameter problems, simulation is often feasible even when the dimension of θ is very large. Moreover, simulation-based inferences can be made about any transformation or function of θ with no special analytic work involved.

Elementwise rates of convergence

Apart from obtaining asymptotic standard errors, it may still be useful to examine rates of convergence corresponding to the individual elements of $\theta = (\theta_1, \theta_2, \ldots, \theta_k)$. These rates may be estimated from the iterations of EM by

$$\hat{\lambda}_j^{(t)} = \frac{\theta_j^{(t+1)} - \theta_j^{(t)}}{\theta_j^{(t)} - \theta_j^{(t-1)}} \tag{3.27}$$

for $j = 1, 2, \ldots, k$ at suitably large values of t. Unlike the eigenvalues of D, which are the fractions of missing information corresponding to the eigenvectors, these elementwise rates pertain to $u_1, u_2, \ldots, u_k$, where u_j is a unit vector with a one in position j and zeroes elsewhere. As noted by Meng and Rubin (1991a), in most cases (3.27) will estimate the largest eigenvalue of D, because u_j will have a nonzero component corresponding to the first eigenvector. If u_j happens to be precisely orthogonal to the first s eigenvectors, then (3.27) will converge to the $(s+1)$st largest eigenvalue of D. Consequently, the elementwise rates of convergence typically provide the first and perhaps a few additional eigenvalues of D, which can be a useful diagnostic for assessing how much information about θ is contained in $P(Y_{mis} | Y_{obs}, \theta)$ relative to Y_{obs}.

For the EM example in Table 3.1, estimates $\hat{\lambda}_1^{(t)}$ and $\hat{\lambda}_2^{(t)}$ of the elementwise rates of convergence corresponding to the mean μ and the variance ψ, respectively, are displayed in Table 3.2. As previously shown, the eigenvalues of D are both equal to $n_0/n = 3/13 = 0.2308$, and the elementwise rates converge to this number quite rapidly. Very close to the mode, successive values of θ are nearly identical and computation of (3.27) becomes numerically unstable. It is generally wise to compute (3.27) using double precision arithmetic and to estimate the rates from the last few iterations before numerical instability becomes evident. Note that in a multiparameter problem these elementwise rates alone are not sufficient

Table 3.5. *Iterations of EM for incomplete uni-variate normal data with estimated elementwise rates of convergence*

t	$\mu^{(t)}$	$\psi^{(t)}$	$\hat{\lambda}_1^{(t)}$	$\hat{\lambda}_2^{(t)}$
0	30.0000	70.0000	—	—
1	43.9231	120.0218	0.2308	−0.8699
2	47.1361	76.5067	0.2308	0.2982
3	47.8776	63.5326	0.2308	0.2428
4	48.0487	60.3825	0.2308	0.2334
5	48.0882	59.6472	0.2308	0.2314
6	48.0973	59.4771	0.2308	0.2309
7	48.0994	59.4378	0.2308	0.2308
8	48.0999	59.4287	0.2308	0.2308
9	48.1000	59.4266	0.2308	0.2308
10	48.1000	59.4261	0.2308	0.2308
11	48.1000	59.4260	0.2308	0.2308
∞	48.1000	59.4260	—	—

to obtain standard errors for the individual elements of $\hat{\theta}$. As seen from (3.25), the variance of a single element of $\hat{\theta}$ generally depends on the entire D matrix, whereas the elementwise rates provide at most only a few eigenvalues of D.

In some problems one or more components of θ may have no missing information at all. In the bivariate normal data depicted in Figure 2.2, for example, there are no missing observations of Y_1 and hence μ_1 and σ_{11} have no missing information. An EM algorithm for these data would converge to the ML estimates for μ_1 and σ_{11} in a single step from any starting value. When one or more components of θ converge immediately, the elementwise rates of convergence from the remaining components still estimate the largest fractions of missing information.

Accelerating convergence

The linear behavior of EM near the mode suggests some potentially useful methods for accelerating convergence. Rearranging (3.16), we can obtain an estimate of $\hat{\theta}$ in terms of two successive iterates $\theta^{(t)}$ and $\theta^{(t+1)}$,

$$\tilde{\theta}^{(t+1)} = \theta^{(t)} + (I - D)^{-1}(\theta^{(t-1)} - \theta^{(t)}), \qquad (3.28)$$

which is typically closer to the mode than $\theta^{(t+1)}$. This technique, commonly known as *Aitken acceleration*, can make a linearly convergent algorithm like EM almost superlinear. When the individual components of θ appear to be converging at the same elementwise rate, (3.24) suggests that

$$\tilde{\theta}^{(t+1)} = \theta^{(t)} + (1 - \lambda_1)^{-1}(\theta^{(t-1)} - \theta^{(t)}) \tag{3.29}$$

may also work well, where λ_1 is the largest eigenvalue of D. These acceleration techniques require an estimate of D or at least its largest eigenvalue, which can be obtained by analytic methods or from the iterations of EM. The use of Aitken-type acceleration methods for EM have been investigated by Louis (1982); Laird, Lange and Stram (1987); and Lansky and Casella (1990). Another technique, proposed by Belin and Diffendal (1991), is to estimate the jth component of θ by

$$\tilde{\theta}_j^{(t+1)} = \theta_j^{(t)} + (1 - \hat{\lambda}_j)^{-1}(\theta_j^{(t-1)} - \theta_j^{(t)}) \tag{3.30}$$

for $j = 1, 2, \ldots, k$, where $\hat{\lambda}_j$ is the estimated elementwise rate of convergence for θ_j given by (3.27). This third method, which may be regarded as intermediate between (3.28) and (3.29), is easier to compute than (3.28) and more appropriate than (3.29) in situations where the elements of θ appear to be converging at different rates.

Care should be taken in the use of these accelerated versions of EM, as they are not guaranteed to increase the loglikelihood at each step. Acceleration should not be employed until $\theta^{(t)}$ is close enough to the mode for (a) the steps of EM to be approximately linear, and (b) the estimated fractions of missing information to be stable. As previously mentioned, slow convergence of EM in an incomplete-data problem should be taken as a warning that certain aspects of θ are being estimated primarily from $P(Y_{mis} \mid Y_{obs}, \theta)$ rather than Y_{obs}. In such problems it is sometimes more reasonable to 'bail out' of the current analysis and fit a simpler model, rather than to continue iterating with a model whose parameters are poorly estimated.

Convergence and prior information

When EM is being used to find a posterior mode rather than an ML estimate, the missing information principle described in Section 3.3.2 applies but in a slightly modified form. The decomposition of (3.19) becomes

$$I_c(\theta) = I_o(\theta) + I_m(\theta) + I_\pi(\theta),$$

where $I_c(\theta)$, $I_o(\theta)$ and $I_m(\theta)$ are defined as above, and the additional term $I_\pi(\theta)$ is the information contained in the prior distribution,

$$I_\pi(\theta) = -\frac{\partial^2}{\partial\theta^2}\,\pi(\theta).$$

This term will be small when π is relatively flat and large when π is sharply peaked. The basic relationship (3.21) between these information quantities and the rate matrix $D = M'(\hat{\theta})$ still applies,

$$D = I_c^{-1}(\hat{\theta})\,I_m(\hat{\theta}),$$

but the complete information matrix $I_c(\hat{\theta})$ now includes prior information. The introduction of a prior may thus be expected to reduce the magnitude of D and accelerate the convergence of EM in most cases. In particular, this will be true when the prior introduces substantial information about those aspects of θ that are most poorly estimated, those that influence the largest eigenvalue of D.

Convergence properties of ECM

The ECM algorithm introduced in Section 3.2.5 shares many of the convergence properties of EM. Like EM, it increases the loglikelihood at each step and converges reliably to a local maximum or (rarely) a saddlepoint of the loglikelihood. Like EM, it also exhibits linear convergence in the vicinity of the mode. ECM can be thought of as a combination of two linearly convergent algorithms: an EM algorithm, which pertains to the incomplete-data aspects of the problem, and a CM or conditional maximization algorithm, which pertains to the maximization of the likelihood in the complete-data case. As pointed out by Meng and Rubin (1992a), there seems to be little advantage to replacing the linearly convergent CM step with one or more steps of a superlinear technique such as Newton-Raphson, because the overall convergence of the combined algorithm will still be linear. Moreover, unless the superlinear algorithm is run to full convergence at each M-step, the loglikelihood would not be guaranteed to increase at each iteration.

With ECM, the global and elementwise rates of convergence cannot immediately be interpreted as fractions of missing information, because the simple identity $D = I_c^{-1}(\hat{\theta})\,I_m(\hat{\theta})$ does not generally hold. Basic results on ECM's rate of convergence, including relationships between the D matrix and information quantities, have been established by Meng (1994). Some of these results are counterintuitive; for instance, examples can be constructed where ECM converges more quickly than EM. A numerical method for obtaining large-sample covariance matrices from ECM, called Supplemented ECM or SECM, is described by Meng and Rubin (1992a).

3.4 Markov chain Monte Carlo

Markov chain Monte Carlo is a collection of techniques for creating pseudorandom draws from probability distributions. In recent years it has been a subject of intense interest among statisticians, spawning a wide range of applications as well as a great deal of innovative theoretical work. In a broad sense, the goal of Markov chain Monte Carlo is to generate one or more values of a random variable Z, which is typically multidimensional. Let $P(Z) = f(Z)$ denote the density of Z, which we call the *target distribution*. Rather than attempting to draw from f directly, we generate a sequence $\{Z^{(1)}, Z^{(2)}, \ldots, Z^{(t)}, \ldots\}$ where each variate in the sequence depends in some fashion on the preceding ones, and where the stationary distribution (i.e. the limiting marginal distribution of $Z^{(t)}$ as $t \to \infty$) is the target f. For a t sufficiently large, $Z^{(t)}$ is approximately a random draw from f. Markov chain Monte Carlo is attractive when f is difficult to draw from directly, but drawing each variate in the sequence is straightforward.

Markov chain Monte Carlo methods have often been classified under 'Bayesian computation' or 'Bayesian posterior simulation' because many of the best known current applications have a strong Bayesian flavor; when viewed strictly as simulation methods, however, there is nothing inherently Bayesian about them. Also, despite the popularity of the term Markovchain Monte Carlo, depending on how the methods are viewed some of them are not strictly Markovian. In this new and rapidly evolving field, the lack of well defined and broadly accepted terminology has sometimes been a source of confusion. The reader should understand that names given to the methods below, and the definitions of these methods, are not universally accepted and may differ somewhat from what other authors have written.

This list of Markov chain Monte Carlo methods is not meant to be exhaustive, but concentrates on some that have proven most useful in the analysis of incomplete multivariate data. Presentations in a more general setting and additional references are given by Gelfand and Smith (1990); the articles by Gelman and Rubin (1992a), Geyer (1992) and Smith and Roberts (1993) with accompanying discussions; and Tierney (1994). Applications of Markov chain Monte Carlo are discussed by Gelfand *et al.* (1990); Casella and George (1992); Smith and Roberts (1993); and Gilks *et al.* (1993), among others. A comprehensive overview including theory and applications appears in the books by Tanner (1993) and Gilks, Richardson, and Spiegelhalter (1996).

3.4.1 Gibbs sampling

Gibbs sampling is the most popular and well known form of Markov chain Monte Carlo. Suppose that a random vector Z is partitioned into J subvectors,

$$Z = (Z_1, Z_2, \ldots, Z_J).$$

Let $P(Z)$ denote the joint distribution of Z, which is also the target distribution to be simulated. In Gibbs sampling, we iteratively draw from the conditional distribution of each subvector given all the others. Given the value of Z at step t, say

$$Z^{(t)} = (Z_1^{(t)}, Z_2^{(t)}, \ldots, Z_J^{(t)}),$$

the value of Z at step $t+1$,

$$Z^{(t+1)} = (Z_1^{(t+1)}, Z_2^{(t+1)}, \ldots, Z_J^{(t+1)}),$$

is obtained by successively drawing from the distributions

$$
\begin{aligned}
Z_1^{(t+1)} &\sim P(Z_1 \,|\, Z_2^{(t)}, Z_3^{(t)}, \ldots, Z_J^{(t)}) \\
Z_2^{(t+1)} &\sim P(Z_2 \,|\, Z_1^{(t+1)}, Z_3^{(t)}, \ldots, Z_J^{(t)}) \\
&\vdots \\
Z_J^{(t+1)} &\sim P(Z_J \,|\, Z_1^{(t+1)}, Z_2^{(t+1)}, \ldots, Z_{J-1}^{(t+1)})
\end{aligned}
\tag{3.31}
$$

in a slight abuse of notation. In other words, we draw from the conditional distributions of Z_1, Z_2, up to Z_J, conditioning each time on the most recently drawn values of all other subvectors. After the full set of subvectors has been drawn, we repeat the whole process to obtain $Z^{(t+2)}$, $Z^{(t+3)}$, and so on. The sequence $\{Z^{(t)} : t = 0, 1, 2, \ldots\}$ forms a Markov chain which, under mild regularity conditions, has a stationary distribution equal to $P(Z)$; that is, $Z^{(t)} \to Z$ in distribution as $t \to \infty$.

The name *Gibbs* is not at all descriptive of this method, but actually refers to a class of probability distributions on lattice systems that have been used in problems of spatial analysis and statistical image reconstruction (Besag, 1974). The first use of Gibbs sampling in this context was made by Geman and Geman (1984), who provided a proof of convergence for a discrete Z with finite state space. The method was independently derived for $J = 2$ by Li (1988), who presented an argument for convergence in the continuous case. Other convergence proofs under various conditions are given by Schervish and Carlin (1992); Liu, Wong, and Kong (1994, 1995); and Tierney (1994).

The regularity conditions necessary to establish convergence of the Gibbs sampler in a general setting are somewhat technical, but they do tend to be satisfied in most problems of practical interest. Informally, one can say that sufficient conditions are (a) that the target distribution $P(Z)$ must be a genuine probability distribution, and the sequence (3.31) must be the actual conditional distributions corresponding to this target; and (b) that the sample space of Z must be 'connected' in the sense that it must be possible to reach any point in the sample space from any other point by repeated sampling from the conditionals in the manner of (3.31); periodicity and absorbing states are not allowed. For more discussion, see Roberts (1996) and Tierney (1996). For some examples of nonconvergence, see Casella and George (1992); Arnold (1993); and Section 3.5.2 below.

As pointed out by Liu, Wong and Kong (1995), the conditional distributions (3.31) in the Gibbs sampler need not be drawn from in any particular order in each iteration, nor do they need to be drawn from equally often. As long as each conditional distribution is visited infinitely often, the stationary distribution will be $P(Z)$. As a practical matter, of course, different visitation schemes will have different properties when only a finite number of iterations are performed. The distributions (3.31) are sometimes called the 'full conditionals' because each one is the distribution of a subvector given all the other subvectors. Other sets of conditional distributions may also be grouped together to form sampling schemes that will converge to $P(Z)$, as described by Gelfand and Smith (1990).

3.4.2 Data augmentation

Closely related to Gibbs sampling is the data augmentation algorithm of Tanner and Wong (1987). Suppose that a random vector z is partitioned into two subvectors, $z = (u, v)$, where the joint distribution $P(z)$ is not easily simulated but the conditional distributions $P(u \mid v) = g(u \mid v)$ and $P(v \mid u) = h(v \mid u)$ are. At iteration

t, let

$$Z^{(t)} = (z_1^{(t)}, z_2^{(t)}, \ldots, z_m^{(t)})$$
$$= ((u_1^{(t)}, v_1^{(t)}), (u_2^{(t)}, v_2^{(t)}), \ldots, (u_m^{(t)}, v_m^{(t)}))$$

be a sample of size m from a distribution that approximates the target distribution $P(z)$. This sample is updated in two steps. First,

$$U^{(t+1)} = (u_1^{(t+1)}, u_2^{(t+1)}, \ldots, u_m^{(t+1)})$$

is created by drawing

$$u_i^{(t+1)} \sim g(u \mid v_i^{(t)})$$

independently for $i = 1, 2, \ldots, m$. Next,

$$V^{(t+1)} = (v_1^{(t+1)}, v_2^{(t+1)}, \ldots, v_m^{(t+1)})$$

is drawn as an iid sample from the equally weighted mixture of the conditionals $h(v \mid u_i^{(t+1)})$,

$$\bar{h}(v \mid U^{(t+1)}) = \frac{1}{m} \sum_{i=1}^{m} h(v \mid u_i^{(t+1)}), \tag{3.32}$$

which completes the new sample

$$Z^{(t+1)} = ((u_1^{(t+1)}, v_1^{(t+1)}), \ldots, (u_m^{(t+1)}, v_m^{(t+1)})).$$

Using functional analysis, Tanner and Wong (1987) show that the distribution of $Z^{(t)}$ converges to $P(z)$ as $t \to \infty$. This result does not require a large value of m; in particular, with $m = 1$ data augmentation reduces to a special case of the Gibbs sampler (3.31) with the random quantities $z = (u, v)$ partitioned into two subvectors, u and v. More generally, if we modify the second step of each iteration by sampling

$$v_i^{(t+1)} \sim h(v \mid u_i^{(t+1)})$$

independently for $i = 1, 2, \ldots, m$ rather than drawing them from the mixture (3.32), then the algorithm becomes m independent, parallel runs of a Gibbs sampler. The mixing of the conditionals $h(v \mid u)$ at each iteration may not provide much practical benefit in speeding the convergence of the $Z^{(t)}$, but when m is large (3.32) provides a good analytic approximation to the marginal density $P(v) = \int P(u, v) \, du$ if such an approximation is desired.

Application to missing-data problems

The name *data augmentation* arose from applications of this algorithm to Bayesian inference with missing data. In many incomplete-data problems, the observed-data posterior $P(\theta | Y_{obs})$ is intractable and cannot easily be summarized or simulated; when Y_{obs} is 'augmented' by an assumed value of the Y_{mis}, however, the resulting complete-data posterior $P(\theta | Y_{obs}, Y_{mis})$ becomes much easier to handle. Consider the following iterative sampling scheme: given a current guess $\theta^{(t)}$ of the parameter, first draw a value of the missing data from the conditional predictive distribution of Y_{mis},

$$Y_{mis}^{(t+1)} \sim P(Y_{mis} | Y_{obs}, \theta^{(t)}). \tag{3.33}$$

Then, conditioning on $Y_{mis}^{(t+1)}$, draw a new value of θ from its complete-data posterior,

$$\theta^{(t+1)} \sim P(\theta | Y_{obs}, Y_{mis}^{(t+1)}). \tag{3.34}$$

Repeating (3.33)–(3.34) from a starting value $\theta^{(0)}$ yields a stochastic sequence $\{(\theta^{(t)}, Y_{mis}^{(t)}) : t = 1, 2, \ldots\}$ whose stationary distribution is $P(\theta, Y_{mis} | Y_{obs})$, and the subsequences $\{\theta^{(t)} : t = 1, 2, \ldots\}$ and $\{Y_{mis}^{(t)} : t = 1, 2, \ldots\}$ have $P(\theta | Y_{obs})$ and $P(Y_{mis} | Y_{obs})$ as their respective stationary distributions. Following the terminology of Tanner and Wong (1987), we will refer to (3.33) as the Imputation or I-step and (3.34) as the Posterior or P-step, because (3.33) corresponds to imputing a value of the missing data Y_{mis} and (3.34) corresponds to drawing a value of θ from a complete-data posterior. For a value of t that is suitably large, we can regard $\theta^{(t)}$ as an approximate draw from $P(\theta | Y_{obs})$; alternatively, we can regard $Y_{mis}^{(t)}$ as an approximate draw from $P(Y_{mis} | Y_{obs})$.

Many particular examples of the algorithm (3.33)–(3.34) will appear throughout the remainder of this book. The first use of this algorithm seems to have been made by Li (1988) who presented an argument for convergence and used it to create imputations of Y_{mis} in incomplete-data problems. The algorithm can be regarded either as a special case of data augmentation with $m = 1$ or as a special case of Gibbs sampling with (Y_{mis}, θ) partitioned into Y_{mis} and θ. Because the former name is more descriptive for incomplete-data problems, we will refer to it as data augmentation rather than Gibbs sampling. For the most part, however, we will use only the special case of data augmentation with $m = 1$. On occasion we will perform $m > 1$ parallel runs of data augmentation, but we will keep the runs independent; that is, we will not employ mixing (3.32) at each iteration.

Data augmentation bears a strong resemblance to the EM algorithm. The E-step of EM calculates the expected complete-data sufficient statistics, whereas the I-step of data augmentation simulates a random draw of the complete-data sufficient statistics. The implementation of an I-step is typically very similar to that of an E-step, usually requiring only minor modifications of the computer code. The M-step of EM is a maximization of a complete-data likelihood, while the P-step of data augmentation is a random draw from a complete-data posterior. The computational requirements of EM and data augmentation are therefore quite similar, as both involve repeated application of complete-data methods to solve an incomplete-data problem.

3.4.3 Examples of data augmentation

Example 1: *Incomplete univariate normal data.* Suppose that $Y = (y_1, y_2, \ldots, y_n)$ is an iid sample from a normal distribution with mean μ and variance ψ which, for the moment, is assumed to be known. If we apply a normal prior distribution to μ with mean μ_0 and variance τ, it follows that the posterior distribution of μ given Y is also normal with mean

$$E(\mu \mid Y) = \left(\frac{n\psi^{-1}}{n\psi^{-1} + \tau^{-1}} \right) \bar{y} + \left(\frac{\tau^{-1}}{n\psi^{-1} + \tau^{-1}} \right) \mu_0 \qquad (3.35)$$

and variance $V(\mu \mid Y) = (n\psi^{-1} + \tau^{-1})^{-1}$, where $\bar{y}$ is the sample mean of $y_1, y_2, \ldots, y_n$. Letting $\tau \to \infty$, the posterior becomes normal with mean $\bar{y}$ and variance $n^{-1}\psi$, which may also be obtained by applying Bayes's formula with the improper diffuse prior $\pi(\mu) \propto c$ where c is a constant (e.g. Box and Tiao, 1992).

Now suppose that only the first n_1 elements of Y are observed and the remaining $n_0 = n - n_1$ are missing. Under ignorability and the diffuse prior $\pi(\mu) \propto c$, the observed-data posterior $P(\mu \mid Y_{obs})$ becomes normal with mean $\bar{y}_{obs} = n_1^{-1} \sum_{i=1}^{n_1} y_i$ and variance $n_1^{-1}\psi$. In this trivial example, values of μ from $P(\mu \mid Y_{obs})$ can be simulated directly using standard routines for generating normal random variates. We can also simulate them iteratively, however, using the data augmentation routine of (3.33)–(3.34). Given a current parameter value $\mu^{(t)}$, the I-step simulates $Y_{mis}^{(t+1)}$ by drawing

$$y_i^{(t+1)} \mid \mu^{(t)}, Y_{obs} \sim N(\mu^{(t)}, \psi) \qquad (3.36)$$

independently for $i = n_1 + 1, \ldots, n$. The P-step then proceeds to draw $\mu^{(t+1)}$ from the complete-data posterior $P(\mu | Y_{obs}, Y_{mis}^{(t+1)})$, a normal distribution with mean

$$\bar{y}^{(t+1)} = n^{-1} \left[\sum_{i=1}^{n_1} y_i + \sum_{i=n_1+1}^{n} y_i^{(t+1)} \right]$$

and variance $n^{-1}\psi$.

In this simple example of data augmentation, one may analytically verify that the distribution of $\mu^{(t)}$ approaches the correct observed-data posterior $N(\bar{y}_{obs}, n_1^{-1}\psi)$ as $t \to \infty$. This is possible because of the following well known property of the normal distribution: If $U \,|\, V \sim N(V, a)$ and $V \sim N(b, c)$ then $U \sim N(b, a+c)$. Applying this property, the conditional distribution of $\mu^{(t)}$ given Y_{obs} and the previous iterate $\mu^{(t-1)}$ is easily seen to be

$$\mu^{(t)} \,|\, \mu^{(t-1)} \sim N(\bar{y}_{obs} + \lambda(\mu^{(t-1)} - \bar{y}_{obs}), n_1^{-1}\psi(1 - \lambda^2)),$$

where $\lambda = n_0/n$ and conditioning on Y_{obs} has been suppressed in the notation. Similarly, the conditional distribution of $\mu^{(t)}$ given Y_{obs} and $\mu^{(t-2)}$ is also normal, with mean

$$
\begin{aligned}
E(\mu^{(t)} | \mu^{(t-2)}) &= E(\, E(\mu^{(t)} | \mu^{(t-1)}) \,|\, \mu^{(t-2)} \,) \\
&= E(\, \bar{y}_{obs} + \lambda(\mu^{(t-1)} - \bar{y}_{obs}) \,|\, \mu^{(t-2)}) \\
&= \bar{y}_{obs} + \lambda^2(\mu^{(t-2)} - \bar{y}_{obs})
\end{aligned}
$$

and variance

$$
\begin{aligned}
V(\mu^{(t)} | \mu^{(t-2)}) &= E(\, V(\mu^{(t)} | \mu^{(t-1)}) \,|\, \mu^{(t-2)} \,) \\
&\quad + V(\, E(\mu^{(t)} | \mu^{(t-1)}) \,|\, \mu^{(t-2)} \,) \\
&= n_1^{-1}\psi(1 - \lambda^2) \\
&\quad + V(\, \bar{y}_{obs} + \lambda(\mu^{(t-1)} - \bar{y}_{obs}) \,|\, \mu^{(t-2)}) \\
&= n_1^{-1}\psi(1 - \lambda^4).
\end{aligned}
$$

Repeating this argument t times gives the marginal distribution of $\mu^{(t)}$ in terms of the starting value $\mu^{(0)}$,

$$\mu^{(t)} \,|\, \mu^{(0)} \sim N(\bar{y}_{obs} + \lambda^t(\mu^{(0)} - \bar{y}_{obs}), n_1^{-1}\psi(1 - \lambda^{2t})), \quad (3.37)$$

which approaches $N(\bar{y}_{obs}, n_1^{-1}\psi)$ as $t \to \infty$ for any fixed $\mu^{(0)}$ as long as $\lambda < 1$. If the starting value $\mu^{(0)}$ is not fixed but drawn from a probability distribution, then we can also investigate the unconditional distribution of $\mu^{(t)}$. In particular, if $\mu^{(0)}$ is drawn from the correct posterior $N(\bar{y}_{obs}, n_1^{-1}\psi)$, then (3.37) implies that $\mu^{(t)}$ will be normal with mean

$$E(\mu^{(t)}) = E(\, E(\mu^{(t)} | \mu^{(0)})) \quad\quad\quad\quad (3.38)$$

$$= E(\bar{y}_{obs} + \lambda^t(\mu^{(0)} - \bar{y}_{obs}))$$
$$= \bar{y}_{obs}$$

and variance

$$V(\mu^{(t)}) = E(V(\mu^{(t)}|\mu^{(0)})) + V(E(\mu^{(t)}|\mu^{(0)})) \qquad (3.39)$$
$$= n_1^{-1}\psi(1 - \lambda^{2t}) + V(\bar{y}_{obs} + \lambda^t(\mu^{(0)} - \bar{y}_{obs}))$$
$$= n_1^{-1}\psi,$$

and stationarity is achieved immediately.

We can also perform data augmentation in this example when the variance ψ is unknown. Under the diffuse prior $\pi(\mu, \psi) \propto \psi^{-1}$, the complete-data posterior is

$$\mu \mid \psi, Y \sim N(\bar{y}, n^{-1}\psi)$$
$$\psi \mid Y \sim (n-1)S^2 \chi_{n-1}^{-2} \qquad (3.40)$$

where S^2 is the sample variance of $y_1, y_2, \ldots, y_n$, and the observed-data posterior is

$$\mu \mid \psi, Y_{obs} \sim N(\bar{y}_{obs}, n_1^{-1}\psi)$$
$$\psi \mid Y_{obs} \sim (n_1 - 1)S_{obs}^2 \chi_{n_1-1}^{-2} \qquad (3.41)$$

where S_{obs}^2 is the sample variance of $y_1, y_2, \ldots, y_{n_1}$. The I-step of data augmentation simulates $Y_{mis}^{(t+1)}$ by drawing

$$y_i^{(t+1)} \mid \mu^{(t)}, \psi^{(t)}, Y_{obs} \sim N(\mu^{(t)}, \psi^{(t)})$$

independently for $i = n_1 + 1, \ldots, n$, and the P-step simulates $\mu^{(t+1)}$ and $\psi^{(t+1)}$ from (3.40) with $Y_{mis}^{(t+1)}$ substituted for Y_{mis}.

In this two-parameter problem, writing down the marginal distribution of $\theta^{(t)} = (\mu^{(t)}, \psi^{(t)})$ at any step t is no longer a simple matter. We can, however, demonstrate empirically that the marginal distribution of $\theta^{(t)}$ approaches the observed-data posterior (3.41) in numerical examples. The algorithm was applied to the univariate sample of size $n_1 = 10$ in Table 3.1 (a), arbitrarily taking $n_0 = 3$ and starting values $\mu^{(0)} = 30$, $\psi^{(0)} = 70$. Simulated marginal densities of $\mu^{(t)}$ and $\psi^{(t)}$ for $t = 1, 2, 3$ are displayed in Figure 3.2. Based on the marginals, it appears that convergence to the observed-data posterior is quite rapid. The densities in Figure 3.2 were simulated by $m = 500$ parallel chains of data augmentation, each starting from $\mu^{(0)}$ and $\psi^{(0)}$. The chains were run independently; no mixing as in (3.32) was used. For plotting purposes, however, the marginal densities were estimated by the 'Rao-Blackwell' method, averaging

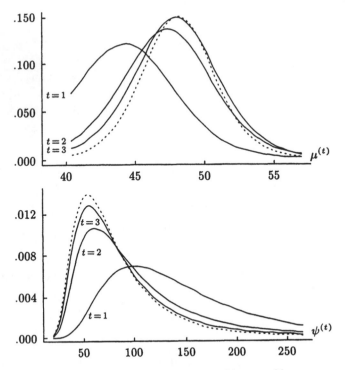

Figure 3.2. *Simulated marginal densities of* $\mu^{(t)}$ *and* $\psi^{(t)}$ *for* $t = 1, 2, 3$, *with dotted lines showing the exact observed-data posteriors.*

formulas for the complete-data marginal posteriors over the 500 iterates of Y_{mis}. This and other techniques for extracting meaningful summaries from Markov chain Monte Carlo runs will be discussed in Chapter 4.

Example 2: *Incomplete binary data.* Let $Y = (y_1, y_2, \ldots, y_n)$ represent the outcomes of n independent Bernoulli trials where $y_i = 1$ with probability θ and $y_i = 0$ with probability $1 - \theta$ for $i = 1, 2, \ldots, n$. The beta prior distribution

$$\pi(\theta) \propto \theta^{\alpha-1}(1 - \theta)^{\beta-1}$$

for $\alpha > 0$, $\beta > 0$, and $0 \leq \theta \leq 1$, denoted by $\theta \sim Beta(\alpha, \beta)$, leads to the complete-data posterior

$$\theta \mid Y \sim Beta(\alpha + \textstyle\sum_{i=1}^{n} y_i, \beta + n - \sum_{i=1}^{n} y_i).$$

For simplicity let us use the limiting form of this prior as $\alpha \to 0$ and $\beta \to 0$, so that the posterior becomes $\theta \mid Y \sim Beta(a, b)$ where

$a = \sum_{i=1}^{n} y_i$ and $b = n - a$; this posterior is proper as long as Y contains at least one success and one failure. Now suppose that the first n_1 elements of Y are observed and the remaining $n_0 = n - n_1$ elements are missing. The observed-data posterior becomes $\theta \mid Y_{obs} \sim Beta(a_1, b_1)$ where $a_1 = \sum_{i=1}^{n_1} y_i$ and $b_1 = n_1 - a_1$, which is proper provided that $1 \le a_1 \le n_1 - 1$.

Applying data augmentation to this example, the I-step fills in the missing trial outcomes by letting $y_i^{(t+1)} = 1$ with probability $\theta^{(t)}$ and 0 otherwise for $i = n_1 + 1, \ldots, n$. The P-step then samples

$$\theta^{(t+1)} \mid Y_{obs}, Y_{mis}^{(t+1)} \sim Beta(a^{(t+1)}, b^{(t+1)}),$$

where

$$
\begin{aligned}
a^{(t+1)} &= a_1 + a_0^{(t+1)} = a_1 + \sum_{i=n_1+1}^{n} y_i^{(t+1)}, \\
b^{(t+1)} &= b_1 + b_0^{(t+1)} = b_1 + n_0 - a_0^{(t+1)}.
\end{aligned}
$$

If data augmentation works properly, then the marginal distribution of $\theta^{(t)}$ as $t \to \infty$ should approach $Beta(a_1, b_1)$, which has mean a_1/n_1. Also, for large t, the distribution of any imputed trial should be Bernoulli with marginal probability of success

$$E(y_i^{(t+1)}) = E(\theta^{(t)}) = a_1/n_1,$$

where conditioning on Y_{obs} is assumed and has been suppressed in the notation. We can algebraically verify that $E(y_i^{(t)})$ does in fact approach a_1/n_1 as $t \to \infty$, because

$$
\begin{aligned}
E(y_i^{(t+1)} \mid Y_{mis}^{(t)}) &= E(\theta^{(t)} \mid Y_{mis}^{(t)}) \\
&= (a_1 + a_0^{(t)})/n \\
&= a_1/n_1 - \lambda(a_0^{(t)}/n_0 - a_1/n_1)
\end{aligned}
$$

where $\lambda = n_0/n$. Similarly,

$$E(y_i^{(t+1)} \mid Y_{mis}^{(1)}) = a_1/n_1 - \lambda^t(a_0^{(1)}/n_0 - a_1/n_1),$$

which implies that

$$E(y_i^{(t+1)} \mid \theta^{(0)}) = a_1/n_1 - \lambda^t(\mu^{(0)} - a_1/n_1). \qquad (3.42)$$

Clearly, (3.42) approaches a_1/n_1 from any starting value $\mu^{(0)}$ as long as $\lambda < 1$. If $\mu^{(0)}$ happens to be equal to a_1/n_1 or is drawn from a probability distribution with mean a_1/n_1, then convergence is immediate. This example was first used by Li (1988).

3.4.4 The Metropolis-Hastings algorithm

An older method of Markov chain Monte Carlo is the algorithm of Metropolis *et al.* (1953) and its generalization by Hastings (1970). The Metropolis-Hastings algorithm will not be needed in the remainder of this book; we briefly mention it, however, because of its usefulness in extending the basic algorithms of Chapters 5-9 to more complicated modeling situations.

In the Hastings version, a Markov chain $\{Z^{(t)} : t = 0, 1, 2, \ldots\}$ with stationary distribution $P(Z) = f(Z)$ is constructed as follows. Given $Z^{(t)}$, a candidate value $\tilde{Z}$ is drawn from a transition distribution $g(Z \mid Z^{(t)})$. Then the ratio

$$R^{(t+1)} = \frac{g(Z^{(t)} \mid \tilde{Z})}{g(\tilde{Z} \mid Z^{(t)})} \frac{f(\tilde{Z})}{f(Z^{(t)})}. \tag{3.43}$$

is calculated. If $R^{(t+1)}$ is greater than 1, we accept the value of the candidate variable and set $Z^{(t+1)} = \tilde{Z}$. If $R^{(t+1)} < 1$, we randomly accept the value of $\tilde{Z}$ as our next iterate $Z^{(t+1)}$ with probability $R^{(t+1)}$, and otherwise keep the current value, $Z^{(t+1)} = Z^{(t)}$. If the transition distribution g allows the process to eventually reach any state in the support of Z, then $Z^{(t)} \to Z$ in distribution as $t \to \infty$.

Metropolis-Hastings is useful when a transition distribution g can be found that (a) is easy to simulate, and (b) leads to acceptance ratios (3.43) that are easy to calculate. Because the target density f enters into the algorithm only through the acceptance ratio, we need only to be able to evaluate f up to a constant of proportionality. This makes Metropolis-Hastings attractive for simulation of Bayesian posterior distributions, for which the densities are typically known only up to a normalizing constant.

From a standpoint of efficiency, it is advantageous for the acceptance ratios to be close to one over the region where $f(Z)$ is appreciable, which occurs when $g(Z \mid Z^{(t)})$ is a good approximation to $f(Z)$. When $g(Z \mid Z^{(t)}) = f(Z)$ for all Z and $Z^{(t)}$, then the acceptance ratio is always one and convergence is immediate. In practical applications, it is wise to choose a g that is somewhat more diffuse (i.e. having heavier tails) than f; otherwise, there may be little opportunity for a candidate value $\tilde{Z}$ to fall in some regions of the sample space where $f(Z)$ is appreciable, and convergence to the target distribution may be too slow for practical use. If g is too diffuse, however, than many of the candidate values will fall outside the range where $f(Z)$ is appreciable, in which case the rejection rate will be very high and convergence will again be slow.

3.4.5 Generalizations and hybrid algorithms

As noted by several authors (Gelman, 1992; Smith and Roberts, 1993; Middleton, 1993; Tierney, 1994), both the Gibbs sampler and the Metropolis-Hastings algorithm may be generalized in a variety of ways. Consider the Gibbs sampler for a random vector $Z = (Z_1, Z_2, \ldots, Z_J)$. In one iteration of ordinary Gibbs, we sample from the full conditionals

$$Z_j^{(t+1)} \sim P(Z_j \mid Z_1^{(t+1)}, \ldots, Z_{j-1}^{(t+1)}, Z_{j+1}^{(t)}, \ldots, Z_J^{(t)}) \qquad (3.44)$$

for $j = 1, 2, \ldots, J$. In practice, however, it is not necessary to generate $Z_j^{(t+1)}$ directly from (3.44), but only from the transition distribution of a Markov chain that has (3.44) as its stationary distribution. In other words, if a Markov chain Monte Carlo scheme can be found that would eventually converge to the local distribution (3.44), we need only to perform one or more cycles of this local algorithm instead of (3.44), and the stationary distribution of the Gibbs sampler will be preserved. In specific examples, it sometimes happens that one (or more) of the full conditional distributions is difficult to simulate directly, but another Gibbs sampler or Metropolis-Hastings algorithm can be found that converges to the desired conditional. By replacing the difficult conditional with one or more iterations of this sampling scheme, we obtain a hybrid algorithm that still converges to the proper target.

Another potential use of these generalized algorithms is in data augmentation with an inconvenient prior. Suppose that a prior distribution $\pi^*(\theta)$ exists that leads to a tractable complete-data posterior $P^*(\theta \mid Y_{obs}, Y_{mis})$, but the prior that we would like to use for inference is $\pi(\theta)$ which leads to a posterior $P(\theta \mid Y_{obs}, Y_{mis})$ that is intractable. In this situation, we can replace the P-step under $\pi(\theta)$ with one or more steps of a Metropolis-Hastings algorithm that draws a candidate value $\tilde{\theta}$ from $P^*(\theta \mid Y_{obs}, Y_{mis})$. The acceptance ratio becomes

$$
\begin{aligned}
R^{(t+1)} &= \frac{P^*(\theta^{(t)} \mid Y_{obs}, Y_{mis})}{P^*(\tilde{\theta} \mid Y_{obs}, Y_{mis})} \frac{P(\tilde{\theta} \mid Y_{obs}, Y_{mis})}{P(\theta^{(t)} \mid Y_{obs}, Y_{mis})} \\
&= \frac{\pi(\tilde{\theta})/\pi^*(\tilde{\theta})}{\pi(\theta^{(t)})/\pi^*(\theta^{(t)})},
\end{aligned}
\qquad (3.45)
$$

which does not depend on Y_{obs} or Y_{mis}. When Metropolis-Hastings is used within data augmentation in this manner, the result is a hybrid algorithm with stationary distribution equal to the correct observed-data posterior under the desired prior. Note that (3.45) requires the evaluation of π and π^* only up to a constant of proportionality, so the acceptance ratios are typically easy to calculate.

3.5 Properties of Markov chain Monte Carlo

3.5.1 The meaning of convergence

Below we discuss some basic properties of Markov chain Monte Carlo, with special emphasis on the data augmentation scheme of (3.33)–(3.34). Unlike optimization methods like EM, which are deterministic and converge to a point in the parameter space, Markov chain Monte Carlo algorithms are stochastic and converge to probability distributions. Yet certain important similarities exist between the convergence behavior of EM and data augmentation.

Assuming the conditions needed for convergence are satisfied, the output of data augmentation is a sequence $\{(\theta^{(t)}, Y_{mis}^{(t)}) : t = 0, 1, 2, \ldots\}$ with stationary distribution $P(\theta, Y_{mis} | Y_{obs})$. For the sequence to have converged, it is sufficient for the distribution of $\theta^{(t)}$ to have converged to $P(\theta | Y_{obs})$, because $\theta^{(t)} \sim P(\theta | Y_{obs})$ implies that $(\theta^{(t+s)}, Y_{mis}^{(t+s)}) \sim P(\theta, Y_{mis} | Y_{obs})$ for all $s > 0$. Equivalently, it is sufficient for the distribution of $Y_{mis}^{(t)}$ to have converged to $P(Y_{mis} | Y_{obs})$. Also, convergence by t iterations means that $\theta^{(s)}$ and $Y_{mis}^{(s)}$ are independent of $\theta^{(s+t)}$ and $Y_{mis}^{(s+t)}$. In applications it is typically more convenient to monitor convergence through the behavior of successive values of θ than successive values of Y_{mis} because the latter is usually of higher dimension. Except in trivial examples like those in Section 3.4.3 for which data augmentation is not needed, summaries of $P(\theta | Y_{obs})$ are not available in closed form, making it difficult to know precisely when convergence has occurred. Techniques for assessing convergence are described in Chapter 4. For now we will discuss only in broad terms some issues surrounding convergence.

3.5.2 Examples of nonconvergence

Nonexistence of a stationary distribution

As mentioned above, convergence of a Gibbs sampler requires that the full conditionals (3.31) are the conditionals of a genuine joint probability distribution. It is possible to construct simple examples in which a set of proper conditional distributions does not define a proper joint distribution (Casella and George, 1992). For data augmentation, Bayes's Theorem guarantees a proper limiting distribution as long as the prior $\pi(\theta)$ is proper. In many real data applications of Bayesian analysis, however, it is convenient to use so-called noninformative priors that are actually improper but lead to proper posteriors when Bayes's formula is applied. Even when an improper π is known to yield a proper posterior in the case of complete data, it may not necessarily do so when some data are missing.

For a very simple example, let $Y = (y_1, y_2)$ represent two independent observations from $N(\mu, \psi)$ with μ and ψ both unknown. Under the standard noninformative prior $\pi(\mu, \psi) \propto \psi^{-1}$, the posterior distribution is given by (3.40) with $n = 2$, $\bar{y} = (y_1 + y_2)/2$ and $S^2 = (y_1 - \bar{y})^2 + (y_2 - \bar{y})^2$. Now suppose that only $y_1 = Y_{obs}$ is observed and $y_2 = Y_{mis}$ is missing. Applying Bayes's formula, the observed-data 'posterior' becomes

$$P(\mu, \psi \mid Y_{obs}) \quad \propto \quad L(\mu, \psi \mid Y_{obs}) \, \pi(\mu, \psi)$$

$$\propto \quad \psi^{-3/2} \exp\left\{ -\frac{(y_1 - \mu)^2}{2\psi}, \right\}$$

which is not a proper probability distribution because the integral

$$\int_0^\infty \int_{-\infty}^\infty \psi^{-3/2} \exp\left\{ -\frac{(y_1 - \mu)^2}{2\psi} \right\} d\mu \, d\psi = \int_0^\infty (2\pi)^{-1/2} \psi^{-2} d\psi$$

does not exist. Yet, one could naively apply data augmentation to this example under the improper prior. The I-step would be

$$y_2^{(t+1)} \sim N(\mu^{(t)}, \psi^{(t)}), \tag{3.46}$$

and the P-step would be

$$\psi^{(t+1)} \mid y_1, y_2^{(t+1)} \quad \sim \quad (S^2)^{(t+1)} \chi_1^{-2}, \tag{3.47}$$

$$\mu^{(t+1)} \mid \psi^{(t+1)}, y_1, y_2^{(t+1)} \quad \sim \quad N(\bar{y}^{(t+1)}, \psi^{(t+1)}/2),$$

where

$$\bar{y}^{(t)} = (y_1 + y_2^{(t)})/2,$$
$$(S^2)^{(t)} = (y_1 - \bar{y}^{(t)})^2 + (y_2^{(t)} - \bar{y}^{(t)})^2.$$

Notice that even though the joint posterior does not exist, both the I-step and the P-step are defined at every iteration. One could naively alternate between (3.46) and (3.47) indefinitely without any clue that the algorithm is not converging.

The fundamental reason why data augmentation fails here is that the mean and variance cannot be jointly estimated on the basis of a single observation y_1. The observed data provide no information on one aspect of $\theta = (\mu, \psi)$, namely ψ, so that unless a proper prior distribution is applied to ψ there is no basis for inference. Although there is no compelling reason to use data augmentation in this trivial example, it is not difficult to construct more realistic multivariate problems where both the I- and P-steps of data augmentation are defined but the stationary distribution does not exist. These would be similar to the examples of Section 3.3.1 where the ML estimate of θ is not unique because the likelihood is maximized over a ridge. Whenever the likelihood has a ridge, certain aspects of the parameter are inestimable, and unless a proper prior is applied to those aspects of θ the posterior will not be proper. Sparse datasets with few observations or high rates of missingness may be prone to these problems. If we suspect that data augmentation may not be converging to a proper posterior, we can switch to a proper prior, thereby guaranteeing that the posterior will be proper as well.

Boundary values and absorbing states

Another basic requirement for the convergence of a Markov chain Monte Carlo algorithm is that the support of the target distribution must be 'connected' in the sense that it must be possible to eventually reach any state from any other state. There must be no periodic states and no absorbing states, i.e. regions where the algorithm could become trapped with zero probability of escape. In the stochastic processes literature, this property is known as *ergodicity*.

Consider again the normal sample $Y = (y_1, y_2)$ where y_1 is observed and y_2 is missing, but now let us suppose that the population mean μ is known, and without loss of generality take $\mu = 0$. Suppose that we apply an improper prior distribution to the variance, $\pi(\psi) \propto \psi^{-(\nu+2)/2}$ where ν is a fixed constant. Given $Y = (y_1, y_2)$, the complete-data posterior is

$$P(\psi | Y) \propto \psi^{-1} \exp\left\{ -\frac{(y_1^2 + y_2^2)}{2\psi} \right\} \psi^{-(\nu+2)/2}$$

or $\psi \mid Y \sim (y_1^2 + y_2^2)\chi_{\nu+2}^{-2}$, which is proper provided that $\nu > -2$. Given only $Y_{obs} = y_1$, the observed-data posterior is

$$P(\psi | Y_{obs}) \propto \psi^{-1/2} \exp\left\{ -\frac{y_1^2}{2\psi} \right\} \psi^{-(\nu+2)/2} \qquad (3.48)$$

or $\psi \mid Y_{obs} \sim y_1^2 \chi_{\nu+1}^{-2}$, which is proper for any $\nu > -1$. If data augmentation were applied to this example, the I-step would be

$$y_2^{(t+1)} \mid \psi^{(t)}, y_1 \sim N(0, \psi^{(t)}),$$

and the P-step would be

$$\psi^{(t+1)} \mid y_1, y_2^{(t+1)} \sim (y_1^2 + (y_2^{(t+1)})^2) \chi_{\nu+2}^{-2}.$$

The algorithm would proceed normally except in the unlikely event that $y_1 = 0$ and $\psi^{(t)}$ happened to become zero at some iteration. If that were to occur, we would obtain $y_2^{(t)} = 0$ and $\psi^{(t)} = 0$ for every iteration thereafter. In other words, $\psi = 0$ would be an absorbing state.

Even if y_1 happened to be zero, absorption would be unlikely because unless we start on the boundary ($\psi^{(0)} = 0$) the event $\psi^{(t)} = 0$ occurs in theory with probability zero. Depending on the computer and random variate generator used, there could be a small chance of falling within machine precision of the boundary, especially if the starting value $\psi^{(0)}$ is very close to zero. The presence of an absorbing state is not the only difficulty in this example, because the observed-data posterior (3.48) is not proper for $y_1 = 0$. In Chapter 8, however, we will see that in some real categorical-data problems absorption onto a boundary becomes a distinct possibility even when the posterior is technically proper, and we will need to handle such situations with care.

3.5.3 Rates of convergence

Assuming that a Markov chain Monte Carlo algorithm does converge to a proper stationary distribution, it is important to consider how quickly this convergence occurs. Convergence rates are typically defined in terms of a distance measure between the marginal distribution of the iterates at any given time and the target distribution. Some interesting theoretical results on convergence rates and further references are given by Schervish and Carlin (1992); Smith and Roberts (1993); Tierney (1994); and Liu, Wong and Kong (1995). This work, although reassuring, does not easily translate into practical guidelines for knowing when convergence has occurred in specific examples. Ongoing research regarding convergence behavior will undoubtedly lead to greater understanding in the future; for now, however, we can informally state a few general principles that apply to incomplete-data problems.

Convergence and missing information

Consider simple data augmentation in which we alternately perform an I-step

$$Y_{mis}^{(t+1)} \sim P(Y_{mis} \,|\, Y_{obs}, \theta^{(t)})$$

and a P-step

$$\theta^{(t+1)} \sim P(\theta \,|\, Y_{obs}, Y_{mis}^{(t+1)}).$$

Intuitively, the rate of convergence should depend on how much information about the parameter is contained in missing data relative to the observed data and the prior. The complete-data posterior may be written

$$P(\theta \,|\, Y_{obs}, Y_{mis}) \propto P(\theta \,|\, Y_{obs}) \, P(Y_{mis} \,|\, Y_{obs}, \theta). \qquad (3.49)$$

In the extreme case where Y_{mis} provides no information about θ beyond that already contained in Y_{obs}, Y_{mis} and θ would be conditionally independent given Y_{obs}; the last term in (3.49) would then be constant with respect to θ, and convergence to the target distribution would be immediate. More generally, if $P(Y_{mis} \,|\, Y_{obs}, \theta)$ as a function of θ is relatively flat over the region of high posterior density (which is typically equivalent to the missing information, as defined in Section 3.3.2, being near zero), then each P-step will be nearly a draw from $P(\theta \,|\, Y_{obs})$ and the algorithm will converge rapidly. On the other hand, if the missing information is a large portion of the total information, then θ will depend heavily on Y_{mis} at each P-step, which will in turn depend on the value of θ used in the previous I-step; successive iterates of θ will tend to be highly correlated and convergence will be slow. Just as with EM, the rate of convergence of data augmentation and the fractions of missing information are fundamentally related.

This relationship between missing information and rate of convergence is difficult to formalize in a general way, but it can be easily demonstrated in simple examples. Consider again the univariate normal data $Y = (y_1, y_2, \ldots, y_n)$ with known variance ψ and unknown mean μ. In Example 1 of Section 3.4.3 we investigated data augmentation under the noninformative prior $\pi(\mu) \propto c$ (a constant), where the first n_1 elements of Y are observed and the remaining $n_0 = n - n_1$ are missing. We found that the stationary distribution of μ is $\mu \,|\, Y_{obs} \sim N(\bar{y}_{obs}, n_1^{-1}\psi)$, and the marginal distribution of $\mu^{(t)}$ is

$$\mu^{(t)} \,|\, \mu^{(0)}, Y_{obs} \sim N(\, \bar{y}_{obs} + \lambda^t (\mu^{(0)} - \bar{y}_{obs}), \; n_1^{-1}\psi(1 - \lambda^{2t}) \,) \quad (3.50)$$

where $\lambda = n_0/n$ is the fraction of missing information. Clearly, the algorithm will approach stationarity rapidly for λ near zero and slowly for λ near one. This example can easily be generalized to an informative prior $\mu \sim N(\mu_0, \tau)$, in which case we would obtain an expression like (3.50) but with the following changes: $\bar{y}_{obs}$ and $n_1^{-1}\psi$ would be replaced by the new observed-data posterior mean and variance, respectively, and λ would be replaced by the new fraction of missing information

$$\lambda^* = \frac{n_0\psi^{-1}}{n\psi^{-1} + \tau^{-1}},$$

where the prior information τ^{-1} now appears in the denominator as a part of the total information.

When the mean and variance are both unknown, the joint distribution of $\mu^{(t)}$ and $\psi^{(t)}$ is intractable, but we can still demonstrate empirically that the rate of convergence depends on n_0/n. Using the $n_1 = 10$ observations in Table 3.1 (a) and the noninformative prior $\pi(\mu, \psi) \propto \psi^{-1}$, we performed data augmentation under various choices of n_0. Independent sample paths for $(\mu^{(t)}, \psi^{(t)})$ beginning from four different starting positions are displayed in Figure 3.3, first for $n_0 = 10$ and again for $n_0 = 90$, with ψ shown on a log scale. The starting values were all chosen to be in the tails of the observed-data posterior, so that the iterates would exhibit an initial trend as they wander into the region of high posterior density. For $n_0 = 10$ the sample paths become heavily intertwined by $t = 8$, suggesting that for most practical purposes the algorithm has probably converged by eight or ten iterations. For $n_0 = 90$, however, the sample paths have still not crossed one another by $t = 25$; the algorithm takes smaller steps and the successive iterates are more highly correlated.

Starting values and starting distributions

In the univariate normal example with known mean, (3.50) reveals that convergence behavior depends not only on the fraction of missing information but also on the choice of a starting value. If we happened to take $\mu^{(0)} = \bar{y}_{obs}$, then the distribution of $\mu^{(t)}$ would have the correct mean (i.e. the same mean as the stationary distribution) for every t. Even though the variance of $\mu^{(t)}$ is always less than the stationary variance, choosing a starting value near the center of the observed-data posterior makes the first moment more nearly correct.

It is also evident from (3.50) that the variance of $\mu^{(t)}$ does not

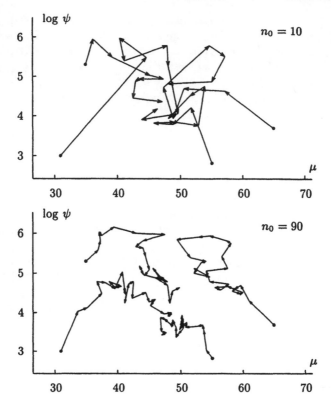

Figure 3.3. *Iterations of data augmentation from various starting values for univariate normal data with $n_0 = 10$ and $n_0 = 90$.*

depend on the starting value $\mu^{(0)}$ as long as $\mu^{(0)}$ is fixed. If we do not use a fixed $\mu^{(0)}$ but draw it from a probability distribution, however, then we can alter the second moment of $\mu^{(t)}$ as well as the first moment. Suppose that $\mu^{(0)}$ is drawn at random from a probability distribution with variance κ. Then (3.39) implies that the unconditional variance of $\mu^{(t)}$ is

$$V(\mu^{(t)}) = n_1^{-1}\psi(1 - \lambda^{2t}) + \lambda^{2t}\kappa,$$

which is equal to the stationary variance $n_1^{-1}\psi$ if $\kappa = n_1^{-1}\psi$; if $\kappa > n_1^{-1}\psi$ then $V(\mu^{(t)}) > n_1^{-1}\psi$ as well. For inferential purposes, it is often wise to draw starting values of parameters at random from a probability distribution that is *overdispersed* relative to (i.e. having variance at least as great as) the target distribution, so that the variance after a finite number of iterations is at least as large as the stationary variance and resulting inferences are conservative (Gelman and Rubin, 1992a). It is also wise to use a starting distribution that is centered at or near the mean of the target distribution, so that the first moment at any iteration will be approximately correct. In Chapter 4 we discuss how one might obtain starting distributions in realistic problems where moments of the stationary distribution are unknown. If a single, fixed starting value is desired, then a point near the center of $P(\theta|Y_{obs})$, e.g. an ML estimate or posterior mode obtained from EM, may be a wise choice.

Difficulties with slow convergence

When Markov chain Monte Carlo converges very slowly in an incomplete-data problem, it is typically for the same reason that EM converges slowly: the fractions of missing information for one or more components of θ are very high. Previous comments about slow convergence of EM apply here as well; it should be taken as a warning that inferences about certain aspects of θ depend heavily on the missing-data model $P(Y_{mis}|Y_{obs},\theta)$. Slow convergence of Markov chain Monte Carlo algorithms can be notoriously difficult to detect (e.g. Gelman and Rubin, 1992b), but when EM is slow it is usually painfully obvious. Consequently, it is good practice to apply EM in addition to Markov chain Monte Carlo, even if merely as a device for diagnosing slow convergence.

Slow convergence of Markov chain Monte Carlo may also be the result of an observed-data posterior that is oddly shaped. If the posterior is poorly connected, e.g. if it has multiple modes that are widely separated by regions of low density, then simulation routines may get stuck in certain regions of the parameter space. Using EM in conjunction with simulation often helps to reveal unusual features of the likelihood or posterior that may be less apparent if only one or the other is applied.

CHAPTER 4

Inference by data augmentation

4.1 Introduction

In a narrow sense, one may define the problem of inference in relation to θ, the unknown parameter of a probability model. The statistician may desire a point estimate for one or more components or functions of θ, summarizing the uncertainty with a confidence interval or confidence region. One may want to test whether θ is equal to some null value or lies in some subset of the natural parameter space, summarizing the evidence with a p-value. With incomplete data, such quantities can be obtained from the observed-data likelihood or posterior, although in practice special computational techniques may be needed.

In a broader sense, however, the problem of inference often goes beyond making statements about a single parameter θ. A data analyst will typically want to apply a variety of exploratory and modeling techniques to a dataset, such as graphical displays, linear regression, factor analysis and so on, to investigate various interesting features of the data. When the data are incomplete, the analyst's task often becomes considerably more difficult. Carrying out procedures that are ordinarily straightforward, such as fitting a satisfactory regression model, may not be straightforward when some data are missing. Analysts need sensible routine methods for analyzing incomplete data, while recognizing and assessing the role of missing-data uncertainty at each step of the analysis.

This chapter addresses inference both in the narrow and broad sense, attacking both through techniques of simulation. Simulation may be used either to make simple inferences about θ or to perform multipurpose data analyses. To accomplish the former, we simulate random values of θ from its observed-data posterior distribution. To accomplish the latter, we generate plausible versions of the unknown Y_{mis}. These complementary techniques will be called, respectively, *parameter simulation* and *multiple imputation*.

In parameter simulation, one creates random but not necessarily independent draws of θ from $P(\theta \,|\, Y_{obs})$. The sample moments of these draws provide estimates of the posterior moments, and the empirical distribution, perhaps smoothed in some fashion, provides estimates of the marginal distributions of individual components or functions of θ. Depending on which features of the posterior distribution are of interest, one may need to generate a large sample to obtain accurate inferences; hundreds or perhaps even thousands of draws of θ may be necessary.

In multiple imputation (Rubin, 1987), one creates m plausible sets of missing values by drawing repeatedly from $P(Y_{mis} \,|\, Y_{obs})$. This results in m simulated complete datasets which are analyzed by complete-data methods. The results of the m complete-data analyses are then formally combined to produce a single overall inference. Exploratory data analyses (e.g. graphical displays) may also be performed on each of the m completed datasets, providing an informal but valuable assessment of how interesting features of the data are affected by missing-data uncertainty. When the fractions of missing information are moderate, as is often the case, only a few imputations (e.g. $m = 3$ or $m = 5$) are usually adequate to provide inferences that are nearly efficient and practically valid.

Data augmentation and related Markov chain Monte Carlo algorithms enable us to perform either parameter simulation, multiple imputation or both; the same algorithm may be used to draw θ from $P(\theta \,|\, Y_{obs})$ and to draw Y_{mis} from $P(Y_{mis} \,|\, Y_{obs})$. Parameter simulation and multiple imputation, to be described in Sections 4.2 and 4.3 respectively, can be viewed merely as two different ways of extracting information from the same Markov chain. Methods for monitoring the convergence of Markov chain Monte Carlo algorithms are discussed in Section 4.4, and Section 4.5 contains practical advice on applying these methods to real data problems.

4.2 Parameter simulation

4.2.1 Dependent samples

A natural way to answer inferential questions concerning particular components or functions of θ is to directly examine and summarize simulated values of θ. Suppose that we run a single series of data augmentation or a related algorithm long enough to achieve approximate stationarity; that is, we choose a t large enough so that $\theta^{(t)}$ is essentially a draw from $P(\theta \,|\, Y_{obs})$. This initial phase, sometimes called the *burn-in period*, is helpful to rid the series of dependence on the starting value or starting distribution. Suppose that we discard the values of θ from the burn-in period and continue for another m iterations, calling the resulting values $\theta^{(1)}, \theta^{(2)}, \ldots, \theta^{(m)}$. These can be regarded as a genuine sample from the observed-data posterior, because stationarity implies that $\theta^{(t)}$ is marginally distributed according to $P(\theta \mid Y_{obs})$ for every t. However, the members of this sample will, in most cases, be dependent upon one another; values of θ that are close to one other in the sequence will tend to be more alike than values that are far apart. Successive values of θ may be highly positively correlated, particularly when convergence is slow.

For many readers, the notion of a dependent sample will be somewhat unfamiliar. Suppose for a moment that we are interested in a particular scalar component or function of the parameter, denoted by $\xi = \xi(\theta)$. If the sample values are independent, then the sample average

$$\bar{\xi} = \frac{1}{m} \sum_{t=1}^{m} \xi^{(t)}, \tag{4.1}$$

where $\xi^{(t)} = \xi(\theta^{(t)})$, $t = 1, 2, \ldots, m$, is the obvious Monte Carlo estimate of the posterior mean

$$E(\xi \mid Y_{obs}) = \int \xi \, P(\xi \mid Y_{obs}) \, d\xi;$$

the sample variance

$$\frac{1}{m-1} \sum_{t=1}^{m} (\xi^{(t)} - \bar{\xi})^2 \tag{4.2}$$

is the obvious estimate of the posterior variance

$$V(\xi \mid Y_{obs}) = \int \xi^2 P(\xi \mid Y_{obs}) \, d\xi - E^2(\xi \mid Y_{obs});$$

and so on. When the sample values are dependent, however, it may not be immediately obvious whether the same types of summaries (averages, etc.) are appropriate. In one important sense, they are. A law of large numbers for Markov chain Monte Carlo (Tierney, 1994) states that under quite general conditions, if $Z^{(1)}, Z^{(2)}, \ldots, Z^{(m)}$ is a realization of a Markov chain Monte Carlo run with target distribution f, then

$$\frac{1}{m} \sum_{t=1}^{m} g(Z^{(t)}) \to E_f[g(Z)] \tag{4.3}$$

(almost surely) for any real-valued function $g(Z)$ as $m \to \infty$, provided that $E_f[g(Z)]$, the expectation of $g(Z)$ under the target distribution, exists. By (4.3) it follows that the sample moments of a dependent sample are consistent estimates of the population moments. A histogram of the sample values will come to resemble the population density for large m. Virtually any summary that is appropriate for an independent random sample is appropriate for a dependent one.

Although the consistency of most empirical summaries is maintained under dependence, however, other familiar properties may be lost. For example, the variance of the sample average (4.1) is not m^{-1} times the variance of a single $\xi^{(t)}$, but also involves the covariances among $\xi^{(1)}, \xi^{(2)}, \ldots, \xi^{(m)}$. If successive iterates are highly positively correlated, then the covariance terms become large and $\bar{\xi}$ becomes substantially less precise than an average from an independent sample of the same size. Moreover, under dependence (4.2) is not in general an unbiased estimate of $V(\xi \mid Y_{obs})$; if successive iterates are positively correlated then (4.2) has a downward bias for any finite m, and the usual justification for using $(m-1)$ in the denominator rather than m no longer applies.

Perhaps the most serious drawback of dependence is that assessing the error of a Monte Carlo estimator is no longer a simple matter. Estimating the error variance internally from a single dependent sample can be difficult. An alternative strategy is to employ *replication*: rather than performing the simulation once, perform it independently k times, and examine the variation among the k replicate values of the estimator. Multiple runs also provide a method for diagnosing lack of convergence of the Markov chain itself (see Section 4.4). In most cases, practitioners would not be interested in Monte Carlo error if they could be assured that it was small enough that their important numerical estimates and conclusions were not in jeopardy. Obtaining accurate measures of Monte Carlo error, therefore, may be a matter of secondary importance when the error is known to be small, and even crude estimates may suffice. On the other hand, if the error is more substantial, then it needs to be assessed more carefully and perhaps even be formally incorporated into p-values and interval estimates.

Subsampling a chain

One way to finesse the issue of dependence in Markov chain Monte Carlo is to subsample the chain: rather than summarizing a posterior by $\theta^{(1)}, \theta^{(2)}, \ldots, \theta^{(m)}$, use $\theta^{(k)}, \theta^{(2k)}, \ldots, \theta^{(mk)}$ where k is chosen large enough to make the sample values approximately independent. Aside from the problem of how to choose k, subsampling obviously requires a greater number of iterations to produce a final sample of the same size. Although the resulting independent sample will tend to give more efficient estimates than a dependent sample, this gain in efficiency will not compensate for the k-fold increase in computation. Moreover, if we run the algorithm for km iterations then we might as well summarize the results using all km iterates, because the average of all km iterates is more precise than the average of every kth iterate (Geyer, 1992; MacEachern and Berliner, 1994). Aside from issues of data storage, if the goal is to obtain direct summaries of a posterior distribution then subsampling the chain is generally not advantageous.

Subsampling and issues of Monte Carlo error will be taken up again in Section 4.4; for now we discuss various ways to extract inferentially meaningful summaries from a single, dependent parameter sample.

4.2.2 Summarizing a dependent sample

Posterior moments

Suppose that we are interested in a particular scalar component or function of the unknown parameter, denoted generically by $\xi = \xi(\theta)$. To the Bayesian, a useful point estimate of ξ is the posterior mean $E(\xi \,|\, Y_{obs})$. From a decision-theoretic standpoint, the posterior mean is the optimal estimate under squared-error loss (e.g. DeGroot, 1970). Even when no explicit loss function is available, the posterior mean is still often regarded as the most natural single-number summary. Another useful quantity is the posterior variance $V(\xi \,|\, Y_{obs})$, which measures uncertainty about the unknown ξ. If $\theta^{(1)}, \theta^{(2)}, \ldots, \theta^{(m)}$ are values from $P(\theta \,|\, Y_{obs})$ produced by a Markov chain Monte Carlo method, then consistent estimates of the posterior mean and variance of ξ are given by

$$\hat{E}(\xi \,|\, Y_{obs}) = \bar{\xi}$$

$$= \frac{1}{m} \sum_{t=1}^{m} \xi^{(t)} \tag{4.4}$$

and

$$\hat{V}(\xi \,|\, Y_{obs}) = \frac{1}{m} \sum_{t=1}^{m} (\xi^{(t)} - \bar{\xi})^2, \tag{4.5}$$

respectively, where $\xi^{(t)} = \xi(\theta^{(t)})$. Higher moments, if desired, may be estimated in a similar fashion.

Posterior distributions and densities

If $\theta^{(1)}, \theta^{(2)}, \ldots, \theta^{(m)}$ are a sample from $P(\theta \mid Y_{obs})$, then it follows that $\xi^{(1)}, \xi^{(2)}, \ldots, \xi^{(m)}$ are a sample from $P(\xi \mid Y_{obs})$, the observed-data marginal distribution of ξ. By (4.3), the posterior cumulative distribution function

$$P(\xi \leq a \mid Y_{obs}) = \int_{-\infty}^{a} P(\xi \mid Y_{obs}) \, d\xi \qquad (4.6)$$

can be consistently estimated for any a by the proportion of sample values $\xi^{(1)}, \xi^{(2)}, \ldots, \xi^{(m)}$ that fall at or below a. Applying this estimate for every a gives the *empirical distribution function*,

$$\hat{F}(a) = \sum_{t=1}^{m} m^{-1} I(\xi^{(t)} \leq a) \qquad (4.7)$$

where $I(\cdot)$ is an indicator function equal to one if the argument is true and zero otherwise. The *empirical density* associated with (4.7) is the discrete probability function that assigns mass $1/m$ to each observed value $\xi^{(t)}$, $t = 1, 2, \ldots, m$.

In most cases the true posterior distribution of $\xi = \xi(\theta)$ is continuous, which suggests that we can improve the empirical density by smoothing it in some fashion. A *histogram* partitions the range of sample values $\xi^{(1)}, \xi^{(2)}, \ldots, \xi^{(m)}$ into a small number of discrete intervals, typically of equal width, and spreads the probability mass of each $\xi^{(t)}$ uniformly over the interval into which it falls. Another important type of density estimator is the class of *kernel estimators*, which have the form

$$\hat{f}(a) = \int_{-\infty}^{\infty} K(a, \xi) \, d\hat{F}(\xi) = \frac{1}{m} \sum_{t=1}^{m} K(a, \xi^{(t)}).$$

The kernel $K(a, \xi)$ is some non-negative function centered at ξ with the property

$$\int_{-\infty}^{\infty} K(a, \xi) \, da = 1.$$

The choice of kernel, which is always somewhat arbitrary, affects the shape of $\hat{f}$ and its degree of smoothness; popular choices are rectangular, triangular and Gaussian kernels with width determined by the number and range of sample values. For more information on kernel estimators see Silverman (1986) or Devroye (1987).

Quantiles

The pth quantile of a random variable with cumulative distribution function F is usually defined as the smallest x for which $F(x) \geq p$. Substituting the empirical distribution function $\hat{F}$ into this definition gives the following method for estimating the quantiles of ξ based on a sample $\xi^{(1)}, \xi^{(2)}, \ldots, \xi^{(m)}$. First, order the sample from smallest to largest; let $\xi^{*(t)}$, $t = 1, 2, \ldots, m$ denote the order statistics,

$$\xi^{*(1)} \leq \xi^{*(2)} \leq \cdots \leq \xi^{*(m)}.$$

If mp happens to be an integer, then the pth quantile is estimated by $\xi^{*(mp)}$; otherwise, it is estimated by $\xi^{*([mp]+1)}$ where $[\cdot]$ denotes the greatest integer function.

In the above method, the estimate of any quantile is restricted to be one of the observed order statistics. A more common practice is to interpolate between the order statistics. Suppose we consider $\xi^{(i)}$ to be an estimate of the pth quantile; there is no universally agreed upon value for p, but common choices include $p = i/(m+1)$ and $p = (i-1)/(m-1)$. Using the former, the estimated pth quantile is the ith order statistic when $i = p(m+1)$ happens to be an integer. When $i = p(m+1)$ is not an integer, we find $i_1 = [p(m+1)]$ and $i_2 = i_1 + 1$ and use the estimate

$$\hat{F}^{-1}(p) = (1-c)\,\xi^{*(i_1)} + c\,\xi^{*(i_2)}, \tag{4.8}$$

where $c = p(m+1) - i_1$. Taking $p = 0.5$, this interpolation method gives the familiar form of a sample median: the middle value if m is odd and the average of the two middle values if m is even.

Interval estimates

A $100(1 - \alpha)\%$ Bayesian posterior region is defined to be any set with posterior probability content at least $1 - \alpha$. That is, A is a $100(1 - \alpha)\%$ posterior region for $\xi = \xi(\theta)$ if

$$P(\xi \in A \,|\, Y_{obs}) \geq 1 - \alpha.$$

Unlike a frequentist confidence region, which has the property that the region will cover ξ with specified long-run frequency over repeated samples, the Bayesian region makes a probability statement about the parameter ξ given the current sample. Given the posterior distribution for a scalar ξ, there are various methods for constructing a Bayesian interval estimate. In the highest posterior density (HPD) method, the interval is chosen so that every value within the interval has posterior density at least as high as every value outside of it (e.g. Box and Tiao, 1992). The HPD method yields the shortest possible interval for ξ, but it is not invariant under nonlinear transformations of the parameter. Another simple technique is the equal-tailed method, in which the endpoints are chosen so that the posterior probability of falling above the upper endpoint and the probability of falling below the lower endpoint are both equal to $\alpha/2$. For example, a 95% equal-tailed interval runs from the 2.5th percentile to the 97.5th percentile of the posterior distribution. Equal-tailed Bayesian posterior intervals can be directly estimated from a sample $\xi^{(1)}, \xi^{(2)}, \ldots, \xi^{(m)}$ by using (4.8). Estimating an HPD interval is more complicated, requiring both a smooth estimate of the posterior density of ξ and its associated cumulative distribution function.

With large datasets and under suitable regularity conditions, the posterior distribution of a parameter ξ tends in many cases to be approximately normally distributed (e.g. Cox and Hinkley, 1974). Under normality the HPD and equal-tailed intervals coincide, and

$$E(\xi \mid Y_{obs}) \pm z_{1-\alpha/2} \sqrt{V(\xi \mid Y_{obs})}, \qquad (4.9)$$

where $z_p = \Phi^{-1}(p)$ denotes the pth quantile of the standard normal distribution, is a $100(1 - \alpha)\%$ posterior interval for ξ. Just as evidence about a parameter in the frequentist case is often summarized by an MLE and an asymptotic variance, Bayesian inferences can also be summarized by a posterior mean and posterior variance, and for large samples and relatively diffuse priors the two answers will tend to be very close. Unlike likelihood-based asymptotic methods, however, Bayesian posterior simulation allows us to readily check the normal approximation, and form alternative interval estimates without recourse to a normality assumption, by examining the simulated density and posterior quantiles directly.

Hypothesis tests

Suppose that we are interested in examining the plausibility of the hypothesis $\xi = \xi_0$ for some specific value ξ_0, versus the alternative that $\xi > \xi_0$ or $\xi < \xi_0$. In the classical framework of hypothesis testing, one defines a test statistic that measures departures from the null hypothesis $\xi = \xi_0$. The evidence against the null is typically measured by a p-value, the probability of observing a test statistic as extreme or more extreme than the one actually observed, calculated under the assumption that the null hypothesis is true. A small p-value indicates either that a rare event must have occurred, or that the null hypothesis must be false.

In the Bayesian framework, the continuity of the posterior distribution for ξ makes $\xi = \xi_0$ an event of zero posterior probability. The probability of a one-sided alternative event $\xi > \xi_0$ or $\xi < \xi_0$, however, is nonzero and is a direct measure of the plausibility of that alternative. The area under the posterior density $P(\xi \mid Y_{obs})$ to the left or to the right of ξ_0 may be thought of as a Bayesian p-value; a very small tail area on either side suggests that ξ_0 is poorly supported and implausible given the observed data. A two-sided Bayesian tail area may be defined as the α for which a $100(1 - \alpha)\%$ Bayesian posterior interval just barely covers ξ_0. With Markov chain Monte Carlo, estimates of these tail areas are directly available from the empirical distribution function of the simulated values (4.7). In large samples, where Bayesian posterior intervals tend to closely agree with their frequentist counterparts, Bayesian p-values will also tend to resemble frequentist p-values.

Beyond scalar quantities

Until this point our discussion has been limited to inference about a single scalar summary of θ. In multiparameter problems (e.g. linear regression modeling), it is common to summarize the results of an analysis by presenting point and interval estimates for a number of scalar quantities (e.g. regression coefficients). It is important to remember, of course, that individual point and interval estimates do not immediately translate into joint inferences, because the quantities of interest are often correlated.

Some of the methods above for summarizing a dependent sample generalize readily to higher dimensions, but others do not. For example, suppose that

$$\xi = (\xi_1(\theta), \xi_2(\theta), \ldots, \xi_d(\theta))^T$$

is a d-dimensional function of θ. The posterior means, variances and covariances for ξ may be estimated by the obvious multivariate extensions of (4.4)–(4.5). Obtaining a $100(1 - \alpha)\%$ Bayesian posterior region, however, is more problematic. The HPD method does extend to $d \geq 2$ dimensions, but estimating an HPD region using a sample-based estimate of the joint density would be difficult at best. Under the simplifying assumption that the posterior is multivariate normal, however (an assumption that may be reasonable if the data sample is large and the parameters are examined on an appropriate scale), the HPD method can be implemented rather easily. Denoting the observed-data posterior mean vector and covariance matrix of ξ by $\hat{\xi}$ and V, respectively, it follows from well-known properties of the multivariate normal distribution that

$$(\xi - \hat{\xi})^T V^{-1}(\xi - \hat{\xi}) \mid Y_{obs} \sim \chi_d^2, \tag{4.10}$$

and a $100(1 - \alpha)\%$ posterior region is the set of all vectors ξ_0 for which

$$(\xi_0 - \hat{\xi})^T V^{-1}(\xi_0 - \hat{\xi}) \le \chi_{d,1-\alpha}^2,$$

where $\chi_{d,p}^2$ denotes the pth quantile of the χ_d^2 distribution. This region is a d-dimensional ellipsoid centered at $\hat{\xi}$. The Bayesian p-value for testing $\xi = \xi_0$ is the choice of α for which the ellipsoid just barely covers ξ_0,

$$P[\chi_d^2 \ge (\xi_0 - \hat{\xi})^T V^{-1}(\xi_0 - \hat{\xi})].$$

Substituting simulation-based estimates of $\hat{\xi}$ and V into these expressions yields simulated posterior regions and p-values. The assumption of multivariate normality may be checked by applying standard multivariate diagnostics to the simulated values of ξ, and, if necessary, transformations may be applied to the individual components of ξ to make normality more plausible.

4.2.3 Rao-Blackwellized estimates

Under certain conditions, it is possible to greatly improve the precision of Monte Carlo estimates by *Rao-Blackwellization* (Gelfand and Smith, 1990; Liu, Wong and Kong, 1994). The name of this method is derived from the well-known Rao-Blackwell theorem of mathematical statistics, which states that if S is an unbiased estimate of a scalar parameter and T is a sufficient statistic, then $S^* = E(S \mid T)$ is also unbiased and has a smaller variance than S (unless S is already a function of T, in which case $S^* = S$ and the two variances are equal).

Suppose that we are interested in estimating the posterior mean of $\xi = \xi(\theta)$. Recall that the output of a data augmentation algorithm is a sequence

$$Y_{mis}^{(1)}, \theta^{(1)}, Y_{mis}^{(2)}, \theta^{(2)}, \ldots, Y_{mis}^{(t)}, \theta^{(t)}, \ldots.$$

If this sequence is preceded by a sufficiently long burn-in period, then $Y_{mis}^{(t)}$ and $\theta^{(t)}$ are distributed according to $P(Y_{mis}|Y_{obs})$ and $P(\theta|Y_{obs})$, respectively for all t. The direct estimate

$$\bar{\xi} = \frac{1}{m} \sum_{t=1}^{m} \xi^{(t)}$$

will be unbiased for $E(\xi|Y_{obs})$. But notice that if an expression for the complete-data posterior mean $E(\xi \mid Y_{obs}, Y_{mis})$ is available in closed form, then we can get another estimate by averaging over the draws of Y_{mis},

$$\tilde{\xi} = \frac{1}{m} \sum_{t=1}^{m} E(\xi|Y_{obs}, Y_{mis}^{(t)}). \tag{4.11}$$

The Rao-Blackwellized estimate $\tilde{\xi}$ is unbiased because

$$\int E(\xi|Y_{obs}, Y_{mis}) \, P(Y_{mis}|Y_{obs}) \, dY_{mis} = E(\xi|Y_{obs}).$$

Moreover, it is at least as efficient as the direct estimate $\bar{\xi}$, because by the key idea of the Rao-Blackwell theorem,

$$V[\,E(\xi^{(t)}|Y_{obs}, Y_{mis}^{(t)})\,|Y_{obs}] \leq V(\xi^{(t)}|Y_{obs}).$$

When the complete-data posterior mean $E(\xi \mid Y_{obs}, Y_{mis})$ is easy to compute, it pays to use the Rao-Blackwellized estimate rather than the direct estimate.

Rao-Blackwellized estimates may also be available for quantities other than the posterior mean. For example, because the posterior density of ξ may be written

$$P(\xi|Y_{obs}) = \int P(\xi|Y_{obs}, Y_{mis}) \, P(Y_{mis}|Y_{obs}) \, dY_{mis},$$

a Rao-Blackwellized density estimate is

$$\frac{1}{m} \sum_{t=1}^{m} P(\xi|Y_{obs}, Y_{mis}^{(t)}), \tag{4.12}$$

a mixture of the complete-data densities over the simulated values of Y_{mis}. It can be shown that (4.12) is superior to direct estimates based on $\xi^{(1)}, \xi^{(2)}, \ldots, \xi^{(m)}$, including kernel estimates (Gelfand and Smith, 1990). Rao-Blackwellized density estimates tend to have a smooth appearance even for small m. Mixtures of complete-data densities were also used by Tanner and Wong (1987) as an essential part of their data augmentation algorithm.

The key idea of Rao-Blackwellization is to make full use of the functional form of complete-data posterior summaries and rely on simulation to solve only the missing-data aspect of the problem. Notice that when there is no missing information about ξ, the complete-data and observed-data posteriors coincide, i.e.

$$P(\xi|Y_{obs}, Y_{mis}) = P(\xi|Y_{obs}).$$

When this happens, Rao-Blackwellized estimates of the posterior moments, posterior density, etc. of ξ do not depend at all on the sample values $Y_{mis}^{(1)}, Y_{mis}^{(2)}, \ldots, Y_{mis}^{(m)}$, and Monte Carlo error is entirely eliminated. Direct estimates based on $\xi^{(1)}, \xi^{(2)}, \ldots, \xi^{(m)}$, however, would still contain random error for finite m even with no missing information. The relative efficiency of the two estimates is closely related to the fraction of missing information for ξ. This relationship is illustrated by the following simple example.

Example: the efficiency of Rao-Blackwellization

Recall Example 1 of Section 3.4.3 in which $Y = (y_1, y_2, \ldots, y_n)$ is an iid sample from $N(\mu, \psi)$, the first n_1 elements of Y are observed and the remaining $n_0 = n - n_1$ elements are missing. When ψ is known, the prior $\pi(\mu) \propto c$ (a constant) leads to the observed-data posterior $\mu \mid Y_{obs} \sim N(\bar{y}_{obs}, n_1^{-1}\psi)$, where $\bar{y}_{obs}$ is the mean of the observed data. Let $\mu^{(1)}, \mu^{(2)}, \ldots, \mu^{(m)}$ be a sample of successive values of μ from a run of data augmentation following a burn-in period. Assuming the burn-in is sufficiently long, the marginal distribution of each member of the sample is the stationary distribution,

$$\mu^{(t)} \sim N(\bar{y}_{obs}, n_1^{-1}\psi) \tag{4.13}$$

for $t = 1, 2, \ldots, m$, where conditioning on Y_{obs} is implicit and has been suppressed in the notation. Using (3.37), we can also find the correlation structure of the dependent sample $\mu^{(1)}, \mu^{(2)}, \ldots, \mu^{(m)}$. The lag-$k$ autocovariance is

$$
\begin{aligned}
\mathrm{Cov}(\mu^{(t)}, \mu^{(t+k)}) &= E[\mathrm{Cov}(\mu^{(t)}, \mu^{(t+k)} \mid \mu^{(t)})] \\
&\quad + \mathrm{Cov}[E(\mu^{(t)}|\mu^{(t)}), E(\mu^{(t+k)}|\mu^{(t)})] \\
&= 0 + \mathrm{Cov}[\mu^{(t)}, \bar{y}_{obs} + \lambda^k(\mu^{(t)} - \bar{y}_{obs})] \\
&= \lambda^k V(\mu^{(t)}) \\
&= \lambda^k n_1^{-1}\psi,
\end{aligned}
$$

where $\lambda = n_0/n$ is the fraction of missing information. It follows that the joint distribution of $\mu^{(1)}, \mu^{(2)}, \ldots, \mu^{(m)}$ is multivariate normal with all means equal to $\bar{y}_{obs}$ and covariance matrix $n_1^{-1}\psi\Lambda$, where

$$
\Lambda = \begin{bmatrix}
1 & \lambda & \lambda^2 & \cdots & \lambda^m \\
\lambda & 1 & \lambda & \cdots & \lambda^{m-1} \\
\lambda^2 & \lambda & 1 & \cdots & \lambda^{m-2} \\
\vdots & \vdots & \vdots & & \vdots \\
\lambda^m & \lambda^{m-1} & \lambda^{m-2} & \cdots & 1
\end{bmatrix}. \tag{4.14}
$$

The direct estimate of the posterior mean $E(\mu|Y_{obs})$ is

$$
\bar{\mu} = \frac{1}{m} \sum_{t=1}^{m} \mu^{(t)},
$$

which has variance

$$
V(\bar{\mu}) = \frac{\psi}{n_1 m^2} \mathbf{1}^T \Lambda \mathbf{1}, \tag{4.15}
$$

where $\mathbf{1} = (1, 1, \ldots, 1)^T$.

Let us now investigate the precision of the Rao-Blackwellized estimate. Recall that the P-step of data augmentation draws $\mu^{(t)}$ from a normal distribution with mean

$$
\begin{aligned}
E(\mu|Y_{obs}, Y_{mis}^{(t)}) &= n^{-1}(n_1 \bar{y}_{obs} + n_0 \bar{y}_{mis}^{(t)}) \\
&= (1-\lambda)\bar{y}_{obs} + \lambda \bar{y}_{mis}^{(t)}
\end{aligned}
$$

and variance $V(\mu|Y_{obs}, Y_{mis}^{(t)}) = n^{-1}\psi$, where

$$
\bar{y}_{mis}^{(t)} = \frac{1}{n_0} \sum_{i=n_1+1}^{n} y_i^{(t)}
$$

is the average of the n_0 responses imputed at the previous I-step. The Rao-Blackwellized estimate of $E(\mu|Y_{obs})$ is therefore

$$
\begin{aligned}
\tilde{\mu} &= \frac{1}{m} \sum_{t=1}^{m} E(\mu|Y_{obs}, Y_{mis}^{(t)}) \\
&= (1-\lambda)\bar{y}_{obs} + \lambda \left(\frac{1}{m} \sum_{t=1}^{m} \bar{y}_{mis}^{(t)} \right).
\end{aligned}
$$

To find the variance of $\tilde{\mu}$, we need to know the covariance structure of the sequence $\bar{y}_{mis}^{(1)}, \bar{y}_{mis}^{(2)}, \ldots, \bar{y}_{mis}^{(m)}$. From (3.36) it follows that

$$
\bar{y}_{mis}^{(t+1)} | \mu^{(t)} \sim N(\mu^{(t)}, n_0^{-1}\psi), \tag{4.16}
$$

where conditioning on Y_{obs} is to be understood. Together, (4.16) and (4.13) imply that $V(\bar{y}_{mis}^{(t)}) \to (n_1^{-1} + n_0^{-1})\psi$ as $t \to \infty$. To derive the lag-k autocovariance, notice that

$$
\begin{aligned}
\mathrm{Cov}(\bar{y}_{mis}^{(t)}, \bar{y}_{mis}^{(t+k)}) &= E[\,\mathrm{Cov}(\bar{y}_{mis}^{(t)}, \bar{y}_{mis}^{(t+k)} \mid \bar{y}_{mis}^{(t)})\,] \\
&\quad + \mathrm{Cov}[\,E(\bar{y}_{mis}^{(t)} \mid \bar{y}_{mis}^{(t)}), \, E(\bar{y}_{mis}^{(t+k)} \mid \bar{y}_{mis}^{(t)})\,] \\
&= \mathrm{Cov}[\,\bar{y}_{mis}^{(t)}, \, E(\bar{y}_{mis}^{(t+k)} \mid \bar{y}_{mis}^{(t)})\,].
\end{aligned}
$$

By repeated application of the conditional expectation rule $E(U) = E[\,E(U \mid V)\,]$, one can show that

$$
E(\bar{y}_{mis}^{(t+k)} \mid \bar{y}_{mis}^{(t)}) = (1 - \lambda^k)\,\bar{y}_{obs} + \lambda^k\,\bar{y}_{mis}^{(t)},
$$

and thus

$$
\begin{aligned}
\mathrm{Cov}(\bar{y}_{mis}^{(t)}, \bar{y}_{mis}^{(t+k)}) &= \lambda^k\, V(\bar{y}_{mis}^{(t)}) \\
&= \lambda^k\, (n_1^{-1} + n_0^{-1})\psi.
\end{aligned}
$$

After a sufficient burn-in period, the covariance matrix for the sample $\bar{y}_{mis}^{(1)}, \bar{y}_{mis}^{(2)}, \dots, \bar{y}_{mis}^{(m)}$ is thus $(n_1^{-1} + n_0^{-1})\psi\Lambda$, where Λ is the patterned matrix shown in (4.14), and the variance of the Rao-Blackwellized estimate is

$$
V(\tilde{\mu}) = \frac{\lambda^2 \psi}{m^2}\,(n_1^{-1} + n_0^{-1})\,\mathbf{1}^T \Lambda \mathbf{1}. \tag{4.17}
$$

Comparing (4.17) with (4.15), we see that the relative efficiency of $\tilde{\mu}$ to $\bar{\mu}$ is

$$
\begin{aligned}
\frac{V(\bar{\mu})}{V(\tilde{\mu})} &= \frac{n_1^{-1}}{\lambda^2(n_1^{-1} + n_0^{-1})} \\
&= \lambda^{-1},
\end{aligned}
$$

the inverse of the fraction of missing information. The advantage of the Rao-Blackwellized estimate over the direct estimate is greatest when the fraction of missing information is small, and diminishes for λ near 1. With 10% missing information, Rao-Blackwellizing the estimate without changing the number of iterations increases precision by a factor of 10. In other words, Rao-Blackwellization allows us to achieve the same precision as with the direct estimate while using only $\sqrt{\lambda}$ times as many iterations.

Now consider density estimation in the two-parameter case where μ and ψ are both unknown. Under the diffuse prior $\pi(\mu, \psi) \propto \psi^{-1}$, the complete-data posterior (3.40) implies that the marginal density for ψ is that of a scaled inverse-χ^2 distribution,

$$
P(\psi \mid Y_{obs}, Y_{mis}) = k^{-1}\, \psi^{-(n+1)/2} \exp\left\{ -\frac{(n-1)S^2}{2\psi} \right\},
$$

where the normalizing constant is

$$k = \Gamma\left(\tfrac{n-1}{2}\right) \left[\frac{2}{(n-1)S^2}\right]^{(n-1)/2}.$$

The marginal distribution for μ can be shown to be

$$\mu \mid Y_{obs}, Y_{mis} \sim \bar{y} + (S/\sqrt{n})\, t_{n-1},$$

for which the density is

$$P(\mu \mid Y_{obs}, Y_{mis}) = \frac{\Gamma\left(\tfrac{n}{2}\right)}{\Gamma\left(\tfrac{n-1}{2}\right)\sqrt{\pi \frac{(n-1)S^2}{n}}} \left[1 + \frac{n(\mu - \bar{y})^2}{(n-1)S^2}\right]^{-n/2}$$

(Section 5.2.2). In this problem, of course, the observed-data marginal posterior densities are also available in closed form; we merely replace n, $\bar{y}$ and S^2 in the complete-data marginals by n_1, $\bar{y}_{obs}$ and S^2_{obs}, respectively. If we simulate the observed-data posterior using data augmentation, however, we can also estimate the observed-data marginal posterior densities, either directly from the iterates of μ and ψ or by Rao-Blackwellization, and compare the estimates with the known true density functions.

To illustrate this, a single run of data augmentation was performed for the univariate sample of size $n_1 = 10$ shown in Table 3.1 (a), assuming that an additional $n_0 = 3$ observations were missing. Beginning with arbitrary starting values for μ and ψ, the chain was run for $m = 500$ iterations following an initial burn-in period of 100 iterations. The true observed-data marginal densities for μ and ψ are displayed in Figure 4.1, along with three simulation-based estimates: histograms of the iterates of μ and ψ, kernel estimates based on the same and Rao-Blackwellized estimates obtained by averaging the expressions for the complete-data marginal densities over the iterates of Y_{mis}. The kernel estimates are based on Gaussian kernels for μ and ψ with standard deviations of 1 and 10, respectively. In this problem, for which the fraction of missing information is $3/13 = 0.23$, the Rao-Blackwellized estimates are nearly indistinguishable from the true densities. The histograms and kernel estimates, however, show a greater amount of random error.

Although these univariate examples are simplistic, we can expect this type of result to hold true in general: Rao-Blackwellization can greatly increase the efficiency of simulation-based estimates, particularly when fractions of missing information are small. Although a Rao-Blackwellized estimate may require some additional analytic

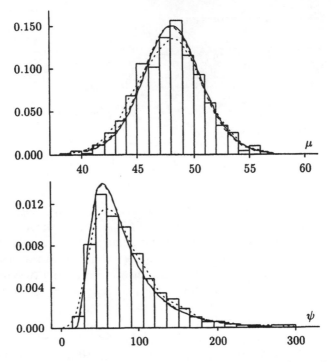

Figure 4.1. *Histograms of $m = 500$ consecutive iterates of μ and ψ with true marginal densities (solid lines), kernel density estimates (dotted lines) and Rao-Blackwellized density estimates (dashed lines).*

work to find a closed-form expression for the complete-data posterior summary, the extra effort is often worthwhile.

4.3 Multiple imputation

Like parameter simulation, multiple imputation is a Monte Carlo approach to the analysis of incomplete data. Described by Rubin (1987) in the context of nonresponse in sample surveys, the technique is quite general and can readily be used in many non-survey applications as well. Multiple imputation shares the same underlying philosophy as EM and data augmentation: solving an incomplete-data problem by repeatedly solving the complete-data version. In multiple imputation, the unknown missing data Y_{mis} are replaced by simulated values $Y_{mis}^{(1)}, Y_{mis}^{(2)}, \ldots, Y_{mis}^{(m)}$. Each of the m completed datasets is analyzed by standard complete-data methods. The variability among the results of the m analyses provides a measure of the uncertainty due to missing data, which, when combined with measures of ordinary sample variation, lead to a single inferential statement about the parameters of interest.

4.3.1 Bayesianly proper multiple imputations

If multiple imputation is to yield valid inferences, the simulated values of Y_{mis} must possess certain properties. Multiple imputations drawn from a distribution possessing these properties are said to be *proper*. Rubin (1987) gives a technical definition for proper multiple imputations; his definition is tied to the frequentist properties of estimators over repeated realizations of a posited response mechanism. For the most part, a thorough understanding of Rubin's definition is not crucial for the purposes of this book, for the following two reasons. First, our statistical procedures are derived primarily from perspectives of likelihood-based or Bayesian inference; we are assuming that valid inferential statements can be obtained through summaries of a likelihood function or posterior distribution arising from a parametric model. Second, because of our ignorability assumption, we will never need to specify a nonresponse mechanism in our analyses. Indeed, with the complicated patterns of missingness often encountered in multivariate datasets, it may be quite difficult to specify any realistic mechanism for the nonresponse, ignorable or otherwise.

Rubin's definition is important for discussing the statistical validity of multiple imputation from frequentist and design-based perspectives. For now, however, let us consider a different concept of what it means for multiple imputations to be proper, which is more suited to the purposes of this book. We will say that multiple imputations are *Bayesianly proper* if they are independent realizations of $P(Y_{mis}|Y_{obs})$, the posterior predictive distribution of the missing data under some complete-data model and prior. Notice that $P(Y_{mis}|Y_{obs})$ may be written as

$$P(Y_{mis}|Y_{obs}) = \int P(Y_{mis}|Y_{obs},\theta)\,P(\theta|Y_{obs})\,d\theta,$$

the conditional predictive distribution of Y_{mis} given θ, averaged over the observed-data posterior of θ. Bayesianly proper multiple imputations thus reflect uncertainty about Y_{mis} given the parameters of the complete-data model, as well as uncertainty about the unknown model parameters. The fact that $P(Y_{mis}|Y_{obs})$ does not rely on the observed response pattern R (Section 2.3) indicates that the resulting multiple imputations are appropriate under an assumption of ignorability.

We will discuss Rubin's definition at the end of this chapter. Except for that brief digression, however, the concept of proper imputations used in the remainder of this book will be that of Bayesianly proper imputations. For brevity, we will usually omit the term Bayesian and refer to the imputations simply as proper; the reader should understand that our usage of the term is not the same as Rubin's.

Proper multiple imputations and data augmentation

It is convenient to create multiple imputations using data augmentation and related algorithms, because the simulated values of Y_{mis} created by these algorithms have $P(Y_{mis}|Y_{obs})$ as their stationary distribution. Because proper multiple imputations must be independent, however, we will not in general be able to use successive iterates of Y_{mis} because they tend to be correlated. Rather, we will have to subsample the chain, e.g. take every kth iterate, where k is chosen large enough so that the dependence will be negligible. Alternatively, we can create proper imputations by simulating m independent chains of length k and retaining the final values of Y_{mis} from each chain, where k is large enough to ensure that the imputations are essentially independent of the starting values or starting distribution. Although this means that creating m imputations requires km iterations, the computational burden will not necessarily be severe, because only a small number of imputations are usually required; in typical applications, we can obtain good results with m as small as 3–5.

Why only a few imputations are needed

For the reader who is unfamiliar with multiple imputation, the claim that $m = 3$ is often adequate may be very surprising; in other applications of Monte Carlo, hundreds or thousands of draws are often needed to achieve an acceptable level of accuracy. In multiple imputation, however, a very small value of m will usually suffice. There are two fundamental reasons for this.

First, like Rao-Blackwellization, multiple imputation relies on simulation to solve only the missing-data aspect of the problem. As with any simulation method, one could effectively eliminate Monte Carlo error by choosing m to be very large, but with multiple imputation the resulting gain in efficiency would typically be unimportant because the Monte Carlo error is a relatively small portion of the overall inferential uncertainty. If the fraction of missing information about a scalar estimand is λ, the relative efficiency (on the variance scale) of a point estimate based on m imputations to one based on an infinite number of imputations is approximately $(1 + \lambda/m)^{-1}$ (Rubin, 1987, p. 114). When $\lambda = 0.2$, for example, an estimate based on $m = 3$ imputations will tend to have a standard error only $\sqrt{1 + 0.2/3} = 1.033$ times as large as the estimate with $m = \infty$. With $\lambda = 0.5$, an estimate based on $m = 5$ imputations will tend to have a standard error only $\sqrt{1 + 0.5/5} = 1.049$ times as large. In most applications, the additional resources that would be required to create and store more than a few imputations would not be well spent.

The second reason why we can often obtain valid inferences with a very small m is that the rules for combining the m complete-data analyses explicitly account for Monte Carlo error. A multiple-imputation interval estimate makes provisions for the fact that both the point and variance estimates contain a predictable amount of simulation error due to the finiteness of m, and the width of the interval is accordingly adjusted to maintain the appropriate probability of coverage.

4.3.2 Inference for a scalar quantity

In Section 4.2 we assumed that the scalar quantity to be estimated was an explicit function of the parameters of the complete-data model, denoting it by $\xi = \xi(\theta)$. Switching now to a notation more consistent with that of Rubin (1987), we denote a generic scalar estimand by Q. In multiple-imputation inference, Q may be an explicit function of the parameters of the *imputation model*, the complete-data model under which the multiple versions of Y_{mis} were created. When this is the case, multiple-imputation estimates of Q are simply Rao-Blackwellized estimates, and the rules for inference given below can be interpreted as Rao-Blackwellized methods that make special provisions for Monte Carlo error incurred by using a small m.

In many other cases, however, Q will not be a parameter of the imputation model. In sample surveys, Q may be a function (a mean, a proportion, a ratio of means, etc.) of data from a finite population. In classical sample-survey methods (e.g. Cochran, 1977), the population data are not modeled but regarded as fixed, and inferences are based purely on the randomization used to draw the sample. Some theoretical justification for using proper multiple imputations from a parametric model in finite-population survey inference is given by Rubin (1987). In other non-survey applications, Q is often a function of parameters of a model tailored to the specific goals of the analysis. This model, which we call the *analyst's model*, may be somewhat different from the imputation model. When the imputation model and analyst's model differ, questions naturally arise about the validity of the inference; these questions will be addressed at the end of this chapter.

Complete-data estimators

To use multiple imputation, we must have a rule for inference about Q in the complete-data case. Let $\hat{Q}$ be the complete-data point estimate for Q, the estimate that we would use if no data were missing. Let U be the variance estimate associated with $\hat{Q}$, so that $\sqrt{U}$ is the complete-data standard error. Because $\hat{Q}$ and U are both functions of $Y = (Y_{obs}, Y_{mis})$, we will sometimes write them as $\hat{Q}(Y_{obs}, Y_{mis})$ and $U(Y_{obs}, Y_{mis})$, respectively. Multiple-imputation inference assumes (a) that $\hat{Q}$ and U are first-order approximations to a posterior mean and variance of Q,

$$\hat{Q}(Y_{obs}, Y_{mis}) \approx E(Q \mid Y_{obs}, Y_{mis}), \qquad (4.18)$$

$$U(Y_{obs}, Y_{mis}) \approx V(Q \mid Y_{obs}, Y_{mis}), \qquad (4.19)$$

under a reasonable complete-data model and prior; and (b) that the complete-data problem is sufficiently regular and the sample size sufficiently large for the asymptotic normal approximation

$$U^{-1/2}(Q - \hat{Q}) \sim N(0, 1) \qquad (4.20)$$

to work well. The approximation (4.20) can be justified either from a frequentist or a Bayesian perspective. To the frequentist, it is a statement about the repeated-sampling properties of $\hat{Q}$ and U for a fixed value of Q; to the Bayesian, it is a statement about the posterior distribution of Q with Y (and hence $\hat{Q}$ and U) held fixed.

Many, but not all, commonly used estimators can be regarded as approximate posterior means, and their variance estimates as approximate posterior variances. MLEs and their asymptotic variances, derived from the curvature of the observed or expected log-likelihood at the mode, typically satisfy (4.18)–(4.20) (Cox and Hinkley, 1974). Estimators that are clearly inefficient, e.g. a sample mean based on only half of the sample, are definitely ruled out, as they do not use all the available information in Y. Certain classes of nonparametric procedures (e.g. methods based only on ranks) should also be ruled out, as they tend to sacrifice some efficiency to avoid specification of a full parametric model. With multiple imputation, just as with complete data, it is good practice to perform the analysis on a scale for which the asymptotic normal approximation is likely to work well; for example, with a correlation coefficient, it is advisable to apply Fisher's transformation (3.14).

Rule for combining complete-data inferences

With m imputations, we can calculate m different versions of $\hat{Q}$ and U. Let

$$\hat{Q}^{(t)} = \hat{Q}(Y_{obs}, Y_{mis}^{(t)})$$

and

$$U^{(t)} = U(Y_{obs}, Y_{mis}^{(t)})$$

be the point and variance estimates using the tth set of imputed data, $t = 1, 2, \ldots, m$. Rubin (1987, Chap. 3) gives the following rule for combining them. The multiple-imputation point estimate for Q is simply the average of the complete-data point estimates,

$$\bar{Q} = \frac{1}{m} \sum_{t=1}^{m} \hat{Q}^{(t)}. \tag{4.21}$$

The variance estimate associated with $\bar{Q}$ has two components. The *within-imputation variance* is the average of the complete-data variance estimates,

$$\bar{U} = \frac{1}{m} \sum_{t=1}^{m} U^{(t)}. \tag{4.22}$$

The *between-imputation variance* is the variance of the complete-data point estimates,

$$B = \frac{1}{m-1} \sum_{t=1}^{m} (\hat{Q}^{(t)} - \bar{Q})^2. \tag{4.23}$$

The *total variance* is defined as

$$T = \bar{U} + (1 + m^{-1})B, \tag{4.24}$$

and inferences are based on the approximation

$$T^{-1/2}(Q - \bar{Q}) \sim t_{\nu}, \tag{4.25}$$

where the degrees of freedom are given by

$$\nu = (m - 1)\left[1 + \frac{\bar{U}}{(1 + m^{-1})B}\right]^2. \tag{4.26}$$

Thus a $100(1 - \alpha)\%$ interval estimate for Q is

$$\bar{Q} \pm t_{\nu, 1-\alpha/2}\sqrt{T}, \tag{4.27}$$

and a p-value for testing the null hypothesis $Q = Q'$ against a two-sided alternative is

$$2P(t_\nu \geq T^{-1/2}|\bar{Q} - Q'|)$$

or, equivalently,

$$P[F_{1,\nu} \geq T^{-1}(\bar{Q} - Q')^2]. \tag{4.28}$$

Missing information

Notice that the degrees of freedom (4.26) depend not only on m, but also on the ratio

$$r = \frac{(1 + m^{-1})B}{\bar{U}}. \tag{4.29}$$

Rubin (1987) calls r the *relative increase in variance due to non-response*, because $\bar{U}$ represents the estimated total variance when there is no missing information about Q (i.e. when $B = 0$). When m is large and/or r is small, the degrees of freedom will be large and (4.25) will be approximately normal.

If we define information as minus one times the average second derivative of the log-posterior density of Q, the information in the approximate posterior (4.25) is $(\nu+1)(\nu+3)^{-1}T^{-1}$. With no missing information, the posterior would become normal with mean $\bar{Q}$ and variance $\bar{U}$, for which the information is $\bar{U}^{-1}$. It follows that

$$\begin{aligned}
\hat{\lambda} &= (\bar{U}^{-1} - (\nu+1)(\nu+3)^{-1}T^{-1})\bar{U} \\
&= \frac{r + 2/(\nu+3)}{r+1} \tag{4.30}
\end{aligned}$$

is an estimate of the fraction of missing information about Q. In applications, calculation of r and $\hat{\lambda}$ is highly recommended, as they are interesting and useful diagnostics for assessing how the missing data contribute to inferential uncertainty about Q.

Heuristic justification

An imprecise but intuitive justification for this procedure is the following. Let us assume that the observed-data posterior for Q is approximately normal, so that if the observed-data posterior moments could be calculated we would use the interval

$$E(Q|Y_{obs}) \pm z_{1-\alpha/2} \sqrt{V(Q|Y_{obs})}. \tag{4.31}$$

Because $E(Q \mid Y_{obs})$ and $V(Q \mid Y_{obs})$ are not readily available, however, we use simulation-based estimates of them provided by the multiple imputations. Notice that by (4.18) and (4.19) we can write

$$E(Q|Y_{obs}) \approx E(\hat{Q}|Y_{obs}) \tag{4.32}$$

and

$$V(Q|Y_{obs}) \approx E(U|Y_{obs}) + V(\hat{Q}|Y_{obs}), \tag{4.33}$$

where the moments on the right-hand sides of (4.32) and (4.33) are calculated over the distribution $P(Y_{mis}|Y_{obs})$ from which the multiple imputations are drawn. By the law of large numbers, $\bar{Q}, \bar{U}$ and B approach $E(\hat{Q}|Y_{obs})$, $E(U|Y_{obs})$, and $V(\hat{Q}|Y_{obs})$, respectively, as $m \to \infty$. Thus, with an infinite number of imputations,

$$\bar{Q} \pm z_{1-\alpha/2} \sqrt{\bar{U} + B} \tag{4.34}$$

would be identical to (4.31). Because m is typically small, however, we need to make two adjustments to (4.34). First, the interval must be widened to reflect the fact that $\bar{Q}$ is randomly different from $E(\hat{Q} \mid Y_{obs})$. With proper imputations, B/m is an unbiased estimate of the variance of $\bar{Q}$, so to account for the error in $\bar{Q}$ we must increase the estimate of the total variance by this amount. Second, because the estimated variance components $\bar{U}$ and B are also estimated with error, we need to widen (4.34) further by replacing the normal quantile with one from a t distribution.

Further justification

Rubin (1987) derives the procedure more formally by Bayesian arguments, showing that (4.25) is an approximate observed-data posterior distribution for Q based on the reduced information in $\hat{Q}^{(1)}, \hat{Q}^{(2)}, \ldots, \hat{Q}^{(m)}$ and $U^{(1)}, U^{(2)}, \ldots, U^{(m)}$ rather than on the infinite number of imputations that one would ideally have. The expression (4.26) for the degrees of freedom ν are obtained by approximately matching the first two moments of the reduced-information posterior to those of a t distribution.

Despite the Bayesian derivation, evaluations have shown that this method leads to inferences that are well calibrated from a frequentist standpoint. Rubin and Schenker (1986) report that multiple-imputation interval estimates tend to have at least the nominal coverage (i.e. a 95% interval covers the true parameter at least 95% of the time) in a variety of scenarios even for m as small as 2. When the actual coverage falls below the nominal coverage, it tends to be either because (a) the fraction of missing information is unusually large, or (b) the complete-data normal approximation (4.20) works poorly. In the former case, we can obtain better results by choosing a larger m. In the latter case, the poor results should be regarded as a inherent shortcoming of the asymptotic approximation for complete data rather than as a failure of the multiple imputation methodology. In many cases, the quality of the complete-data normal approximation can be improved by a suitable reparameterization.

In addition to simulation studies, further theoretical justification for this method is provided by Schenker and Welsh (1988), who established frequentist consistency of multiple-imputation inferences for linear regression analysis with an incomplete response variable. The result was later extended by Brownstone (1991) to incomplete predictors. Additional references supporting the use of (4.25) are given by Rubin (1996).

4.3.3 Inference for multidimensional estimands

Several extensions of the above method have been developed for estimands that are multidimensional. Suppose now that Q is a $k \times 1$ vector. Rather than finding confidence regions for Q, which are often difficult to interpret (especially when k is large), we will focus on finding a p-value for testing the hypothesis that Q equals a particular value of interest Q_0. In practice, this typically arises because one is interested in comparing two models for the data, M_0 and M_1, where M_1 is more general than M_0 and reduces to M_0 when $Q = Q_0$. We now discuss three alternative rules for calculating a p-value from multiply-imputed data.

Combining point estimates and covariance matrices

Let $\hat{Q}$ be a complete-data point estimate of Q, and U an asymptotic covariance matrix associated with $\hat{Q}$. The following method assumes that, with complete data, the distribution of $(\hat{Q} - Q)$ is sufficiently close to $N(0, U)$ that an accurate p-value may be obtained from the multivariate Wald statistic and a chisquare reference distribution,

$$P[\chi_k^2 \geq (\hat{Q} - Q_0)^T U^{-1}(\hat{Q} - Q_0)]. \qquad (4.35)$$

With large samples, (4.35) is a valid p-value both in the frequentist and the Bayesian sense.

With incomplete data we cannot calculate (4.35) and need a new test statistic that is a function only of Y_{obs}. As in the scalar case, with m imputations we calculate m estimates $\hat{Q}^{(1)}, \hat{Q}^{(2)}, \ldots, \hat{Q}^{(m)}$ and m covariance matrices $U^{(1)}, U^{(2)}, \ldots, U^{(m)}$. The multivariate analogues of (4.21)–(4.24) are

$$\bar{Q} = \frac{1}{m} \sum_{t=1}^{m} \hat{Q}^{(t)},$$

$$\bar{U} = \frac{1}{m} \sum_{t=1}^{m} U^{(t)},$$

$$B = \frac{1}{m-1} \sum_{t=1}^{m} (\hat{Q}^{(t)} - \bar{Q})(\hat{Q}^{(t)} - \bar{Q})^T,$$

$$T = \bar{U} + (1 + m^{-1})B.$$

Using the natural multivariate extension of (4.28), one might suppose that

$$P[F_{k,\nu} \geq (\bar{Q} - Q_0)^T T^{-1}(\bar{Q} - Q_0)/k]$$

would be an appropriate p-value, where ν depends on the precision with which T estimates the observed-data posterior variance of Q,

$$V(Q|Y_{obs}) \approx E(U|Y_{obs}) + V(\hat{Q}|Y_{obs}).$$

It turns out, however, that finding an adequate reference distribution for the statistic

$$(\bar{Q} - Q_0)^T T^{-1}(\bar{Q} - Q_0)/k$$

is not a simple matter. The main problem is that for small m, the between-imputation covariance matrix B is a very noisy estimate of $V(\hat{Q}|Y_{obs})$, and does not even have full rank if $m \leq k$.

One way out of this difficulty is to make the simplifying assumption that the population between- and within-imputation covariance matrices are proportional to one another,

$$V(\hat{Q}|Y_{obs}) \propto E(U|Y_{obs}),$$

which is equivalent to assuming that the fractions of missing information for all components of Q are equal. Under this assumption, a more stable estimate of total variance is

$$\tilde{T} = (1 - r_1)\,\bar{U},$$

where

$$r_1 = (1 + m^{-1})\,\text{tr}(B\bar{U}^{-1})/k \tag{4.36}$$

is the average relative increase in variance due to nonresponse across the components of Q. Using $\tilde{T}$ rather than T, the test statistic becomes

$$D_1 = (\bar{Q} - Q_0)^T \tilde{T}^{-1}(\bar{Q} - Q_0)/k, \tag{4.37}$$

and a p-value for testing $Q = Q_0$ is

$$p = P(F_{k,\nu_1} \geq D_1).$$

The best approximation to date for the degrees of freedom ν_1 is given by Li, Raghunathan and Rubin (1991),

$$\nu_1 = 4 + (t - 4)\left[1 + (1 - 2t^{-1})\,r_1^{-1}\right]^2, \tag{4.38}$$

where $t = k(m - 1)$. This procedure requires $t > 4$; when $t \leq 4$, we may use an alternative expression given by Rubin (1987),

$$\nu_1 = t\,(1 + k^{-1})\,(1 + r_1^{-1})^2/2.$$

Although (4.37) and (4.38) are derived under the strong assumption that the fractions of missing information for all components of Q are equal, Li, Raghunathan and Rubin (1991) report encouraging results even when this assumption is violated. In a simulation study, they examined the performance of this procedure using values of m between 2 and 10 and average fractions of missing information up to 0.5, in problems with up to $k = 35$ parameters. At worst the procedure tends to be somewhat conservative (overstating the p-values), and there is a small loss of power relative to the ideal case with $m = \infty$. These simulations support the use of this procedure in many situations of practical interest. It is important to note, however, that the simulations assume the appropriateness of (4.35), the chisquare approximation for the complete-data Wald statistic. For the procedure to work well in practice, we need a large sample and an appropriate scale for Q to ensure validity of the usual complete-data asymptotic approximations.

Combining p-values

Calculation of the statistic D_1 and its associated degrees of freedom requires access to the point estimates and covariance matrices from the m complete-data analyses. Software packages for common procedures, e.g. linear or logistic regression, typically allow the user to examine and save the covariance matrices for further analysis. When k is large, however, this procedure may be somewhat cumbersome, particularly when a large number of tests are to be performed. One might ask whether it is possible to obtain a valid inference using only the m complete-data p-values, or, equivalently, the m complete-data Wald statistics

$$d_W^{(t)} = (Q^{(t)} - Q_0)^T (U^{(t)})^{-1}(Q^{(t)} - Q_0), \qquad (4.39)$$

$t = 1, 2, \ldots, m$. Such a procedure is described by Li $et\ al.$ (1991), who propose the statistic

$$D_2 = \frac{\bar{d}_W k^{-1} - (m+1)(m-1)^{-1}r_2}{1 + r_2}, \qquad (4.40)$$

where

$$\bar{d}_W = \frac{1}{m} \sum_{t=1}^{m} d_W^{(t)}$$

is the average of the Wald statistics, and

$$r_2 = (1 + m^{-1}) \left[\frac{1}{m-1} \sum_{t=1}^{m} \left(\sqrt{d_W^{(t)}} - \overline{\sqrt{d_W}} \right)^2 \right]$$

is $(1 + m^{-1})$ times the sample variance of their square roots. The quantity r_2 is a clever estimate of r_1, the average relative increase in variance due to nonresponse, based only on the Wald statistics. Notice that with no missing information, $r_2 = 0$ and (4.40) reduces to the average of the Wald statistics divided by k. The combined p-value for testing $Q = Q_0$ is

$$p = P(F_{k,\nu_2} \geq D_2),$$

where the degrees of freedom are

$$\nu_2 = k^{-3/m}(m-1)(1 + r_2^{-1})^2. \qquad (4.41)$$

This procedure was developed partly using theoretical arguments and partly through the results of simulation studies for $m = 3$, so it should be expected to work best with $m = 3$ imputations. Li $et\ al.$ (1991) examined the behavior of this procedure in problems with up to $k = 25$ parameters, with m ranging from 2 to 10 and the average fraction of missing information $\bar{\lambda}$ up to 0.5 both when the individual fractions of missing information are equal and unequal. For a nominal 5%-level test, the procedure tends to be conservative for $\bar{\lambda} < 0.2$ and anticonservative for $\bar{\lambda} > 0.2$. In what we might expect to be one of the worst cases ($k = 25$, $m = 2$ and $\bar{\lambda} = 0.5$) the actual level of the 5% test is about 8%. Overall, the results seem to be best with $m = 3$, which is not surprising because the procedure was developed with $m = 3$ in mind. In simulations D_2 was not highly correlated with the more nearly optimal statistic D_1, so there appears to be a substantial loss in power when using D_2 rather than D_1. Li *et al.* (1991) suggest that this procedure be used only as a rough guide, and that the analyst should interpret it as providing a range of p-values between one half and twice the calculated value.

Combining likelihood-ratio test statistics

A third procedure for multivariate estimands, which may be regarded as intermediate between the previous two, is described by Meng and Rubin (1992b). Making use of the well known fact that the Wald statistic is asymptotically equivalent to that of the likelihood-ratio test, they propose a method for combining the complete-data likelihood-ratio test statistics. The resulting statistic, D_3, is typically easier to compute than D_1 although not quite as convenient as D_2. It is, however, asymptotically equivalent to D_1 for any m, so it should retain the good performance of D_1 in a wide variety of scenarios.

Let ψ denote the vector of unknown parameters in the analyst's model, and $Q = Q(\psi)$ a k-dimensional function of ψ that is of interest; specifically, we wish to test the hypothesis that $Q = Q_0$ for a given Q_0. Let $l(\psi \,|\, Y_{obs}, Y_{mis})$ denote the complete-data log-likelihood function, $\hat{\psi}$ the MLE or maximizer of $l(\psi \,|\, Y_{obs}, Y_{mis})$, and $\hat{\psi}_0$ the maximizer of $l(\psi \,|\, Y_{obs}, Y_{mis})$ subject to the constraint $Q(\psi) = Q_0$. In regular problems, the complete-data likelihood-ratio test statistic

$$
\begin{aligned}
d_L &= d_L(\hat{\psi}, \hat{\psi}_0 \,|\, Y_{obs}, Y_{mis}) \\
&= 2[\, l(\hat{\psi} \,|\, Y_{obs}, Y_{mis}) - l(\hat{\psi}_0 \,|\, Y_{obs}, Y_{mis})\,]
\end{aligned}
$$

is asymptotically distributed as χ_k^2 under the null hypothesis, and is asymptotically equivalent to the Wald statistic (4.35). Let

$$d_L^{(t)} = d_L(\hat{\psi}^{(t)}, \hat{\psi}_0^{(t)} | Y_{obs}, Y_{mis}^{(t)})$$

be the likelihood-ratio test statistic from the tth imputed dataset, $t = 1, 2, \ldots, m$, where $\hat{\psi}^{(t)}$ is the maximizer of $l(\psi | Y_{obs}, Y_{mis}^{(t)})$ and $\hat{\psi}_0^{(t)}$ is the maximizer of $l(\psi | Y_{obs}, Y_{mis}^{(t)})$ subject to $Q(\psi) = Q_0$. Let

$$\bar{d}_L = \frac{1}{m} \sum_{t=1}^{m} d_L^{(t)}$$

be the average of these likelihood-ratio statistics, and

$$\bar{\psi} = \frac{1}{m} \sum_{t=1}^{m} \hat{\psi}^{(t)}, \tag{4.42}$$

$$\bar{\psi}_0 = \frac{1}{m} \sum_{t=1}^{m} \hat{\psi}_0^{(t)} \tag{4.43}$$

the averages of the complete-data estimates of ψ across imputations. Finally, let

$$\tilde{d}_L = \frac{1}{m} \sum_{t=1}^{m} d_L(\bar{\psi}_0, \bar{\psi} | Y_{obs}, Y_{mis}^{(t)})$$

be the average of the likelihood-ratio statistics evaluated at $\bar{\psi}_0$ and $\bar{\psi}$, rather than at the imputation-specific parameter estimates. The test statistic proposed by Meng and Rubin (1992b) is

$$D_3 = \frac{\tilde{d}_L}{k(1 + r_3)}, \tag{4.44}$$

where

$$r_3 = \frac{m+1}{k(m-1)} (\bar{d}_L - \tilde{d}_L) \tag{4.45}$$

is an alternative estimate of the average relative increase due to nonresponse that is asymptotically equivalent to (4.36). The p-value associated with D_3 is

$$p = P(F_{k,\nu_3} \geq D_3) \tag{4.46}$$

with degrees of freedom calculated in the same manner as for D_1,

$$\nu_3 = \begin{cases} 4 + (t - 4) \left[1 + \left(1 - 2t^{-1} \right) r_3^{-1} \right]^2 & \text{if } t = k(m - 1) > 4, \\ t \left(1 + k^{-1} \right) (1 + r_3^{-1})^2 / 2 & \text{otherwise.} \end{cases}$$

In addition to the usual likelihood-ratio test statistics for each imputed dataset, this procedure also requires evaluation of the complete-data likelihood ratio at $(\bar{\psi}, \bar{\psi}_0)$ for each dataset. Implementation of this procedure thus requires code for evaluating the complete-data loglikelihood at user-specified values of the parameter, something which is not typically provided in standard statistical software. For many commonly used models, however, the complete-data loglikelihood is straightforward to derive and compute, and with a little effort on the part of the analyst the procedure can often be implemented without difficulty. Because this method is asymptotically equivalent for any m to the one that uses D_1, the properties of the two methods should be very similar.

Notice that a Wald test depends on the particular choice of scale for the unknown quantity Q, whereas a likelihood-ratio test is invariant to changes in scale. For this reason, some prefer the likelihood-ratio test in certain cases, believing it to be somewhat more trustworthy than the Wald test when the normality of $(\hat{Q}-Q)$ is in doubt. The likelihood-ratio procedure for multiply-imputed datasets described above may, at first glance, appear to be scale-invariant, but it is not; in particular, the averaging of the parameter estimates (4.42)–(4.43) will lead to somewhat different results under nonlinear transformations of ψ. The derivation of this procedure does assume the approximate complete-data normality of $(\hat{\psi} - \psi)$, so for best results the parameter estimates should probably be averaged on a scale for which the normality assumption is reasonable. Care must be taken, however, to ensure that the averages of parameter estimates lie within the parameter space, which will not necessarily happen if the averaging is done on an arbitrary scale. The sensitivity of this procedure to alternative parameterizations is not entirely clear and is worthy of further investigation.

4.4 Assessing convergence

In the last two sections, we examined techniques for extracting inferentially meaningful quantities from the output of Markov chain Monte Carlo. Responsible use of these methods requires some formal or informal assessment of the simulation algorithm's convergence properties; we need to know whether the algorithm has run 'long enough' for the results to be reliable. The meaning of convergence, and the diagnostic tools for assessing it, will vary according to the method of inference being used. In parameter simulation, we must choose a number of iterations to ensure that the resulting summaries (sample moments, quantiles, etc.) are sufficiently close to the posterior quantities they estimate; in this case, we need to assess convergence in the sense given by the law of large numbers (4.3). With multiple imputation, however, the goal is to simulate approximately independent draws from $P(Y_{mis}|Y_{obs})$; in that case, we need to assess convergence of the distribution of the iterates to their stationary distribution. Because these two concepts of convergence are quite different, the relevant diagnostic tools for assessing them are necessarily different. Convergence to stationarity, the weaker of the two concepts, is discussed in Sections 4.4.1–4.4.3; convergence of estimated posterior summaries is discussed in Section 4.4.4.

4.4.1 Monitoring convergence in a single chain

We now address the question, 'How long do I have to run my algorithm before it converges to the stationary distribution?'. The answer, of course, is that it depends. The rate of convergence depends on the fractions of missing information (Section 3.5.3) which vary from application to application. Even within a single application, the number of iterations required to achieve approximate stationarity depends on the starting value or starting distribution. For example, convergence will be faster from a starting value near the center of the observed-data posterior than from a starting value in the tails. In practice, it is helpful to know roughly how large a value k is needed for $\theta^{(t+k)}$ to be essentially independent of $\theta^{(t)}$ for any $\theta^{(t)}$ within the range of appreciable posterior density. If such a value were known, then a burn-in period of length k would be sufficient to achieve stationarity provided that the starting value was not highly unusual with respect to $P(\theta|Y_{obs})$. Moreover, after the burn-in period, every kth iterate of θ could then be taken as an independent draw from $P(\theta|Y_{obs})$, and every kth iterate of Y_{mis} could be used for proper multiple imputation.

Various methods for approximating k have appeared in the literature. The most accessible of these involve *output analysis*, examining the iterates of θ from one or more simulation runs. When θ is multidimensional, we can monitor the behavior of various components or scalar functions of θ. The marginal distributions of the components will often converge at different rates, however, and convergence by the kth iteration for every component or function that we examine does not necessarily imply that the joint posterior has converged; there is always a possibility that the distribution of some unknown function has not yet converged. Several methods have been proposed for choosing a value of k pertinent to the convergence of the entire joint distribution (Ritter and Tanner, 1992; Roberts, 1992; Liu and Liu, 1993), but these can be difficult to implement in practice. In typical missing-data scenarios addressed by this book, fractions of missing information are moderate and data augmentation algorithms tend to converge quickly. Pathological behavior such as slow convergence or nonexistence of a stationary distribution usually means that the model is too complicated (i.e. has too many parameters) to be supported by the observed data, and the problem should probably be reformulated. For our purposes, the most sensible diagnostics are those that can be implemented quickly and easily, providing an informal but reliable assessment of whether the situation is normal or pathological. Convergence diagnostics have been and will probably continue to be the subject of vigorous research efforts, and improved methods may be available soon. Further discussion and references on convergence are given by Smith and Roberts (1993); Tanner (1993); and Gilks, Richardson and Spiegelhalter (1996).

Time-series plots and autocorrelation

For an individual component or function $\xi = \xi(\theta)$, plotting the iterates of ξ from a single run can be a quick and easy way to assess convergence for that component. Recall Example 1 of Section 3.4.3 in which the first n_1 values of a univariate normal sample are observed and the remaining $n_0 = n - n_1$ are missing, and consider data augmentation for the two-parameter case in which $\theta = (\mu, \psi)$ is unknown. Using the $n_1 = 10$ data values in Table 3.1 (a), we performed runs of data augmentation for two different cases: $n_0 = 3$, corresponding to 23% missing information, and $n_0 = 90$, corresponding to 90% missing information. In each case, we used the starting value $(\mu^{(0)}, \psi^{(0)}) = (30, 70)$ and ran a single chain. Time-series plots of μ and ψ over the first 100 iterations are shown in Figure 4.2. The variance ψ is plotted on a log scale, for which the posterior distribution is more nearly symmetric.

Because $\mu^{(0)} = 30$ is located in the distant tails of the observed-data posterior (see Figure 4.1), Figure 4.2 (a) and (c) show initial trends as μ wanders back into the region of high posterior density. Had the starting value been located near the center of the distribution (e.g. at an observed-data MLE or posterior mode) this trend would not have been evident. Once the parameters are in the region of appreciable density, serial correlation provides evidence about how fast the algorithm converges. For 23% missing informa-

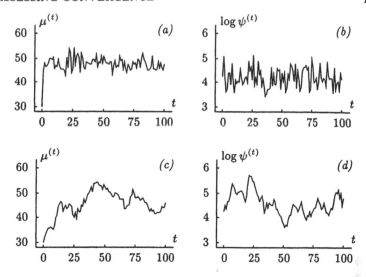

Figure 4.2. *First 100 parameter iterates from single runs of data augmentation: (a) μ and (b) $\log \psi$ with $n_0 = 3$, corresponding to 23% missing information; (c) μ and (d) $\log \psi$ with $n_0 = 90$, corresponding to 90% missing information.*

tion, (a) and (b) reveal no discernible trends; the plots resemble horizontal bands, indicating a low ratio of signal to noise. For 90% missing information, however, (c) and (d) reveal important trends lasting for 25 iterations or more, indicating that successive iterates are highly correlated. The plots in (a) and (b) are typical of situations in which the fractions of missing information are low to moderate, for which data augmentation is known to converge rather quickly. Long-term trends and high serial correlation, as in (c) and (d), are typical when the fractions of missing information are high and data augmentation converges slowly.

To investigate relationships among successive iterates, we could examine scatterplots of $\mu^{(t)}$ versus $\mu^{(t+k)}$ and $\psi^{(t)}$ versus $\psi^{(t+k)}$ for various choices of k. A more concise way to represent these relationships, however, is through the *autocorrelation function* (ACF). The lag-k autocorrelation for a stationary series $\{\xi^{(t)} : t = 1, 2, \ldots, m\}$ is defined to be

$$\rho_k = \frac{\text{Cov}(\xi^{(t)}, \xi^{(t+k)})}{V(\xi^{(t)})}. \tag{4.47}$$

Notice that by stationarity $V(\xi^{(t)}) = V(\xi^{(t+k)})$. A sample estimate

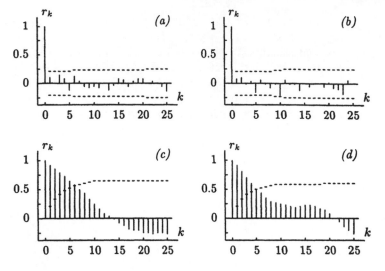

Figure 4.3. *Sample ACFs for the series in Figure 4.2 (a)-(d) estimated from iterations 11 to 100, with dashes indicating approximate 0.05-level critical values for testing* $\rho_k = \rho_{k+1} = \rho_{k+2} = \cdots = 0$.

of ρ_k is given by

$$r_k = \frac{\sum_{t=1}^{m-k}(\xi^{(t)} - \bar{\xi})(\xi^{(t+k)} - \bar{\xi})}{\sum_{t=1}^{m}(\xi^{(t)} - \bar{\xi})^2}, \qquad (4.48)$$

where $\bar{\xi}$ is the mean of the series (e.g. Box and Jenkins, 1976). A plot of r_k versus k for relevant values of k, known as a sample ACF plot or correlogram, provides a useful summary of linear serial dependence. Sample ACFs for the four series in Figure 4.2 are shown in Figure 4.3. To prevent the estimates from being unduly influenced by initial trends due to the implausible starting value, the first 10 values from each series were omitted from the calculation of the sample ACFs. Because the four series in Figure 4.2 are actually two bivariate series, we could also have estimated cross-correlation functions to assess the relationships between $\mu^{(t)}$ and $\psi^{(t+k)}$ and between $\mu^{(t+k)}$ and $\psi^{(t)}$, but for brevity these are omitted.

Variability of the sample autocorrelation

The sample ACFs in Figure 4.3 (a) and (b) show that serial dependence in the first series ($n_0 = 3$) dies out very quickly; the estimated correlations are below 0.2 even at lag 1. The second series, represented by (c) and (d), however, exhibits a high degree of serial dependence, and the correlations are still large beyond lag 10. Notice that in (c) and (d), as k increases r_k drops below zero. In general, one would not expect negative autocorrelations; the negative estimates are fluctuations due to the small sample size. Sample ACFs can be quite noisy, especially when the true serial correlation is high, and adjacent autocorrelation estimates are themselves highly correlated. For this reason, it is helpful to calculate estimates of variability associated with a sample ACF. For a stationary normal process that dies out after lag k' (i.e. $\rho_k = 0$ for all $k > k'$), the variance of r_k for $k > k'$ is approximately

$$V(r_k) \approx \frac{1}{m} \left(1 + 2 \sum_{t=1}^{k'} \rho_t^2 \right), \qquad (4.49)$$

where m is the sample size or length of the series (Bartlett, 1946). Moreover, when $\rho_k = 0$ the distribution of r_k is approximately normal (Anderson, 1942). Therefore, an approximate α-level test of the null hypothesis of no correlation at lag k or beyond,

$$\rho_k = \rho_{k+1} = \rho_{k+2} = \cdots = 0, \qquad (4.50)$$

versus the alternative hypothesis $\rho_k \neq 0$, rejects the null if

$$|r_k| \geq z_{1-\alpha/2} \left[\frac{1}{m} \left(1 + 2 \sum_{t=1}^{k-1} r_t^2 \right) \right]^{1/2}.$$

Critical values for 0.05-level tests of (4.50) for each k are shown in Figure 4.3 as dashed lines. In (a) and (b), none of the correlations for lag 1 or beyond are significantly different from zero. In (c) and (d), the correlations do not differ significantly from zero beyond lag 6, but the large standard errors indicate that the estimates are very noisy. To accurately estimate the true correlation structure for (c) and (d), we obviously need a much larger sample size. Figure 4.4 shows sample ACFs based on simulation runs of length $m = 10\,000$, for which the standard errors are negligibly small. From these plots, it is apparent that the autocorrelations are effectively zero by lag 3 for (a) and (b), and by lag 40 for (c) and (d).

As demonstrated by this example, long-term trends or drifts in scalar summaries of θ indicate slow convergence to stationarity, whereas the absence of such trends suggests rapid convergence. Time-series plots may also help diagnose pathological situations in which the algorithm does not converge at all because the posterior

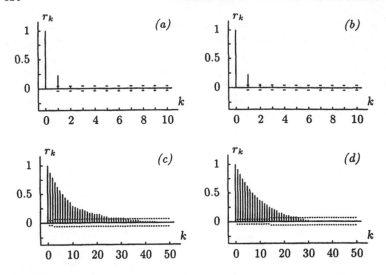

Figure 4.4. *Sample autocorrelation functions for the series in Figure 4.2 (a)–(d) estimated from 10 000 iterations, with dashes indicating approximate 0.05-level critical values for testing* $\rho_k = \rho_{k+1} = \rho_{k+2} = \cdots = 0$.

distribution does not exist. Recall the example of Section 3.5.2 in which a single value y_1 from $N(\mu, \psi)$ is observed but a second value y_2 is missing, and we apply the improper prior $\pi(\mu, \psi) \propto \psi^{-1}$. The I- and P-steps of data augmentation (3.46)–(3.47) are well defined, but the observed-data posterior is not proper because y_1 alone provides no information about ψ. Figure 4.5 shows time-series plots from a single run of data augmentation for this example with $y_1 = 0$, $\mu^{(0)} = 1$ and $\psi^{(0)} = 1$. In the first 100 iterations, the range of the observed values of $\log \psi$ exceeds 35, which means that ψ itself varies over more than 15 orders of magnitude. With more iterations, ψ continues to drift unless the program halts due to numeric overflow or underflow. Whenever ψ wanders close to zero, μ is constrained to be very close to $y_1 = 0$, but when ψ is large μ can become large in either the positive or negative direction. Such highly erratic behavior in time-series plots suggests that one or more components of θ are nearly or entirely inestimable from Y_{obs}.

Warnings about time series and autocorrelation

Time-series plots and autocorrelation are easy to understand and implement, but they are not foolproof. Suppose that for all the

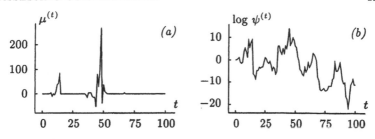

Figure 4.5. *First 100 iterates of (a) μ and (b) log ψ from a single run of data augmentation with a nonexistent posterior.*

scalar summaries of θ we examine, the autocorrelations have effectively died out after lag k. Should we conclude that the algorithm effectively converges to stationarity after k steps? The answer is no, for several reasons. First, zero correlation is not precisely the same as independence, and nonlinear associations may exist beyond lag k. In practice this is probably not a major concern, particularly when the components or functions of θ have been scaled to approximate normality. More importantly, the possibility always exists that the algorithm has not converged with respect to some component or function of θ that we have not examined. For this reason, it is always wise to monitor scalar functions that are suspected to converge slowly, i.e. functions for which the fractions of missing information are thought to be high. Practical suggestions for finding such functions are given in Section 4.4.3.

A final reason why time-series plots and sample ACFs can mislead is that the observed-data posterior distribution may be oddly shaped, and the algorithm may have inadequate opportunity to visit certain regions of the parameter space for reasonable choices of m. For example, if the posterior is multimodal and the modes are separated by regions of low density, an algorithm could 'get stuck' near one of the modes for a large number of iterations. If we had the misfortune of starting near a local mode that was far from the others, we could be misled into thinking that the algorithm had converged when, in fact, it had never left the vicinity of the local mode. Multiple modes and oddly-shaped posteriors are typically associated with datasets that are sparse, i.e. having a small sample size, high rates of missingness, and a large number of parameters to be estimated. In many cases these difficulties can be detected a priori by thoughtful examination of the data and missingness patterns. Multiple modes and high fractions of missing information can also be detected by the behavior of EM (Section 3.3), or by repeated simulation runs from a variety of starting values.

4.4.2 Monitoring convergence with parallel chains

Another group of methods for diagnosing convergence to stationarity involves running multiple independent chains from a common starting value or starting distribution (Tanner and Wong, 1987; Gelfand et al., 1990; Gelman and Rubin, 1992a). Suppose that we choose R starting values of θ from a distribution f_0. If we simulate a single chain of length m from each starting value, then the iterates of θ form an array,

$$\theta^{(1:0)}, \quad \theta^{(1:1)}, \quad \theta^{(1:2)}, \quad \ldots, \quad \theta^{(1:m)},$$
$$\theta^{(2:0)}, \quad \theta^{(2:1)}, \quad \theta^{(2:2)}, \quad \ldots, \quad \theta^{(2:m)},$$
$$\vdots$$
$$\theta^{(R:0)}, \quad \theta^{(R:1)}, \quad \theta^{(R:2)}, \quad \ldots, \quad \theta^{(R:m)},$$

where value t from run r is denoted by $\theta^{(r:t)}$. If f_0 assigns all its mass to a single point, then the starting values $\theta^{(r:0)}$ will be identical; otherwise they may be different. Denote the replicate values of θ at iteration t collectively by

$$\theta^{(*:t)} = \{\theta^{(r:t)} : r = 1, 2, \ldots, R\}.$$

If stationarity has been achieved by step t, then $\theta^{(*:t)}$ will be an iid sample from the target distribution $P(\theta \mid Y_{obs})$. Examination of summaries of $\theta^{(*:t)}$ for $t = 1, 2, \ldots$ thus provide evidence about how rapidly the process converges to stationarity from f_0.

As with previous methods, one needs to decide which summaries of the distribution of θ to monitor at each iteration. Some obvious choices are sample moments, quantiles and density estimates for scalar functions of θ. Note that even when stationarity is achieved, these sample quantities could vary considerably across iterations simply due to the finiteness of R. Unless R is very large we may have difficulty in deciding whether the discrepancy between summaries of $\theta^{(*:t)}$ and $\theta^{(*:t+1)}$ is due to non-stationarity or ordinary sampling fluctuation. It may be possible to reduce the sampling fluctuation in the estimates by Rao-Blackwellization. Suppose that rather than retaining the iterates of θ from the multiple runs, we retain iterates of Y_{mis}. Let

$$Y_{mis}^{(*:t)} = \{Y_{mis}^{(r:t)} : r = 1, 2, \ldots, R\},$$

where $Y_{mis}^{(r:t)}$ denotes the tth value of Y_{mis} from simulation run r. A comparison of Rao-Blackwellized moment or marginal density estimates based on $Y_{mis}^{(*:t)}$ and $Y_{mis}^{(*:t+1)}$ suggests whether convergence has been attained by iteration t. Use of this technique in a univariate normal example is illustrated in Figure 3.2.

Overdispersed starting values

Multiple-chain methods help diagnose how many iterations are required for convergence from a particular starting distribution. This is somewhat different from our working notion of convergence given at the beginning of Section 4.4.1, however, which requires a k large enough so that $\theta^{(t+k)}$ is essentially independent of $\theta^{(t)}$ for any $\theta^{(t)}$ within the region of appreciable posterior density. To check convergence in the latter sense, one would need to try a variety of starting values over the region where $P(\theta \mid Y_{obs})$ is appreciable. In general, one would expect to achieve stationarity more rapidly from a starting value near the center of the posterior (e.g. an MLE or posterior mode) than from a starting value in the tails. For this reason, Gelman and Rubin (1992a) recommend multiple runs from starting values that are overdispersed relative to (i.e. exhibiting greater variability than) the target distribution $P(\theta \mid Y_{obs})$, because this will result in a conservative estimate of the number of iterations needed to achieve stationarity. Moreover, it will greatly reduce our chance of being misled if the posterior is so oddly shaped that single runs tend to get stuck in small regions.

Obtaining starting values that are overdispersed relative to the target distribution $P(\theta \mid Y_{obs})$ may not be a simple matter, because in applications $P(\theta \mid Y_{obs})$ is the intractable distribution that the algorithm is intended to simulate. Gelman and Rubin (1992a) recommend drawing starting values from a multivariate t-distribution with tails heavier than the normal (e.g. a multivariate t with few degrees of freedom) centered at the posterior mode, with covariances determined by the second derivative matrix of the log-posterior at the mode. If multiple modes are found, they recommend using a mixture of multivariate distributions centered at each mode. In practice this method would be tedious to implement for many of the problems in this book, because the observed-data loglikelihoods are often complicated and difficult to differentiate. Numerical estimates of a second-derivative matrix can be obtained with the SEM algorithm (Section 3.3.4), but when the dimension of θ is high this can be computationally prohibitive as well. If the prior distribution being applied to θ is proper, then the prior may serve as a handy source of starting values, particularly if it is easy to simulate. When the prior is improper, however, this will not be possible.

One simple method for obtaining an overdispersed starting distribution that may work well in a variety of problems is *bootstrap resampling* (Efron and Tibshirani, 1993). Suppose that the observed multivariate data matrix Y_{obs} has n rows corresponding to n sample units, some of which have missing values on one or more variables. Let $\hat{\theta} = \hat{\theta}(Y_{obs})$ denote the MLE or posterior mode of θ, which can be found, for example, via the EM algorithm. Suppose that we construct a new observed data matrix Y_{obs}^* by drawing a simple random sample of n^* rows from Y_{obs} with replacement, and calculate $\hat{\theta}^* = \hat{\theta}(Y_{obs}^*)$, e.g. by applying the EM algorithm to Y_{obs}^*. If we take $n^* = n$, then $\hat{\theta}^*$ will be an approximate draw from the sampling distribution of $\hat{\theta}$, and in well-behaved problems for which the observed-data posterior is approximately normal, the distribution of $\hat{\theta}^*$ will not be far from the observed-data posterior. If we use a value of n^* considerably smaller than n, say $n^* = n/2$, then $\hat{\theta}^*$ may tend to be overdispersed relative to $P(\theta \mid Y_{obs})$. Approximating the posterior distribution of a parameter by the sampling distribution of its MLE is not, in general, a practice to be recommended for purposes of inference (e.g. Hill, 1987). For the mere purpose of finding starting values for a Markov chain Monte Carlo algorithm, however, a high degree of accuracy is not required, and boostrap resampling with $n^* < n$ may be perfectly adequate.

4.4.3 Choosing scalar functions of the parameter

The methods we have discussed for diagnosing stationarity pertain to individual components or scalar functions of θ. When the dimension of θ is very high, it may not be feasible to monitor convergence for every component of θ, much less all the functions of θ that seem relevant. If the goal of the analysis is to draw inference about one particular function $\xi = \xi(\theta)$, then we may not need to worry about convergence in the global sense; convergence with respect to the marginal distribution of ξ may be good enough. In the analysis of real datasets, however (and particularly when we are trying to create multiple imputations for a variety of future analyses) it may be difficult to pre-specify all of the functions of θ that are relevant, and achieving stationarity with respect to the entire joint distribution of θ becomes more important.

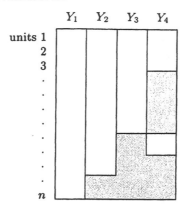

Figure 4.6. *Incomplete multivariate dataset with four variables.*

In high-dimensional situations, we should pay particular attention to components or functions of θ for which convergence is likely to be slow. Because convergence rates are closely related to missing information, it makes sense to focus on aspects of θ for which the fractions of missing information are high. Often some of these functions of θ can be identified a priori by examining the observed data and missingness patterns. For example, an incomplete multivariate dataset with four variables is depicted in Figure 4.6, with shaded areas indicating missing data. Because Y_1 is fully observed and Y_2 is nearly so, we expect the parameters governing the joint distribution of Y_1 and Y_2 to converge rapidly. The parameters governing the marginal distribution of Y_4, however, will probably converge more slowly, as will the parameters describing the relationships of Y_4 to the other variables (e.g. correlations and partial correlations). A high rate of missing observations for a variable does not automatically translate into high rates of missingness for its marginal parameters, because the variable may be highly correlated with other variables that are more fully observed. In practice, however, rates of missing observations are usually suggestive of rates of missing information.

Worst linear function of the parameter

If we could find a scalar function of θ that is 'worst' in the sense that its marginal distribution converges most slowly, then convergence with respect to this function would strengthen the evidence for global convergence. Locating such a function would be difficult,

and in general that function would depend on the starting value
or starting distribution. If we restrict attention to linear functions,
however, functions of the form $v^T\theta$ for some constant vector v, then
a plausible choice for v can often be found from the convergence
behavior of EM. Recall that in the vicinity of the mode the iterations of EM are approximately linear, with rate governed by the
largest eigenvalue of the asymptotic rate matrix (Section 3.3.2).
Suppose that we rotate the axes of the parameter space to form a
new orthogonal coordinate system whose first axis is v_1, the eigenvector of the rate matrix corresponding to this largest eigenvalue.
The first coordinate of a point θ in this new system would then be
proportional to the inner product of v_1 with θ.

From a standpoint of convergence, it makes sense to regard $v_1^T\theta$
as the worst linear function of θ, because among all linear functions
its asymptotic rate of missing information is the highest. Moreover,
use of this function is attractive from a computational standpoint
because a numerical estimate of v_1 is readily obtained from the
trajectory of EM. It follows from (3.23) that near the mode, $\theta^{(t)} -$
$\hat{\theta}$ is approximately proportional to v_1. Therefore, an estimate of
v_1 can be obtained simply by taking the difference between the
convergent value $\hat{\theta}$ and any of the final iterates of EM, e.g. the
estimate of θ one step prior to convergence. The suggested worst
linear function of θ is then

$$\xi(\theta) = \hat{v}_1^T(\theta - \hat{\theta}), \qquad (4.51)$$

where $\hat{v}_1$ is the numerical estimate of v_1. Although it is not necessary to subtract $\hat{\theta}$ from θ in (4.51), it seems useful to do so because
the sign of $\xi(\theta)$ then indicates whether we are positioned to the left
or to the right of the mode with respect to $\hat{v}_1$. We can interpret
$\xi(\theta)$ as a weighted sum of the components of θ, where the weights
are equal to the perturbations from the mode in the final iterations
of EM. Any components with no missing information will drop out
of this sum, because for them EM converges immediately.

Some limited experience with (4.51) in real-data problems suggests that this function is among the slowest to approach stationarity when the observed-data posterior is nearly normal. When the
posterior is very non-normal, however (e.g. if it has multiple modes)
then other functions may converge more slowly. With some oddly-
shaped posteriors, we have found functions other than (4.51) for
which the ACFs take twice as many iterations to die out than for
(4.51). We should be careful, therefore, not to attach undue significance to apparent stationarity for this function, particularly when

some parameters are very poorly estimated. In problems for which the posterior is nearly normal, however, monitoring this function can be very helpful.

Observed-data loglikelihood

Another useful scalar function of θ to monitor is the observed-data loglikelihood function $l(\theta \mid Y_{obs})$, or, for easier interpretation, the likelihood-ratio statistic

$$d_L(\theta) = 2[\, l(\hat{\theta} \mid Y_{obs}) - l(\theta \mid Y_{obs})\,],$$

where $\hat{\theta}$ is the MLE or posterior mode. For large samples, the observed-data posterior distribution of this function tends to be approximately χ^2 with degrees of freedom equal to the dimension of θ. If a single chain is started at the mode, and after a number of iterations the value of this function has not yet risen above the dimension of θ, then there is powerful evidence that stationarity has not yet been achieved. Unless evaluation of the observed-data loglikelihood is computationally burdensome, monitoring the behavior of this statistic is also highly recommended.

4.4.4 Convergence of posterior summaries

Thus far we have discussed methods for diagnosing convergence of the distribution of the iterates of θ to $P(\theta \mid Y_{obs})$. This is the type of convergence necessary for generating proper multiple imputations of Y_{mis}. If the goal is to make direct inferences about functions of θ, however, we need to assess convergence in a different sense; we need to ensure that our Monte Carlo estimates of summaries of the posterior distribution (moments, quantiles, densities, etc.) are sufficiently close to the targets they estimate. More generally, we need methods for measuring the Monte Carlo error in these summaries, and perhaps even adjusting interval estimates and p-values to account for the error.

Methods based on a single chain

Let $\theta^{(1)}, \theta^{(2)}, \ldots, \theta^{(M)}$ denote the output from a single simulation run of length M, possibly after discarding the iterates from an initial burn-in period, and let

$$\bar{\xi} = \frac{1}{M} \sum_{t=1}^{M} \xi^{(t)}$$

denote the sample average of $\xi^{(t)} = \xi(\theta^{(t)})$ for a scalar function ξ. Notice that many of the single-run estimators described in Section 4.2, e.g. marginal moments, cumulative distribution and density estimates, can be written in this form. Rao-Blackwellized estimates can also be written in this form if we let Y_{mis} play the role of θ. Estimating the variance of $\bar{\xi}$ from the sequence $\xi^{(1)}, \xi^{(2)}, \ldots, \xi^{(M)}$ is not a trivial matter, because members of the sequence are correlated; the sample variance of $\xi^{(1)}, \xi^{(2)}, \ldots, \xi^{(M)}$ divided by M may grossly underestimate $V(\bar{\xi})$.

In most cases, a conservative upper bound for $V(\bar{\xi})$ can be estimated by subsampling the chain. Suppose that we average over every bth iterate,

$$\bar{\xi}_{(b)} = \frac{1}{m} \sum_{t=1}^{m} \xi^{(tb)},$$

where $m = M/b$. If $\xi^{(b)}, \xi^{(2b)}, \ldots, \xi^{(mb)}$ are uncorrelated, which can often be ascertained by inspection of the sample ACF, then an unbiased estimate of $V(\bar{\xi}_{(b)})$ is m^{-1} times the sample variance of $\xi^{(b)}, \xi^{(2b)}, \ldots, \xi^{(mb)}$. This estimate is also a crude upper bound for the variance of $\bar{\xi} = \bar{\xi}_{(1)}$, because $V(\bar{\xi}_{(b)})$ generally exceeds $V(\bar{\xi})$.

More efficient techniques are available for obtaining consistent estimates of $V(\bar{\xi})$ based on $\xi^{(1)}, \xi^{(2)}, \ldots, \xi^{(M)}$. Methods involving autocovariance and spectral analysis are described by Geweke (1992) and Geyer (1992), and an overview is also given by Ripley (1987). Care must be taken when applying these variance estimates based on a single chain; although they are theoretically consistent, some of them may grossly underestimate the actual variance in problems for which convergence to stationarity is slow (Raftery and Lewis, 1992a).

Methods based on multiple chains

Simple and reliable estimates of Monte Carlo error can also be obtained through the use of multiple chains (Gelman and Rubin, 1992a). Suppose that we perform R replicate runs from a common starting value or starting distribution, and, perhaps after a burn-in period, obtain a sample of size m from each run. Denote the tth value of θ from the rth run by $\theta^{(r:t)}$. Let $\xi^{(r:t)} = \xi(\theta^{(r:t)})$ be some scalar function,

$$\bar{\xi}^{(r)} = \frac{1}{m} \sum_{t=1}^{m} \xi^{(r:t)}$$

the sample average of ξ within the rth run, and

$$\bar{\xi} = \frac{1}{Rm} \sum_{r=1}^{R} \sum_{t=1}^{m.} \xi^{(r:t)}$$

the pooled average from all runs. Then the between-run variance

$$B = \frac{1}{R-1} \sum_{r=1}^{R} (\bar{\xi}^{(r)} - \bar{\xi})^2$$

unbiasedly estimates the variance of a single $\bar{\xi}^{(r)}$, and B/R estimates the variance of the pooled estimate $\bar{\xi}$. These variances being estimated are conditional upon the starting value or starting distribution. If the starting distribution is equal to $P(\theta \mid Y_{obs})$, or if there is a burn-in period long enough to guarantee stationarity, then B/R will also be an unbiased estimate of the unconditional variance of $\bar{\xi}$. If the burn-in period is not long enough, then B/R will tend to be conservative (i.e. upwardly biased) if the starting values are overdispersed relative to $P(\theta \mid Y_{obs})$, otherwise it could be biased downward. Unless one is relatively certain that stationarity will be achieved by the end of the burn-in period, it would be safer to start the chains from R different, preferably overdispersed starting values than from a single value.

Interval estimation for a scalar summary

Gelman and Rubin (1992a) propose that this estimate of Monte Carlo error be formally incorporated into a Bayesian interval estimate for the unknown $\xi = \xi(\theta)$. Let

$$W = \frac{1}{R(m-1)} \sum_{r=1}^{R} \sum_{t=1}^{m} (\xi^{(r:t)} - \bar{\xi}^{(r)})^2$$

be the average of the R within-run variances. Viewing the data as a balanced one-way layout, the analysis of variance for the random-effects model leads to

$$\hat{\sigma}^2 = \frac{m-1}{m} W + B$$

as an estimate of the posterior variance $V(\xi \mid Y_{obs})$. Unlike the moment estimator (4.5) based on a single run, $\hat{\sigma}^2$ is an unbiased estimate of $V(\xi \mid Y_{obs})$, assuming the burn-in period for each run is sufficient to ensure stationarity. Combining $\hat{\sigma}^2$ with the estimated Monte Carlo error associated with $\bar{\xi}$ leads to the estimated total variance

$$\hat{T} = \hat{\sigma}^2 + B/R,$$

and a $100(1 - \alpha)\%$ posterior interval for ξ is

$$\bar{\xi} \pm t_{\nu,1-\alpha/2}\sqrt{\hat{T}}, \qquad (4.52)$$

where $t_{\nu,p}$ denotes the pth quantile of the t distribution with ν degrees of freedom. The assumption underlying (4.52) is that the posterior distribution of ξ is normal, and the use of a t distribution accounts for the fact that the components of variance are estimated rather than known. Gelman and Rubin (1992a) provide an expression for ν based on an estimated variance of $\hat{T}$, using a method similar to that of Satterthwaite (1946). When m is large enough so that the within-run estimates $\bar{\xi}^{(r)}$ are very close, ν is large and $t_{\nu,1-\alpha/2}$ becomes essentially a normal quantile.

The use of (4.52) for inference has limitations, most notably the assumption of normality of the posterior distribution for ξ. When m is large and the distribution of the iterates appears to be non-normal, it may be more reasonable to combine the runs and base an interval estimate on quantiles of the pooled sample of Rm observations. Whether or not one formally incorporates estimates of Monte Carlo error into the inference, however, the use of multiple runs and evaluation of the between-run variance can be very useful. Note also that multiple runs can be used to estimate the Monte Carlo variance of an estimator that does not have the form of a sample average, e.g. a sample quantile, for which a variance estimate based on a single run would be difficult to derive. Whenever a simulation run is replicated R times, there will automatically be $R-1$ degrees of freedom available for estimating the variance of any statistic calculated from a single run, regardless of its functional form.

4.5 Practical guidelines

Sections 4.2–4.4 may leave the uninitiated reader with a bewildering array of choices and questions regarding almost every aspect of analyzing an incomplete dataset: whether to use parameter simulation or multiple imputation, which convergence diagnostics to monitor, and how to carry out the simulation in an efficient manner while avoiding potential pitfalls. We conclude this chapter with some suggestions on how to choose between methods and implement them in real-data problems.

4.5.1 Choosing a method of inference

In many incomplete-data problems, it will be possible to conduct inference either by (a) calculating appropriate summaries of the iterates of θ, or by (b) generating multiple imputations of Y_{mis} and combining the results of repeated complete-data analyses. A third set of techniques, briefly discussed in Chapter 3, is based on direct evaluation of the observed-data likelihood function, e.g. likelihood-ratio tests (Section 3.2.4). For a single, well defined inferential question, likelihood methods are in principle the most efficient because they do not involve simulation at all. They do require, however (as does multiple imputation), a sample sufficiently large for the usual asymptotic approximations to work well. Moreover, likelihood methods can be somewhat less versatile than simulation in that special computational algorithms may be needed to answer specific questions. Likelihood methods can readily yield a p-value for testing nested hypotheses, when maxima can be found under both the null and alternative hypotheses. In some problems, however, finding the maximum under one or both hypotheses may require a specially designed EM algorithm. Obtaining interval estimates can also be difficult, requiring analytic or numerical differentiation of the loglikelihood. A likelihood-based p-value, when available, is a useful benchmark against which to compare the results of a simulation-based method, and in large-sample problems it may be regarded as the best answer. When the likelihood answer is less reliable or difficult to obtain, however, we will need to depend on parameter simulation or multiple imputation. Below are some important considerations in choosing among the simulation-based methods.

Nature of the inferential question. Is there a well defined parameter or group of parameters of interest, or is the analysis more exploratory in nature? In the latter case, multiple imputation may be best; one good set of, say, $m = 5$ imputations may suffice for a variety of analyses, whereas parameter simulation could require hundreds or thousands of draws per analysis. Care must be taken, however, to ensure that the model used to create the imputations is general enough to encompass all of the analyses being contemplated (Section 4.5.4). Particularly when the dataset is large and simulation runs are expensive, multiple imputation may be the most practical approach, because generating and storing, say, five versions of Y_{mis} will tend to be cheaper than generating and storing a thousand or more iterates of a high-dimensional θ. On the other hand, if interest truly does focus on a single parameter or small group of parameters, then parameter simulation may be quite reasonable, especially in smaller problems for which the simulations run quickly and the relevant summaries of θ are easily stored.

Asymptotic considerations. In multiple imputation, the rules for combining complete-data inferences all assume that the sample is large enough for the usual asymptotic approximations to hold. For smaller samples, when the asymptotic methods break down, simulation-based summaries of the posterior distribution of θ may be preferable, provided that one keeps in mind their Bayesian interpretation and dependence upon a prior.

Rates of missing information. When fractions of missing information are low, methods that average over simulated values of Y_{mis} (i.e. Rao-Blackwellized and multiple-imputation estimates) can be much more efficient than methods that average over simulated values of θ. With low rates of missing information, multiple-imputation estimates based on, say, $m = 5$ imputations may be nearly as precise as averages over hundreds of draws of θ. With high rates of missing information, however, a larger number of imputations may be necessary.

Robustness. With parameter simulation, the form of the parametric complete-data model often plays a crucial role in the inference. If the model's assumptions are seriously violated, then the observed-data likelihood or posterior may be a poor summary of the data's evidence about θ; indeed, if the modeling assumptions do not hold, then the interpretation of θ itself may be questionable. In multiple-imputation inferences, however, the impact of the complete-data model may be less crucial; rather than being applied to the complete data, the model is used only to predict the missing part. Imputations created under a false model may not have a disastrous effect on the final inference, provided that the analyses of the imputed datasets are carried out under more plausible assumptions; this is particularly true when the amounts of missing data are not large. For this reason, in many realistic scenarios multiple imputation may tend to be more robust to departures from the data model than parameter simulation.

4.5.2 Implementing a parameter-simulation experiment

Exploration. The best way to avoid pitfalls is to gain some basic understanding of the problem at the outset. How much information is missing? Do the observed-data likelihood and posterior seem well behaved, or are they oddly shaped with multiple modes, ridges, or suprema on the boundary? Sometimes these questions can be nearly answered through previous experience with similar datasets, and through prior examination of the observed data and patterns of missingness. The EM algorithm can also be an excellent diagnostic tool. Running EM from a variety of starting values and evaluating the loglikelihood function or log-posterior density at the stationary points can reveal multiple modes, ridges and boundary suprema. The iterations of EM give quick estimates of the largest rates of missing information and the worst linear functions of θ. If the highest rates of missing information are extremely high, say 90% or more, we should expect a data augmentation algorithm to converge very slowly. If the rates are high, say 50–80%, convergence may not be too difficult to attain, but we should remember that inferences about certain aspects of θ may rely heavily upon unverifiable assumptions about the missingness mechanism (see Section 3.3.4). If the likelihood and posterior seem well behaved and rates of missing information are moderate, say 40% or less, we may expect the simulations to proceed without much difficulty.

Preliminary runs. Preliminary simulation runs are necessary to give us an idea of how many iterations are needed to achieve stationarity. In these runs, important functions of θ should be saved and plotted. Unfortunately, the single-chain diagnostic methods of Section 4.4.1 tend to work best when they are actually needed the least, when algorithms converge reliably and rapidly from any reasonable starting value. Performing a variety of exploratory runs from different starting values, preferably overdispersed relative to $P(\theta \mid Y_{obs})$, is highly recommended to avoid the pitfalls associated with oddly shaped posteriors. Time-series plots that overlay the output of multiple runs on the same set of axes are useful; they help us to identify pathological situations in which the algorithm appears to 'converge' quickly from each starting value, but the convergence is illusory because the iterates from the different runs do not overlap.

Single versus multiple chains. Whether the simulation should be carried out using a single chain or multiple chains has been the subject of lively debate in the Markov chain Monte Carlo literature (Gelman and Rubin, 1992a; Geyer, 1992; Raftery and Lewis, 1992b; Smith and Roberts, 1993). Given that Rm iterations are to be performed, is it better to use a single run of length Rm, or R

parallel runs of length m? If the cost of the two methods is the same, then the single-chain method may be somewhat more precise for estimating a single quantity such as posterior mean, because fewer burn-in iterations will be discarded. On the other hand, the cost of the two methods may not be the same; multiple chains might be convenient and perhaps even less expensive if multiple computers or parallel processing are available. If we are confident that the algorithm converges reliably and in a reasonable amount of time from a particular starting value (e.g. a mode), then running a single chain from this starting value is not a bad strategy. Such confidence, however, can probably be gained only through multiple runs from a variety of starting values at the preliminary stage. Moreover, the use of multiple chains is arguably the simplest and most reliable way to assess the Monte Carlo error of an estimate.

The importance of reproducibility. When analyzing data by simulation, one must recognize that a simulation is an *experiment* and should be conducted according to well accepted practices of scientific inquiry. Before considering a result to be reliable, we should have confidence that another knowledgeable analyst, carrying out an independent analysis with the same data and the same model, would be led to essentially the same conclusions. Short of finding another analyst to reproduce the results, the best way to gain such confidence is through replication. Before completely trusting the results from a single run, we should, if at all possible, try to verify them by repeating the experiment with a new random number generator seed and a new starting value of θ.

4.5.3 Generating multiple imputations

If the immediate goal of the simulation is to create proper multiple imputations of Y_{mis}, then the comments above regarding exploration of the observed-data likelihood or posterior, preliminary runs and convergence diagnostics still apply. If the imputations are to be used in a wide variety of analyses, we should strive for global convergence to the joint posterior distribution of θ, rather than convergence of the marginal distributions of scalar functions of θ, because we may not know which functions of θ will be the subject of future analyses. In preliminary runs, we should pay close attention to those functions for which the rates of missing information are high. In judging how many iterations are needed to achieve approximate global stationarity, we should choose a number k large enough that the ACFs of the worst functions of θ are effectively zero by lag k, and perhaps even double or triple that number, if possible, to provide an extra margin of safety.

Once we have decided on the number of iterations k needed for stationarity, we can proceed to generate the m multiple imputations. One way to do this is to run a single chain for mk iterations, taking every kth iterate of Y_{mis}. With a single chain, there is a danger in choosing a value of k that is too small; the multiple imputations could be correlated and understate the missing-data uncertainty. This danger can be avoided by running m parallel chains of length k from overdispersed starting values, and taking the final value of Y_{mis} from each chain. If the starting values are truly overdispersed, then choosing k too small will overstate the missing-data uncertainty and cause inferences to be conservative. If overdispersed starting values are difficult to obtain, then running a single chain of length mk, or m parallel chains of length k emanating from a common starting value (e.g. a mode), are acceptable provided that we are relatively certain that the choice of k is large enough.

4.5.4 Choosing an imputation model

Inference by multiple imputation proceeds in two distinct phases: first, the missing data are filled in m times; second, the m versions of the complete data are analyzed and the results are combined into a single inferential statement. These two phases may be carried out on different occasions and even by different persons. This temporal separation of the phases is one of the most important advantages of multiple-imputation inference, because the missing-data aspects of the problem are confined entirely to the first phase; after imputation, no special incomplete-data techniques are needed to complete the second phase. Consequently, one good set of m imputations can effectively solve the missing-data problems for a large number of future analyses. Multiple imputation is especially attractive for large datasets (e.g. public-use files from censuses or sample surveys) that will be analyzed in a variety of ways by a variety of people, many of whom may not have the technical knowledge or resources needed to analyze the incomplete version of the data. Multiple imputations can be created by a person or organization having special expertise in missing-data techniques; in many cases, the imputer will have detailed knowledge or even additional data that cannot be made available to the analysts but which may be relevant to the prediction of Y_{mis} (Rubin, 1987).

Because the imputation and analysis phases are distinct, it is natural to ask whether multiple imputation leads to valid inferences when the imputer's model and the analyst's model differ. The rules for combining complete-data inferences were derived under some implicit assumptions of agreement between the two models. For example, the validity of (4.32)–(4.33) requires that the imputation and analysis phases condition on the same set of observed data Y_{obs}. If the imputed datasets are distributed to a variety of users, however, it is possible or even likely that inconsistencies will arise between the imputer's and analyst's models. The validity of multiple-imputation inferences when the imputer's and analyst's models differ has been the subject of recent controversy (Fay, 1992; Kott, 1992; Meng, 1995; Rubin, 1996). A basic understanding of the implications of discrepant models is important, even for the imputer who produces imputations solely for personal use, because discrepancies are common and can impact the multiple-imputation inferences either positively or negatively. We now discuss in broad terms some types of discrepancies and their potential impact on multiple-imputation inferences.

When the analyst assumes more than the imputer

One possible inconsistency is that the analyst's and imputer's models differ, but that the analyst's model can be regarded as a special case of the imputer's. For example, suppose that a dataset contains three variables, Y_1, Y_2 and Y_3, that only Y_3 has missing values and that proper multiple imputations are simulated under a linear regression of Y_3 on Y_1 and Y_2,

$$Y_3 = \beta_0 + \beta_1 Y_1 + \beta_2 Y_2 + \varepsilon, \qquad (4.53)$$

where the error ε is normally distributed. Furthermore, suppose that the analyst subsequently models Y_3 as a linear regression given only Y_1, omitting Y_2 from the model. The analyst's model is then a special case of the imputer's with $\beta_2 = 0$.

The practical implication of the discrepancy depends on whether the analyst's extra assumption is true. Note that $\beta_2 = 0$ being true does not invalidate the imputer's model at all; (4.53) still applies. Therefore, inferences derived from multiple imputation will be valid, although probably somewhat conservative, because the imputations will reflect an extra degree of uncertainty due to the fact that the imputer's procedure estimates β_2 rather than setting it to zero. For example, predictions for future observations of Y_3 at specified values of Y_1 will be unbiased, but interval estimates will be somewhat wider than they would have been if the imputer had assumed $\beta_2 = 0$.

On the other hand, suppose that in reality β_2 is not zero. The predictions of Y_3 given by the analyst's model will then be biased. This bias, however, will be the fault of the analyst rather than the imputer. In this case there is nothing wrong with the imputed datasets, and an analysis under an appropriate model will lead to appropriate conclusions. Biases and inappropriate conclusions that arise because an analyst uses an inappropriate model should not be regarded as a shortcoming of the imputation method, just as inappropriate analyses of a complete dataset are not the fault of the data collector.

When the imputer assumes more than the analyst

Another type of inconsistency arises when the analyst's model is more general than the imputer's; that is, the imputer applies assumptions to the complete data that the analyst does not. Once again, the practical implications of this inconsistency will depend on whether the extra assumptions are true, so we consider the two possibilities in turn.

The case where the imputer's additional assumptions are true has investigated by Fay (1992), Meng (1995) and Rubin (1996). Fay (1992) shows by example that when $m = \infty$, the total variance T for a scalar estimand Q given by (4.24) may be larger than the variance of $\bar{Q}$ over repeated realizations of the sampling and imputation procedure. This does not, however, invalidate the method for combining complete-data inferences about Q described in Section 4.3.2. In fact, as demonstrated by Meng (1995) and Rubin (1996), the point estimate $\bar{Q}$ is more efficient than an observed-data estimate derived purely from the analyst's model, because it incorporates the imputer's superior knowledge about the state of nature, a property that Rubin (1996) calls *superefficiency*. Moreover, the multiple-imputation interval estimate (4.27) has an average width that is shorter than a confidence interval derived purely from the observed data and the analyst's model, even though it is conservative, having frequency coverage greater than the nominal $100(1 - \alpha)\%$. Meng (1995) demonstrates that under fairly general conditions, the addition of true prior information to an imputation model can only increase the efficiency of $\bar{Q}$ while, at the same time, decrease the width and increase the coverage of the multiple-imputation interval estimate. Thus there is no real sense in which an imputer's superior knowledge can invalidate the inference; on the contrary, additional information can only help.

Reversing the three-variable example used above, suppose that the imputer creates imputations for Y_3 under the reduced model

$$Y_3 = \beta_0 + \beta_1 Y_1 + \varepsilon, \tag{4.54}$$

which we assume to be true, but the analyst fits the more general model (4.53). Under ignorability, the analyst can obtain valid inferences without imputation by basing the regression analysis only on those units for which Y_3 is observed. Alternatively, he or she can also perform a multiple-imputation analysis using the imputations created under (4.54). If the imputation model is true, the latter approach will be superior to the former, because it will provide point and interval estimates for β_2 that are more tightly concentrated around the true value of zero; the extra information conveyed in the imputations results in a more efficient procedure than one based on the observed data alone.

Now consider the situation where the imputer assumes more than the analyst, but the additional assumptions are false. Clearly, in this case multiple-imputation inferences can be erroneous. In the regression example, imputations created under the mistaken assumption that $\beta_2 = 0$ will bias the analyst's estimates of β_2 toward zero. Multiple imputations created under an erroneous model can lead to erroneous conclusions, just as a faulty model for complete data can lead to faulty conclusions when no data are missing.

Sometimes the nature of the analysis and the pattern of missing values force the imputer to make certain assumptions that the analyst apparently does not need to make. For example, consider a regression analysis with predictor variables that are partially missing. In order to impute the missing values, the imputer must posit a joint distribution for all variables in the dataset, including the predictors. The analyst, however, makes no distributional assumptions about the predictors in the completed datasets, and specifies only the conditional distribution of the response given the predictors. At first glance, it appears that a discrepancy exists between the imputer's and analyst's models, with the imputer's model being the more restrictive of the two. This discrepancy is illusory, however, because if the analyst had been given only Y_{obs} then he or she could not proceed to make an efficient inference without imposing some kind of similar distributional assumptions on the predictors. In situations of this type, the additional assumptions used by the imputer should not be viewed in a negative light, because the same kind of restrictions would have to be imposed by an analyst who did not have access to the imputed values.

4.5.5 Further comments on imputation modeling

From the above discussion, we see that the major danger of inconsistency between the imputer's and analyst's models arises when the imputer makes poorly grounded assumptions but the analyst does not. For this reason, it is important that the imputation model does not impose restrictions on unknown parameters that will later be the subject of the analyst's inquiry. For example, if the analyst is going to investigate the correlation between two variables Y_1 and Y_2, then both variables need to be present in the multivariate imputation model even if only one of them has missing values, and the correlation between them should be left unspecified. Design variables (see Section 2.6.2) should be included in the imputation model if at all possible. To produce high-quality imputations for a particular variable Y_1, the imputation model should include variables that are (a) potentially related to Y_1, and (b) potentially related to missingness of Y_1. A general guideline is that the imputer should use a model that is general enough to preserve any associations among variables (two-, three-, or even higher-way associations) that may be the target of subsequent analyses.

Balanced against the theoretical advantages of a large, general imputation model are practical limitations in computing resources, or inherent limitations of the observed data Y_{obs}, which may prevent us from using an imputation model as general as we would like. As the number of variables and parameters grows, we may find that the ideal model may be too large to implement in the available computing environment. Moreover, we may find that the model has more parameters than can be estimated from Y_{obs}, particularly when the prior distribution is diffuse; we may not be able to use the model without an informative prior. When the imputer is producing imputations purely for personal use, he or she may be able to tailor an imputation model for the intended analyses. An organization that must impute a large public-use data file, however, must try to anticipate the analyses of many future data users and build the imputation model accordingly. In some cases compromises will have to be made: the imputer may have to sacrifice some of the imputation model's generality to stay within the constraints of what the computing environment and the observed data can support. Construction of imputation models that are appropriate for specific analyses will be illustrated by the real-data examples of Chapters 5–9. Further discussion of practical considerations in choosing an imputation model for a large multipurpose database is given by Schafer, Khare and Ezzati-Rice (1993).

Robustness

It is important to remember that failure of an imputation model does not damage the integrity of the entire dataset, but only the portion that is imputed. Unless large amounts of data are imputed, biases introduced by an inappropriate imputation method may not be disastrous because they can be mitigated by the non-imputed data. In contrast, however, inferences by methods that do not separate the imputation phase from the analysis phase (e.g. methods of parameter simulation described in Section 4.2) will suffer more greatly under model failure, because the erroneous modeling assumptions will then be applied to the entire dataset rather than just the missing part. Once a missing-data problem is solved through imputation, an analyst tends to have greater freedom to investigate alternative models than would otherwise be possible if he or she had access to the observed data alone.

Analyses not based on full parametric models

The basic methods of multiple-imputation inference (Section 4.3) were derived under the assumption that the complete-data estimators $\hat{Q}$ and U are first-order approximations to the posterior mean and variance, respectively, of the estimand Q. Some methods of statistical inference, however, are not readily interpretable as approximate Bayesian procedures under any known parametric model. Examples of this include: nonparametric methods such as those based on ranks or permutation distributions; some of the classical design-based estimators for complex sample surveys, and their associated variance estimates calculated by methods such as the jackknife and balanced repeated replication (Wolter, 1985); and estimates and standard errors from generalized linear models based on quasilikelihood (McCullagh and Nelder, 1989). Is it acceptable to use multiple imputation in the context of any of these procedures? A partial answer is provided by Rubin (1987, pp. 118–199), who states conditions under which a multiple-imputation procedure will yield inferences with frequentist validity without reference to any specific parametric model. Multiple imputations that possess this property are said to be *proper*.

Rubin's definition of proper basically means that the summary statistics $\bar{Q}$, $\bar{U}$ and B, defined in (4.21)–(4.23), yield approximately valid inferences for the complete-data statistics $\hat{Q}$ and U over repeated realizations of the missing-data mechanism. The three conditions necessary for imputations to be proper are:

1. As the number of imputations becomes large, $(\bar{Q} - \hat{Q})/\sqrt{B}$ should become approximately $N(0,1)$ over the distribution of the response indicators R with Y held fixed.

2. As the number of imputations becomes large, $\bar{U}$ should be a consistent estimate of U, with R regarded as random and Y regarded as fixed.

3. The true between-imputation variance (i.e. the variance of $\bar{Q}$ over an infinite number of multiple imputations) should be stable over repeated samples of the complete data Y, with variability of a lower order than that of $\hat{Q}$.

Rubin (1987) shows that if (a) the complete-data inference based on $\hat{Q}$ and U is valid over repeated samples, and (b) the imputation method is proper, then the multiple imputation will yield inferences that are valid from a purely frequentist standpoint.

Except in trivial cases (e.g. univariate data missing completely at random), it can be extremely difficult to determine whether a multiple-imputation method is proper according to this definition. The most elaborate examples to date are given by Binder and Sun (1996). These lend important insights into the behavior of multiple imputation in inferential settings that are nonparametric and non-Bayesian. For the complicated multivariate situations described in this book, however, we have little hope of analytically demonstrating that Bayesian, model-based imputation methods are proper. From a practical standpoint, knowing whether an imputation method is technically proper for a particular analysis is less important than knowing whether it actually behaves well or poorly over repeated samples. The latter question can be addressed through simulation studies with realistic complete-data populations and realistic response mechanisms. Examples of simulation studies will be given in Sections 6.4 and 9.5.3.

CHAPTER 5

Methods for normal data

5.1 Introduction

The most common probability model for continuous multivariate data is the multivariate normal distribution. Many standard methods for analyzing multivariate data, including factor analysis, principal components and discriminant analysis, are based upon an assumption of multivariate normality. Moreover, the classical techniques of linear regression and analysis of variance assume conditional normality of the response variables given linear functions of the predictors, which is the conditional distribution implied by a multivariate normal model for all the variables. Because statistical methods motivated by assumptions of normality are in such widespread use, it is natural to seek general techniques for inference from incomplete normal data.

Datasets encountered in the real world often deviate from multivariate normality, but in many cases the normal model will be useful even when the actual data are nonnormal. There are several important reasons for this. First, one can often make the normality assumption more tenable by applying suitable transformations to one or more of the variables. Second, if some variables in a dataset are clearly nonnormal (e.g. discrete) but are completely observed, then the multivariate normal model may still be used for inference provided that (a) it is plausible to model the incomplete variables as conditionally normal given a linear function of the complete ones, and (b) the parameters of inferential interest pertain only to this conditional distribution (Section 2.6.2).

Finally, even if some of the incompletely observed variables are clearly nonnormal, it may still be reasonable to use the normal model as a convenient device for creating multiple imputations. As pointed out in Section 4.5.4, inference by multiple imputation may be robust to departures from the imputation model if the amounts of missing information are not large, because the imputation model is effectively applied not to the entire dataset but only to its missing part. For example, it may be quite reasonable to use a normal model to impute a variable that is ordinal (consisting of a small number of ordered categories), provided that the amount of missing data is not extensive and the marginal distribution is not too far from being unimodal and symmetric. When using the normal model to impute categorical data, however, the continuous imputes should be rounded off to the nearest category to preserve the distributional properties as fully as possible and to make them intelligible to the analyst. We have found that the normal model, when used in this fashion, can be an effective tool for imputing ordinal and even binary data in instances where constructing a more elaborate categorical-data model would be impractical (Schafer, Khare and Ezzati-Rice, 1993).

5.2 Relevant properties of the complete-data model

5.2.1 Basic notation

We begin by establishing some notational conventions that will be used throughout the chapter. The dataset, as depicted in Figure 2.1, is assumed to be a matrix of n rows and p columns, with rows corresponding to observational units and columns corresponding to variables. Denote the complete data by $Y = (Y_{obs}, Y_{mis})$, where Y_{obs} and Y_{mis} are the observed and missing portions of the matrix, respectively. Let y_{ij} denote an individual element of Y, $i = 1, 2, \ldots, n$, $j = 1, 2, \ldots, p$. The ith row of Y, expressed as a column vector (all vectors will be regarded as column vectors), is

$$y_i = (y_{i1}, y_{i2}, \ldots, y_{ip})^T.$$

We assume that $y_1, y_2, \ldots, y_n$ are independent realizations of a random vector, denoted symbolically as $(Y_1, Y_2, \ldots, Y_p)^T$, which has a multivariate normal distribution with mean vector μ and covariance matrix Σ; that is,

$$y_1, y_2, \ldots, y_n \mid \theta \sim \text{iid } N(\mu, \Sigma),$$

where $\theta = (\mu, \Sigma)$ is the unknown parameter. Throughout the chapter, we assume no prior restrictions on θ other than the positive definiteness of Σ ($\Sigma > 0$); that is, we allow θ to lie anywhere within its natural parameter space. Because the density of a single row is

$$P(y_i \mid \theta) = |2\pi\Sigma|^{-\frac{1}{2}} \exp\left\{ -\tfrac{1}{2}(y_i - \mu)^T \Sigma^{-1}(y_i - \mu) \right\},$$

the complete-data likelihood is, discarding a proportionality constant,

$$L(\theta|Y) \propto |\Sigma|^{-\frac{n}{2}} \exp\left\{-\frac{1}{2}\sum_{i=1}^{n}(y_i - \mu)^T \Sigma^{-1}(y_i - \mu)\right\}. \quad (5.1)$$

Maximum-likelihood estimates

By expanding the exponent in (5.1) and using the fact that

$$\begin{aligned} y_i^T \Sigma^{-1} y_i &= \operatorname{tr} y_i^T \Sigma^{-1} y_i \\ &= \operatorname{tr} \Sigma^{-1} y_i y_i^T, \end{aligned}$$

it follows that the complete-data loglikelihood can be written as

$$\begin{aligned} l(\theta|Y) = {}&-\tfrac{n}{2}\log |\Sigma| - \tfrac{n}{2}\mu^T \Sigma^{-1}\mu \\ &+ \mu^T \Sigma^{-1} T_1 - \tfrac{1}{2}\operatorname{tr} \Sigma^{-1} T_2, \end{aligned} \quad (5.2)$$

where

$$T_1 = \sum_{i=1}^{n} y_i = Y^T \mathbf{1}, \quad (5.3)$$

$$T_2 = \sum_{i=1}^{n} y_i y_i^T = Y^T Y \quad (5.4)$$

are the complete-data sufficient statistics, and $\mathbf{1} = (1, 1, \ldots, 1)^T$. Note that T_1 is the vector of column sums,

$$T_1 = \left(\ \textstyle\sum_{i=1}^{n} y_{i1}, \quad \sum_{i=1}^{n} y_{i2}, \quad \ldots, \quad \sum_{i=1}^{n} y_{ip}\ \right)^T,$$

and T_2 is the matrix of columnwise sums of squares and cross-products,

$$T_2 = \begin{bmatrix} \sum_{i=1}^{n} y_{i1}^2 & \sum_{i=1}^{n} y_{i1}y_{i2} & \cdots & \sum_{i=1}^{n} y_{i1}y_{ip} \\ \sum_{i=1}^{n} y_{i2}y_{i1} & \sum_{i=1}^{n} y_{i2}^2 & \cdots & \sum_{i=1}^{n} y_{i2}y_{ip} \\ \vdots & \vdots & & \vdots \\ \sum_{i=1}^{n} y_{ip}y_{i1} & \sum_{i=1}^{n} y_{ip}y_{i2} & \cdots & \sum_{i=1}^{n} y_{ip}^2 \end{bmatrix}.$$

Because the multivariate normal is a regular exponential family and the loglikelihood is linear in the elements of T_1 and T_2, we can maximize the likelihood by equating the realized values of T_1 and T_2 with their expectations, $E(T_1) = n\mu$ and $E(T_2) = n(\Sigma + \mu\mu^T)$. This leads immediately to the well known result that the MLEs for

μ and Σ are the sample mean vector

$$\bar{y} = n^{-1} \sum_{i=1}^{n} y_i, \qquad (5.5)$$

and the sample covariance matrix

$$\begin{aligned} S &= n^{-1} Y^T Y - \bar{y}\bar{y}^T \\ &= n^{-1} \sum_{i=1}^{n} (y_i - \bar{y})(y_i - \bar{y})^T, \qquad (5.6) \end{aligned}$$

respectively. Note that S is a biased estimate of Σ, and in practice it is more common to use the unbiased version $n(n-1)^{-1}S$. Further details on estimation and frequentist inference for the multivariate normal model can be found in standard texts on multivariate analysis (e.g. Anderson, 1984).

5.2.2 Bayesian inference under a conjugate prior

The simplest way to conduct Bayesian inference in the complete-data case is to apply a parametric family or class of prior distributions that is *conjugate* to the likelihood function (5.1). A conjugate class has the property that any prior $\pi(\theta)$ in the class leads to a posterior $P(\theta \mid Y) \propto \pi(\theta) L(\theta \mid Y)$ that is also in the class. When both μ and Σ are unknown, the most natural conjugate class for the multivariate normal data model is the normal inverted-Wishart family.

The inverted-Wishart distribution

If X is an $m \times p$ data matrix whose rows are iid $N(0, \Lambda)$, then the matrix of sums of squares and cross-products $A = X^T X$ is said to have a Wishart distribution, and we write

$$A \sim W(m, \Lambda). \qquad (5.7)$$

The parameters m and Λ are often called the *degrees of freedom* and *scale*, respectively. The dimension of A ($p \times p$) is not explicitly reflected in the notation (5.7) because it is conveyed by the dimension of Λ.

The Wishart distribution arises in frequentist theory as the sampling distribution of S. For our purposes it will be more convenient to work with the inverted-Wishart distribution. If $A \sim W(m, \Lambda)$

then $B = A^{-1}$ is said to be inverted-Wishart, and we write

$$B \sim W^{-1}(m, \Lambda).$$

Omitting normalizing constants, the inverted-Wishart density for $m \geq p$ can be shown to be

$$P(B|m, \Lambda) \propto |B|^{-\left(\frac{m+p+1}{2}\right)} \exp\left\{ -\tfrac{1}{2} \operatorname{tr}\Lambda^{-1}B^{-1} \right\} \qquad (5.8)$$

over the region where $B > 0$. For $m < p$, the matrix A is singular and $B = A^{-1}$ does not exist. Notice that (5.8) is a proper density function for any choice of $m \geq p$ and $\Lambda > 0$; we need not restrict ourselves to integer values of m. The mean of the inverted-Wishart distribution is

$$E(B|m, \Lambda) = \frac{1}{m - p - 1} \Lambda^{-1} \qquad (5.9)$$

provided that $m \geq p+2$. In the special case of $p = 1$, the inverted-Wishart reduces to a scaled inverted-chisquare, $c\chi_m^{-2}$, with $c = \Lambda^{-1}$. These and other well-known properties of the Wishart and inverted-Wishart distributions are discussed in many texts on multivariate analysis; an excellent reference is Muirhead (1982).

For our purposes, it will also be useful to know that the mode of the inverted-Wishart density is

$$\operatorname{mode}(B|m, \Lambda) = \frac{1}{m + p + 1} \Lambda^{-1}. \qquad (5.10)$$

Demonstrating this fact involves maximizing the logarithm of (5.8), an exercise which is nearly identical to deriving the ML estimates for the multivariate normal distribution by maximizing the loglikelihood (5.2). We omit details of this calculation, but for a thorough demonstration in the case of the loglikelihood the interested reader may refer to Mardia, Kent and Bibby (1979, pp. 103–105).

The normal inverted-Wishart prior and posterior

Returning to the problem of Bayesian inference for $\theta = (\mu, \Sigma)$ under a multivariate normal model, let us apply the following prior distribution. Suppose that, given Σ, μ is assumed to be conditionally multivariate normal,

$$\mu \,|\, \Sigma \sim N(\mu_0, \tau^{-1}\Sigma), \qquad (5.11)$$

where the hyperparameters $\mu_0 \in \mathcal{R}^p$ and $\tau > 0$ are fixed and known. Moreover, suppose that Σ is inverted-Wishart,

$$\Sigma \sim W^{-1}(m, \Lambda) \qquad (5.12)$$

for fixed hyperparameters $m \geq p$ and $\Lambda > 0$. The prior density for θ is then

$$\pi(\theta) \propto |\Sigma|^{-\left(\frac{m+p+2}{2}\right)} \exp\left\{ -\tfrac{1}{2}\operatorname{tr}\Lambda^{-1}\Sigma^{-1}\right\}$$

$$\times \exp\left\{ -\tfrac{\tau}{2}(\mu - \mu_0)^T \Sigma^{-1}(\mu - \mu_0)\right\}. \qquad (5.13)$$

Following some matrix algebra, the complete-data likelihood function (5.1) can be rewritten as

$$L(\theta|Y) \propto |\Sigma|^{-\frac{n}{2}} \exp\left\{ -\tfrac{n}{2}\operatorname{tr}\Sigma^{-1}S\right\}$$

$$\times \exp\left\{ -\tfrac{n}{2}(\bar{y} - \mu)^T \Sigma^{-1}(\bar{y} - \mu)\right\}. \qquad (5.14)$$

Multiplying this likelihood by (5.13) and performing some algebraic manipulation, it follows that $P(\theta|Y)$ has the same form as (5.13) but with new values for $(\tau, m, \mu_0, \Lambda)$; that is, the complete-data posterior is normal inverted-Wishart,

$$\mu \mid \Sigma, Y \sim N(\mu_0', (\tau')^{-1}\Sigma), \qquad (5.15)$$

$$\Sigma \mid Y \sim W^{-1}(m', \Lambda'), \qquad (5.16)$$

where the updated hyperparameters are

$$\tau' = \tau + n,$$

$$m' = m + n,$$

$$\mu_0' = \left(\frac{n}{\tau + n}\right)\bar{y} + \left(\frac{\tau}{\tau + n}\right)\mu_0,$$

and

$$\Lambda' = \left[\Lambda^{-1} + nS + \left(\frac{\tau n}{\tau + n}\right)(\bar{y} - \mu_0)(\bar{y} - \mu_0)^T\right]^{-1}.$$

In the special case of $p = 1$, the posterior becomes

$$\mu \mid \Sigma, Y \sim N(\mu_0', (\tau')^{-1}\Sigma),$$

$$\Sigma \mid Y \sim c'\chi_{m'}^{-2},$$

where

$$c' = c + \sum_{i=1}^n (y_i - \bar{y})^2 + \left(\frac{\tau n}{\tau + n}\right)(\bar{y} - \mu_0)^2$$

and $c = \Lambda^{-1}$ is the prior scale for Σ.

Existence of the prior distribution requires $\tau > 0$, $m \geq p$ and $\Lambda > 0$. Notice, however, that we may apply the updating formulas and still obtain acceptable values of τ', m', and Λ' for certain

$\tau \leq 0$ and $m < p$. Under ordinary circumstances it would not make sense to use a negative value for τ, because μ_0' would then become a weighted average of $\bar{y}$ and μ_0 with negative weight for μ_0. Taking $\tau = 0$, however, may be quite sensible when little or no prior information about μ is available, because it results in a posterior distribution for μ centered about $\bar{y}$. Moreover, in some cases a choice of $m < p$ may be attractive as well: see Section 5.2.3 below.

Inferences about the mean vector

By integrating the normal inverted-Wishart density function (5.13) over Σ, one can show that the marginal prior distribution of μ implied by (5.11)–(5.12) is a multivariate t distribution centered at μ_0 with $\nu = m - p + 1$ degrees of freedom. The mean of this distribution is μ_0 provided that $\nu > 1$, and the covariance matrix is $(\nu - 2)^{-1}\tau^{-1}\Lambda^{-1}$ provided that $\nu > 2$. Other properties of this multivariate t distribution are discussed in many texts on multivariate analysis; a good reference is Press (1982). In particular, the marginal prior distribution of any scalar component or linear function of the components of μ is univariate t. Suppose that $\xi = a^T\mu$, where a is a constant vector of length p. The marginal prior distribution of ξ implied by (5.11)–(5.12) is then $(\xi - \xi_0)/\sigma \sim t_\nu$ where $\nu = m - p + 1$, $\xi_0 = a^T\mu_0$, and

$$\sigma = \sqrt{\frac{a^T\Lambda^{-1}a}{\tau\nu}}.$$

The marginal prior density is

$$P(\xi) = \frac{\Gamma\left(\frac{\nu+1}{2}\right)}{\Gamma\left(\frac{\nu}{2}\right)\sqrt{\pi\nu\sigma^2}}\left[1 + \frac{(\xi - \xi_0)^2}{\nu\sigma^2}\right]^{-(\nu+1)/2}, \qquad (5.17)$$

where $\Gamma(\cdot)$ denotes the gamma function. After observing Y we can obtain $P(\xi|Y)$, the marginal posterior distribution of ξ, simply by replacing the hyperparameters $(\tau, m, \mu_0, \Lambda)$ in the above expressions with their updated values $(\tau', m', \mu_0', \Lambda')$.

Inferences about the covariance matrix

In many problems the parameters of interest are functions of μ, and Σ is best regarded as a nuisance parameter. On occasion, however, an estimate of Σ is needed. From a Bayesian standpoint there is no universally accepted 'best' estimate of Σ. The optimal estimate depends on the choice of a loss function, and in practice it tends to be difficult or impossible to choose among the various loss functions. Bayesian estimation of a covariance matrix raises some interesting theoretical problems that have yet to be resolved (Dempster, 1969a). If the current state of knowledge about Σ is described by $\Sigma \sim W^{-1}(m, \Lambda)$, then competing estimates include the mean (5.9) and the mode (5.10). To complicate matters further, suppose that the mean μ and the covariance matrix Σ are both of interest, and the current state of knowledge about $\theta = (\mu, \Sigma)$ is represented by the normal inverted-Wishart distribution

$$\mu \mid \Sigma \sim N(\mu_0, \tau^{-1}\Sigma),$$
$$\Sigma \sim W^{-1}(m, \Lambda).$$

By a calculation that is essentially equivalent to maximizing the multivariate-normal loglikelihood function, one can then show that the joint mode is achieved at $\mu = \mu_0$ and

$$\Sigma = \frac{1}{m + p + 2} \Lambda^{-1}.$$

Note that maximizing the joint density for μ and Σ is not equivalent to maximizing the marginal densities for μ and Σ separately.

When a Bayesian estimate of Σ is needed, we will adopt the following rule-of-thumb: if the current state of knowledge about Σ is described by $\Sigma \sim W^{-1}(m, \Lambda)$ irrespective of μ, then estimate Σ by $m^{-1}\Lambda^{-1}$. This represents a compromise between the mean (5.9) and the marginal mode (5.10).

5.2.3 Choosing the prior hyperparameters

A noninformative prior

When no strong prior information is available about θ, it is customary to apply Bayes's theorem with the improper prior

$$\pi(\theta) \propto |\Sigma|^{-\left(\frac{p+1}{2}\right)}, \tag{5.18}$$

which is the limiting form of the normal inverted-Wishart density (5.11)–(5.12) as $\tau \to 0$, $m \to -1$ and $\Lambda^{-1} \to 0$. Notice that μ does not appear on the right-hand side of (5.18); the prior 'distribution' of μ is assumed to be uniform over the p-dimensional real space. Under this improper prior, the complete-data posterior becomes

$$\mu \mid \Sigma, Y \sim N(\bar{y}, n^{-1}\Sigma), \tag{5.19}$$
$$\Sigma \mid Y \sim W^{-1}(n-1, (nS)^{-1}). \tag{5.20}$$

A non-Bayesian justification for the use of this prior is that the posterior distribution of the pivotal quantity

$$T^2 = (n-1)(\bar{y} - \mu)^T S^{-1}(\bar{y} - \mu)$$

becomes $(n-1)p(n-p)^{-1}F_{p,n-p}$, the same as its sampling distribution conditionally upon θ (DeGroot, 1970). The ellipsoidal $(1-\alpha)100\%$ HPD region for μ under this prior is identical to the classical $(1-\alpha)100\%$ confidence region for μ from sampling theory, and for inferences about μ the Bayesian and frequentist answers coincide. The improper prior (5.18) also arises by applying the Jeffreys invariance principle to μ and Σ (Box and Tiao, 1992).

If our primary interest is not in μ but in Σ, then the frequentist justification for using (5.18) as a noninformative prior is not as strong because of the ambiguities involved in estimation of Σ. Notice, however, that if we use our rule-of-thumb that a reasonable estimate for $\Sigma \sim W^{-1}(m, \Lambda)$ is $m^{-1}\Lambda^{-1}$, then (5.20) leads to the point estimate $(n-1)^{-1}nS$. This is the estimate of Σ that is most widely used in practice, because it is unbiased for fixed θ over repetitions of the sampling procedure. For these reasons, we will accept (5.18) as a reasonable prior distribution when prior information about θ is scanty.

Informative priors

When an informative prior distribution is needed, it is often possible to choose reasonable values for the hyperparameters by appealing to the device of *imaginary results*. Suppose that we regard the improper prior (5.18) as representing a state of complete ignorance about θ. After observing a sample of n observations with mean $\bar{y}$ and covariance matrix S, the new state of knowledge is represented by (5.19)–(5.20). By this logic, we can interpret the hyperparameters in (5.11)–(5.12) as a summary of the information provided by an imaginary set of data: μ_0 represents our best guess as to what μ might be (the imaginary $\bar{y}$); τ represents the number of imaginary prior observations on which the guess μ_0 is based; $m^{-1}\Lambda^{-1}$ represents our best guess as to what Σ might be (the imaginary S); and $m = \tau - 1$ represents the number of imaginary prior degrees of freedom on which the guess $m^{-1}\Lambda^{-1}$ is based.

A ridge prior

It sometimes happens that the sample covariance matrix S is singular or nearly so, either because the data are sparse (e.g. n is not substantially larger than p), or because such strong relationships exist among the variables that certain linear combinations of the columns of Y exhibit little or no variability. When this happens, it may be difficult to obtain sensible inferences about μ unless we introduce some prior information about Σ. The following is a suggestion for choosing a prior distribution to stabilize the inference when little is known a priori about μ or Σ.

Suppose that we adopt the limiting form of the normal inverted-Wishart prior (5.13) as $\tau \to 0$ for some m and Λ. The posterior becomes

$$\mu \mid \Sigma, Y \quad \sim \quad N(\bar{y}, n^{-1}\Sigma), \tag{5.21}$$

$$\Sigma \mid Y \quad \sim \quad W^{-1}(m + n, [\Lambda^{-1} + nS]^{-1}), \tag{5.22}$$

which is proper provided that $m + n \geq p$ and $(\Lambda^{-1} + nS) > 0$. Notice that this posterior is very similar to the posterior distribution (5.19)–(5.20) obtained under the standard noninformative prior, except that the covariance matrix Σ has been 'smoothed' toward a matrix proportional to Λ^{-1}. If we take $m = \epsilon$ for some $\epsilon > 0$ and $\Lambda^{-1} = \epsilon S^*$ for some covariance matrix S^*, then our rule-of-thumb estimate of Σ is

$$\frac{1}{m + n}(\Lambda^{-1} + nS) = \left(\frac{\epsilon}{n + \epsilon}\right)S^* + \left(\frac{n}{n + \epsilon}\right)S,$$

a weighted average of S and S^* with weights determined by the relative sizes of n and ϵ.

When S is singular or nearly so, it makes sense to choose S^* to move the weighted average of the two matrices away from the boundary of the parameter space. One effective way to do this is to set the diagonal elements of S^* equal to those of S and the off-diagonal elements equal to zero,

$$S^* = \text{Diag } S. \tag{5.23}$$

The resulting 'prior', which is not really a prior in the Bayesian sense because it is partly determined by the data, has the practical effect of allowing the means and variances to be estimated from the data alone, but smooths the correlation matrix slightly toward the identity. The degree of smoothing is determined by the relative sizes of ϵ and n, and ϵ can be regarded as an imaginary number of prior degrees of freedom added to the inference. Note that ϵ need not be an integer, and in some cases even a small fractional value of ϵ may be sufficient to overcome computational difficulties associated with singular covariance matrices. Use of this prior is closely related to the technique of ridge regression (e.g. Draper and Smith, 1981), and can be regarded as a form of empirical Bayes inference (e.g. Berger, 1985). This prior can be very helpful for stabilizing inferences about μ when some aspects of Σ are poorly estimated.

5.2.4 Alternative parameterizations and sweep

Suppose that z is a $p \times 1$ random vector distributed as $N(\mu, \Sigma)$, which we partion as $z^T = (z_1^T, z_2^T)$ where z_1 and z_2 are subvectors of lengths p_1 and $p_2 = p - p_1$, respectively. It is well known that the marginal distributions of z_1 and z_2 are $N(\mu_1, \Sigma_{11})$ and $N(\mu_2, \Sigma_{22})$, where $\mu^T = (\mu_1^T, \mu_2^T)$ and

$$\Sigma = \left[\begin{array}{cc} \Sigma_{11} & \Sigma_{12} \\ \Sigma_{21} & \Sigma_{22} \end{array} \right]$$

are the partitions of μ and Σ corresponding to $z^T = (z_1^T, z_2^T)$. Moreover, the conditional distributions are also normal; in particular, the distribution of z_2 given z_1 is normal with mean

$$\begin{aligned} E(z_2 | z_1) &= \mu_2 + B_{2 \cdot 1}(z_1 - \mu_1) \\ &= \alpha_{2 \cdot 1} + B_{2 \cdot 1} z_1 \end{aligned}$$

and covariance matrix $\Sigma_{22 \cdot 1}$, where

$$\begin{aligned} \alpha_{2 \cdot 1} &= \mu_2 - \Sigma_{21}\Sigma_{11}^{-1}\mu_1, \\ B_{2 \cdot 1} &= \Sigma_{21}\Sigma_{11}^{-1}, \\ \Sigma_{22 \cdot 1} &= \Sigma_{22} - \Sigma_{21}\Sigma_{11}^{-1}\Sigma_{12} \end{aligned} \tag{5.24}$$

are the vector of intercepts, matrix of slopes and matrix of residual covariances, respectively, from the regression of z_2 on z_1.

Because specifying the joint distribution of z_1 and z_2 is equivalent to specifying the marginal distribution of z_1 and the conditional distribution of z_2 given z_1, we can characterize the parameters of the distribution of z either by $\theta = (\mu, \Sigma)$ or by $\phi = (\phi_1, \phi_2)$, where $\phi_1 = (\mu_1, \Sigma_{11})$ and $\phi_2 = (\alpha_{2 \cdot 1}, B_{2 \cdot 1}, \Sigma_{22 \cdot 1})$. It is easy to show that the transformation $\phi = \phi(\theta)$ is one-to-one, with the inverse transformation $\theta = \phi^{-1}(\phi)$ given by

$$\begin{aligned} \mu_2 &= \alpha_{2 \cdot 1} + B_{2 \cdot 1}\mu_1, \\ \Sigma_{12} &= \Sigma_{11} B_{2 \cdot 1}^T, \\ \Sigma_{22} &= \Sigma_{22 \cdot 1} + B_{2 \cdot 1} \Sigma_{11} B_{2 \cdot 1}^T. \end{aligned} \tag{5.25}$$

Moreover, the parameters ϕ_1 and ϕ_2 are distinct in the sense that the parameter space of ϕ is the Cartesian cross-product of the individual parameter spaces of ϕ_1 and ϕ_2; that is, any choice of $\alpha_{2 \cdot 1}$, $B_{2 \cdot 1}$ and $\Sigma_{22 \cdot 1} > 0$ will produce a valid $\theta = (\mu, \Sigma)$ with $\Sigma > 0$.

When a probability distribution is applied to $\theta = (\mu, \Sigma)$, it is occasionally necessary to find the density function for ϕ. Let $f(\theta)$ be the density of θ, and $g(\phi)$ the density of $\phi = \phi(\theta)$ induced by f. The relationship between g and f is

$$g(\phi) = f(\phi^{-1}(\phi)) \, \|J\|^{-1},$$

where J is the Jacobian or first-derivative matrix of the transformation from θ to ϕ, and $\|J\|$ means the absolute value of the determinant of J. Notice that $\alpha_{2 \cdot 1}$, $B_{2 \cdot 1}$ and $\Sigma_{22 \cdot 1}$ are of the same dimension as μ_2, Σ_{21} and Σ_{22}, respectively, so J can be partitioned as

$$J = \begin{bmatrix} \dfrac{\partial \mu_1}{\partial \mu_1} & \dfrac{\partial \mu_1}{\partial \Sigma_{11}} & \dfrac{\partial \mu_1}{\partial \mu_2} & \dfrac{\partial \mu_1}{\partial \Sigma_{21}} & \dfrac{\partial \mu_1}{\partial \Sigma_{22}} \\[2mm] \dfrac{\partial \Sigma_{11}}{\partial \mu_1} & \dfrac{\partial \Sigma_{11}}{\partial \Sigma_{11}} & \dfrac{\partial \Sigma_{11}}{\partial \mu_2} & \dfrac{\partial \Sigma_{11}}{\partial \Sigma_{21}} & \dfrac{\partial \Sigma_{11}}{\partial \Sigma_{22}} \\[2mm] \dfrac{\partial \alpha_{2 \cdot 1}}{\partial \mu_1} & \dfrac{\partial \alpha_{2 \cdot 1}}{\partial \Sigma_{11}} & \dfrac{\partial \alpha_{2 \cdot 1}}{\partial \mu_2} & \dfrac{\partial \alpha_{2 \cdot 1}}{\partial \Sigma_{21}} & \dfrac{\partial \alpha_{2 \cdot 1}}{\partial \Sigma_{22}} \\[2mm] \dfrac{\partial B_{2 \cdot 1}}{\partial \mu_1} & \dfrac{\partial B_{2 \cdot 1}}{\partial \Sigma_{11}} & \dfrac{\partial B_{2 \cdot 1}}{\partial \mu_2} & \dfrac{\partial B_{2 \cdot 1}}{\partial \Sigma_{21}} & \dfrac{\partial B_{2 \cdot 1}}{\partial \Sigma_{22}} \\[2mm] \dfrac{\partial \Sigma_{22 \cdot 1}}{\partial \mu_1} & \dfrac{\partial \Sigma_{22 \cdot 1}}{\partial \Sigma_{11}} & \dfrac{\partial \Sigma_{22 \cdot 1}}{\partial \mu_2} & \dfrac{\partial \Sigma_{22 \cdot 1}}{\partial \Sigma_{21}} & \dfrac{\partial \Sigma_{22 \cdot 1}}{\partial \Sigma_{22}} \end{bmatrix},$$

where the submatrices along the diagonal are square. By inspection of (5.24), we see that this matrix has the pattern

$$J = \begin{bmatrix} I & 0 & 0 & 0 & 0 \\ 0 & I & 0 & 0 & 0 \\ \times & \times & I & \times & 0 \\ 0 & \times & 0 & \times & 0 \\ 0 & \times & 0 & \times & I \end{bmatrix},$$

where I denotes an identity matrix, 0 denotes a zero matrix and $\times$ denotes a matrix that is neither I nor 0. It is a well-known property of determinants that

$$\begin{vmatrix} A & B \\ 0 & C \end{vmatrix} = |A|\,|C| \qquad (5.26)$$

for square A and C. Applying (5.26) repeatedly, the determinant of J reduces to

$$|J| = \left| \dfrac{\partial B_{2 \cdot 1}}{\partial \Sigma_{21}} \right|. \qquad (5.27)$$

With Σ_{11} held fixed, $B_{2\cdot1} = \Sigma_{21}\Sigma_{11}^{-1}$ is a linear transformation of Σ_{21}. It can be shown that the Jacobian of the linear transformation from W $(p \times q)$ to $Z = WB$ for nonsingular B $(q \times q)$ is $|B|^p$ (e.g. Mardia, Kent and Bibby, 1979, Table 2.4.1), and thus

$$\|J\| = |\Sigma_{11}|^{-p_2}. \tag{5.28}$$

The sweep operator

The algorithms presented in this chapter will require repeated use of the transformations (5.24) and (5.25). To simplify both the notation and implementation of these algorithms, we will rely heavily on a device known as the sweep operator. First introduced by Beaton (1964), the sweep operator is commonly used in linear model computations and stepwise regression. Dempster (1969b) describes its relationship to methods of successive orthogonalization, and Little and Rubin (1987) demonstrate the usefulness of sweep in ML estimation for multivariate missing-data problems. Further information and references are given by Thisted (1988).

Suppose that G is a $p \times p$ symmetric matrix with elements g_{ij}. The sweep operator SWP[k] operates on G by replacing it with another $p \times p$ symmetric matrix H,

$$H = \mathrm{SWP}[k]\,G,$$

where the elements of H are given by

$$
\begin{aligned}
h_{kk} &= -1/g_{kk}, \\
h_{jk} &= h_{kj} = g_{jk}/g_{kk} \quad \text{for } j \neq k, \\
h_{jl} &= h_{lj} = g_{jl} - g_{jk}g_{kl}/g_{kk} \quad \text{for } j \neq k \text{ and } l \neq k.
\end{aligned}
\tag{5.29}
$$

After application of (5.29), the matrix is said to have been *swept on position* k. In a computer program, sweep can be carried out as follows: first, replace g_{kk} with $h_{kk} = -1/g_{kk}$; next, replace the remaining elements $g_{jk} = g_{kj}$ in row and column k with $h_{jk} = -g_{jk}h_{kk}$; and finally, replace the remaining elements $g_{jl} = g_{lj}$ in the other rows and columns by $h_{jl} = g_{jl} - g_{kl}h_{jk}$. This method is efficient both in terms of computation time and memory, because no storage locations other than the matrix itself are necessary. Because both G and H are symmetric, further savings can be achieved by computing and retaining only the upper-triangular portion of the matrix.

Suppose that a $p \times p$ matrix G is partitioned as

$$G = \begin{bmatrix} G_{11} & G_{12} \\ G_{21} & G_{22} \end{bmatrix},$$

where G_{11} is $p_1 \times p_1$. After sweeping on positions $1, 2, \ldots, p_1$, the matrix becomes

$$\mathrm{SWP}[1, 2, \ldots, p_1]\, G = \begin{bmatrix} -G_{11}^{-1} & G_{11}^{-1} G_{12} \\ G_{21} G_{11}^{-1} & G_{22} - G_{21} G_{11}^{-1} G_{12} \end{bmatrix},$$

which is recognizable as a matrix version of (5.29). The notation $\mathrm{SWP}[1, 2, \ldots, p_1]$ indicates successive application of (5.29),

$$\mathrm{SWP}[1, 2, \ldots, p_1]\, G = \mathrm{SWP}[p_1] \cdots \mathrm{SWP}[2]\, \mathrm{SWP}[1]\, G.$$

Sweeps on multiple positions need not be carried out in any particular order, because the sweep operator is commutative,

$$\mathrm{SWP}[k_2]\, \mathrm{SWP}[k_1]\, G = \mathrm{SWP}[k_1]\, \mathrm{SWP}[k_2]\, G.$$

Sweeping a $p \times p$ matrix G on positions $1, 2, \ldots, p$ has the effect of replacing G by $-G^{-1}$. This inverse exists if and only if none of the attempted sweeps involve division by zero. When inverting a matrix with sweep, we can also readily obtain the determinant. Let γ_k denote the kth diagonal element of the matrix after it is swept on positions $1, 2, \ldots, k-1$,

$$\gamma_k = \left(\mathrm{SWP}[1, 2, \ldots, k-1]\, G \right)_{kk}.$$

Then

$$|G| = \prod_{k=1}^{p} \gamma_k, \tag{5.30}$$

where γ_1 is taken to be g_{11}, the first element of G. Thus the determinant can be found by computing the product of the pivots (i.e. the diagonal elements of the matrix) as they appear immediately before the matrix is swept on them (Dempster, 1969b).

It is also convenient to define a *reverse-sweep* operator that returns a swept matrix to its original form. The reverse-sweep operator, denoted by

$$H = \mathrm{RSW}[k]\, G,$$

replaces the elements of G with

$$\begin{aligned}
h_{kk} &= -1/g_{kk}, \\
h_{jk} &= h_{kj} = -g_{jk}/g_{kk} \text{ for } j \neq k, \\
h_{jl} &= h_{lj} = g_{jl} - g_{jk}g_{kl}/g_{kk} \text{ for } j \neq k \text{ and } l \neq k.
\end{aligned} \tag{5.31}$$

Notice that reverse sweep is remarkably similar to sweep, with the only difference being a minus sign in the calculation of $h_{jk} = h_{kj}$. It is easy to verify that reverse sweep is indeed the inverse of sweep,

$$\mathrm{RSW}[k]\,\mathrm{SWP}[k]\,G \;=\; G,$$

and that reverse sweep is commutative,

$$\mathrm{RSW}[k_2]\,\mathrm{RSW}[k_1]\,G \;=\; \mathrm{RSW}[k_1]\,\mathrm{RSW}[k_2]\,G.$$

Computing alternative parameterizations

From a statistical viewpoint, the sweep operator is highly useful for the following reason: when applied to the parameters of the multivariate normal model, sweep converts a variable from a response to a predictor. Suppose that z is a $p \times 1$ random vector distributed as $N(\mu, \Sigma)$, and we partition it as $z^T = (z_1^T, z_2^T)$ where z_1 has length p_1. Let us arrange the parameters $\theta = (\mu, \Sigma)$ as a $(p+1) \times (p+1)$ matrix in the following manner,

$$\theta = \begin{bmatrix} -1 & \mu^T \\ \mu & \Sigma \end{bmatrix} = \begin{bmatrix} -1 & \mu_1^T & \mu_2^T \\ \mu_1 & \Sigma_{11} & \Sigma_{12} \\ \mu_2 & \Sigma_{21} & \Sigma_{22} \end{bmatrix}. \tag{5.32}$$

The reason for placing -1 in the upper-left corner will be explained shortly. To simplify book-keeping, we will allow the row and column indices to run from 0 to p rather than from 1 to $p+1$, so that the parameters pertaining to the jth variable will appear in row and column j. Suppose that we sweep this θ-matrix on positions $1, 2, \ldots, p_1$; the result will be, by the matrix analogue of (5.29),

$$\begin{bmatrix} -1 - \mu_1^T \Sigma_{11}^{-1} \mu_1 & \mu_1^T \Sigma_{11}^{-1} & \mu_2^T - \mu_1^T \Sigma_{11}^{-1} \Sigma_{12} \\ \Sigma_{11}^{-1} \mu_1 & -\Sigma_{11}^{-1} & \Sigma_{11}^{-1} \Sigma_{12} \\ \mu_2 - \Sigma_{21} \Sigma_{11}^{-1} \mu_1 & \Sigma_{21} \Sigma_{11}^{-1} & \Sigma_{22} - \Sigma_{21} \Sigma_{11}^{-1} \Sigma_{12} \end{bmatrix}.$$

Comparing this to (5.24), we see that the last $p - p_1$ rows and columns contain $\alpha_{2\cdot 1}$, $B_{2\cdot 1}$, and $\Sigma_{22\cdot 1}$, the parameters of the conditional distribution of z_2 given z_1,

$$\mathrm{SWP}[1, \ldots, p_1]\,\theta = \begin{bmatrix} -1 - \mu_1^T \Sigma_{11}^{-1} \mu_1 & \mu_1^T \Sigma_{11}^{-1} & \alpha_{2\cdot 1}^T \\ \Sigma_{11}^{-1} \mu_1 & -\Sigma_{11}^{-1} & B_{2\cdot 1}^T \\ \alpha_{2\cdot 1} & B_{2\cdot 1} & \Sigma_{22\cdot 1} \end{bmatrix}.$$

Moreover, the upper-left $(p_1 + 1) \times (p_1 + 1)$ submatrix contains in swept form the parameters of the marginal distribution of z_1,

$$
\begin{bmatrix} -1 & \mu_1^T \\ \mu_1 & \Sigma_{11} \end{bmatrix} = \text{RSW}[1,\ldots,p_1] \begin{bmatrix} -1 - \mu_1^T \Sigma_{11}^{-1} \mu_1 & \mu_1^T \Sigma_{11}^{-1} \\ \Sigma_{11}^{-1} \mu_1 & -\Sigma_{11}^{-1} \end{bmatrix}.
$$

We have thus shown that $\phi = (\mu_1, \Sigma_{11}, \alpha_{2\cdot1}, B_{2\cdot1}, \Sigma_{22\cdot1})$, expressed in matrix form as

$$
\phi = \begin{bmatrix} -1 & \mu_1^T & \alpha_{2\cdot1}^T \\ \mu_1 & \Sigma_{11} & B_{2\cdot1}^T \\ \alpha_{2\cdot1} & B_{2\cdot1} & \Sigma_{22\cdot1} \end{bmatrix}, \tag{5.33}
$$

can be computed from the θ-matrix by first sweeping the full matrix on positions $1, 2, \ldots, p_1$, and then reverse-sweeping the upper-left $(p_1 + 1) \times (p_1 + 1)$ submatrix on the same positions.

The reason for placing -1 in the upper-left corner of the θ-matrix (5.32) is that this matrix can be considered to be already swept on position 0. Notice that if we reverse-sweep θ on position 0, we obtain

$$
\text{RSW}[0] \begin{bmatrix} -1 & \mu^T \\ \mu & \Sigma \end{bmatrix} = \begin{bmatrix} 1 & \mu^T \\ \mu & \Sigma + \mu\mu^T \end{bmatrix}, \tag{5.34}
$$

the parameters of the multivariate normal distribution expressed in terms of the first two moments of z about the origin. This unswept version of θ is quite useful because it is the natural representation for computing ML estimates. Suppose that Y is an $n \times p$ data matrix whose rows are independent realizations of the random vector z. If we arrange the sufficient statistics $T_1 = Y^T \mathbf{1}$ and $T_2 = Y^T Y$ into a $(p + 1) \times (p + 1)$ matrix

$$
T = [\mathbf{1}, Y]^T [\mathbf{1}, Y] = \begin{bmatrix} n & T_1^T \\ T_1 & T_2 \end{bmatrix}, \tag{5.35}
$$

then the moment equations for ML estimation set (5.34) equal to $n^{-1}T$. Hence the ML estimate of θ may be computed from the sufficient statistics by

$$
\hat{\theta} = \text{SWP}[0]\, n^{-1}T.
$$

Because ML estimates are invariant under transformations of the parameter, the MLE for an alternative parameterization ϕ can be obtained by sweeping $\hat{\theta}$ on the appropriate positions.

variables

	Y_1	Y_2	Y_3	$\ldots$	Y_p
patterns $s = 1$	1	1	1		1
2	0	1	1		1
.	1	0	1		1
.	0	0	1		1
.	1	1	0		1
.	.	.	.		.
.	.	.	.		.
.	.	.	.		.
.	0	1	0		0
S	1	0	0		0

Figure 5.1. *Matrix of missingness patterns associated with* Y, *with 1 denoting an observed variable and 0 denoting a missing variable.*

5.3 The EM algorithm

When portions of the data matrix Y are missing, ML estimates cannot in general be obtained in closed form; we must resort to iterative computation. The EM algorithm for a multivariate normal data matrix with an arbitrary pattern of missing values was described by Orchard and Woodbury (1972); Beale and Little (1975); Dempster, Laird and Rubin (1977); and Little and Rubin (1987). Because of its usefulness and its similarities to the simulation algorithms that follow, we describe in detail one possible implementation of EM for incomplete multivariate normal data.

5.3.1 Preliminary manipulations

To simplify notation and facilitate computations, it is helpful at the outset to group the rows of Y by their missingness patterns. A matrix of missingness patterns corresponding to Y is shown in Figure 5.1. We will index the missingness patterns by $s = 1, 2, \ldots, S$, where S is the number of unique patterns appearing in the data matrix. The trivial pattern with all variables missing should be omitted from consideration. Rows of Y that are completely missing contribute nothing to the observed-data likelihood and would only slow the convergence of EM by increasing the fractions of missing information (Section 3.3.2).

For book-keeping purposes it will be helpful to define the following quantities. Let R be an $S \times p$ matrix of binary indicators with typical element r_{sj}, where

$$r_{sj} = \begin{cases} 1 & \text{if } Y_j \text{ is observed in pattern } s, \\ 0 & \text{if } Y_j \text{ is missing in pattern } s. \end{cases}$$

The matrix R is shown in Figure 5.1. For each missingness pattern s, let $\mathcal{O}(s)$ and $\mathcal{M}(s)$ denote the subsets of the column labels $\{1, 2, \ldots, p\}$ corresponding to variables that are observed and missing, respectively,

$$\mathcal{O}(s) = \{j : r_{sj} = 1\},$$

$$\mathcal{M}(s) = \{j : r_{sj} = 0\}.$$

Finally, let $\mathcal{I}(s)$ denote the subset of $\{1, 2, \ldots, n\}$ corresponding to the rows of Y that exhibit pattern s. For example, suppose that the data matrix has ten rows with no missing values, and after sorting these rows are labeled $1, \ldots, 10$; the first row of R is then $(1, 1, \ldots, 1)$, and

$$\mathcal{O}(1) = \{1, 2, \ldots, p\},$$
$$\mathcal{M}(1) = \emptyset,$$
$$\mathcal{I}(1) = \{1, 2, \ldots, 10\}.$$

5.3.2 The E-step

Recall that in the E-step of EM, one calculates the expectation of the complete-data sufficient statistics over $P(Y_{mis} \mid Y_{obs}, \theta)$ for an assumed value of θ. These statistics are of the form $\sum_i y_{ij}$ and $\sum_i y_{ij} y_{ik}$, so to perform the E-step we need to find the expectations of y_{ij} and $y_{ij} y_{ik}$ over $P(Y_{mis} \mid Y_{obs}, \theta)$.

Because the rows $y_1, y_2, \ldots, y_n$ of Y are independent given θ, we can write

$$P(Y_{mis} \mid Y_{obs}, \theta) = \prod_{i=1}^{n} P(y_{i(mis)} \mid y_{i(obs)}, \theta),$$

where $y_{i(obs)}$ and $y_{i(mis)}$ denote the observed and missing subvectors of y_i, respectively. The distribution $P(y_{i(mis)} \mid y_{i(obs)}, \theta)$ is a multivariate normal linear regression of $y_{i(mis)}$ on $y_{i(obs)}$, and the parameters of this regression can be calculated by sweeping the θ-matrix on the positions corresponding to the variables in $y_{i(obs)}$. If row i is in missingness pattern s, then the parameters of

$P(y_{i(mis)}\,|\,y_{i(obs)},\theta)$ are contained in $\mathrm{SWP}[\mathcal{O}(s)]\,\theta$ in the rows and columns labeled $\mathcal{M}(s)$. Let A denote the swept parameter matrix

$$A = \mathrm{SWP}[\mathcal{O}(s)]\,\theta,$$

and let a_{jk} denote the (j,k)th element of A, $j,k = 0,1,\ldots,p$. Using the results of Section 5.2.4, the reader may verify that the first two moments of $y_{i(mis)}$ with respect to $P(Y_{mis}\,|\,Y_{obs},\theta)$ are given by

$$E(y_{ij}\,|\,Y_{obs},\theta) = a_{0j} + \sum_{k\in\mathcal{O}(s)} a_{kj}y_{ik},$$
$$\mathrm{Cov}(y_{ij},y_{ik}\,|\,Y_{obs},\theta) = a_{jk}$$

for each $i \in \mathcal{I}(s)$ and $j,k \in \mathcal{M}(s)$. For any $j \in \mathcal{O}(s)$, of course, the moments are

$$E(y_{ij}\,|\,Y_{obs},\theta) = y_{ij},$$
$$\mathrm{Cov}(y_{ij},y_{ik}\,|\,Y_{obs},\theta) = 0,$$

because y_{ij} is regarded as fixed. Applying the relation

$$E(y_{ij}y_{ik}\,|\,Y_{obs},\theta) = \mathrm{Cov}(y_{ij},y_{ik}\,|\,Y_{obs},\theta)$$
$$+ E(y_{ij}\,|\,Y_{obs},\theta)\,E(y_{ik}\,|\,Y_{obs},\theta),$$

it follows that

$$E(y_{ij}\,|\,Y_{obs},\theta) = \begin{cases} y_{ij} & \text{for } j \in \mathcal{O}(s), \\ y_{ij}^{*} & \text{for } j \in \mathcal{M}(s), \end{cases}$$

and

$$E(y_{ij}y_{ik}\,|\,Y_{obs},\theta) = \begin{cases} y_{ij}y_{ik} & \text{for } j,k \in \mathcal{O}(s), \\ y_{ij}^{*}y_{ik} & \text{for } j \in \mathcal{M}(s), k \in \mathcal{O}(s), \\ a_{jk} + y_{ij}^{*}y_{ik}^{*} & \text{for } j,k \in \mathcal{M}(s), \end{cases}$$

where

$$y_{ij}^{*} = a_{0j} + \sum_{k\in\mathcal{O}(s)} a_{kj}y_{ik}. \tag{5.36}$$

The E-step consists of calculating and summing these expected values of y_{ij} and $y_{ij}y_{ik}$ over i for each j and k. The output of an E-step can then be written as $E(T\,|\,Y_{obs},\theta)$, where T is the matrix of complete-data sufficient statistics

$$
T = \begin{bmatrix} n & 1^T Y \\ Y^T 1 & Y^T Y \end{bmatrix} = \sum_{i=1}^{n} \begin{bmatrix} n & y_{i1} & y_{i2} & \cdots & y_{ip} \\ & y_{i1}^2 & y_{i1}y_{i2} & \cdots & y_{i1}y_{ip} \\ & & y_{i2}^2 & \cdots & y_{i2}y_{ip} \\ & & & \ddots & \vdots \\ & & & & y_{ip}^2 \end{bmatrix}.
$$

The elements below the diagonal are not shown and may be omitted from the calculations because they are redundant. Notice that the matrix $A = \mathrm{SWP}[\mathcal{O}(s)]\,\theta$ needed for the E-step depends on the missingness pattern s, and thus in practice the elements of $E(T \mid Y_{obs}, \theta)$ must be calculated by first summing expected values of y_{ij} and $y_{ij}y_{ik}$ for $i \in \mathcal{I}(s)$, and then summing across patterns $s = 1, 2, \ldots, S$, with a new A-matrix being calculated for each missingness pattern.

5.3.3 Implementation of the algorithm

Once $E(T \mid Y_{obs}, \theta)$ has been found, carrying out the M-step is relatively trivial. For a given value of T the complete-data MLE is $\hat{\theta} = \mathrm{SWP}[0]\,n^{-1}T$, and the M-step merely carries out this same operation on $E(T \mid Y_{obs}, \theta)$ rather than T. A single iteration of EM can thus be written succinctly as

$$
\theta^{(t+1)} = \mathrm{SWP}[0]\,n^{-1}E(T \mid Y_{obs}, \theta^{(t)}). \tag{5.37}
$$

In principle the EM algorithm for incomplete multivariate normal data is completely defined by (5.37), but from a practical standpoint we should still consider how to implement the algorithm in an efficient manner. It is beneficial to keep both processing time and memory usage down, but tradeoffs between the two are inevitable; one can always reduce processing time at the expense of additional memory by storing rather than recomputing quantities that must be used repeatedly. The implementation suggested here stores rather than recomputes the portions of $E(T \mid Y_{obs}, \theta)$ that do not depend on θ and thus remain the same for every E-step. This method may not be optimal for any particular dataset, but it is not difficult to program and seems to perform well in a wide variety of situations.

Observed and missing parts of the sufficient statistics

We can express the matrix T as the sum of matrices corresponding to the individual missingness patterns. Let

$$T(s) = \begin{bmatrix} n_s & \sum y_{i1} & \sum y_{i2} & \cdots & \sum y_{ip} \\ & \sum y_{i1}^2 & \sum y_{i1} y_{i2} & \cdots & \sum y_{i1} y_{ip} \\ & & \sum y_{i2}^2 & \cdots & \sum y_{i2} y_{ip} \\ & & & \ddots & \vdots \\ & & & & \sum y_{ip}^2 \end{bmatrix},$$

where all sums are taken over $i \in \mathcal{I}(s)$, and $n_s = \sum_{i \in \mathcal{I}(s)} 1$ is the sample size in missingness pattern s; then

$$T = \sum_{s=1}^{S} T(s).$$

Each $T(s)$ can be further partitioned into an observed part and a missing part. Notice that the elements of $T(s)$ in the rows and columns labeled $\mathcal{M}(s)$ are functions of Y_{mis} and perhaps Y_{obs}, whereas the remaining elements of $T(s)$ are functions of Y_{obs} only. Define a new matrix $T_{mis}(s)$ which has the same elements as $T(s)$ in the rows and columns labeled $\mathcal{M}(s)$, but with all other elements set to zero, and define $T_{obs}(s)$ to be $T(s) - T_{mis}(s)$. For example, consider a dataset with $p = 3$ variables, and suppose that missingness pattern s has Y_1 and Y_3 observed but Y_2 missing; then

$$T_{obs}(s) = \begin{bmatrix} n_s & \sum y_{i1} & 0 & \sum y_{i3} \\ & \sum y_{i1}^2 & 0 & \sum y_{i1} y_{i3} \\ & & 0 & 0 \\ & & & \sum y_{i3}^2 \end{bmatrix},$$

$$T_{mis}(s) = \begin{bmatrix} 0 & 0 & \sum y_{i2} & 0 \\ & 0 & \sum y_{i1} y_{i2} & 0 \\ & & \sum y_{i2}^2 & \sum y_{i2} y_{i3} \\ & & & 0 \end{bmatrix},$$

where all sums are taken over $i \in \mathcal{I}(s)$. Finally, define

$$T_{obs} = \sum_{s=1}^{S} T_{obs}(s) \quad \text{and} \quad T_{mis} = \sum_{s=1}^{S} T_{mis}(s),$$

```
T := T_obs
for s:= 1 to S do
    for j:= 1 to p do
        if r_sj = 1 and θ_jj > 0 then θ := SWP[j] θ
        if r_sj = 0 and θ_jj < 0 then θ := RSW[j] θ
        end do
    for i ∈ I(s) do
        for j ∈ M(s) do
            c_j := θ_0j
            for k ∈ O(s) do c_j := c_j + θ_kj y_ik
            end do
        for j ∈ M(s) do
            T_0j := T_0j + c_j
            for k ∈ O(s) do T_kj := T_kj + c_j y_ik
            for k ∈ M(s) and k ≥ j do T_kj := T_kj + θ_kj + c_k c_j
            end do
        end do
    end do
end do
θ := SWP[0] n^{-1} T
```

Figure 5.2. *Single iteration of EM for incomplete multivariate normal data, written in pseudocode.*

so that $T = T_{obs} + T_{mis}$. The E-step may then be written

$$
\begin{aligned}
E(T | Y_{obs}, \theta) &= T_{obs} + E(T_{mis} | Y_{obs}, \theta) \\
&= \sum_{s=1}^{S} T_{obs}(s) + \sum_{s=1}^{S} E(T_{mis}(s) | Y_{obs}, \theta).
\end{aligned}
$$

The elements of T_{obs} can be calculated once at the outset of the program and stored for all future iterations of EM.

An implementation in pseudocode

One possible implementation of an iteration of EM is shown in Figure 5.2. It is written in *pseudocode*, a shorthand language that can be understood by anyone with programming experience and is easily converted into standard languages like Fortran or C. In this pseudocode, the symbol ':=' indicates the operation of assignment; for example, '$a := b$' means 'set a equal to b.' This implementation requires two $(p+1) \times (p+1)$ matrix workspaces: T, into which the expected sufficient statistics are accumulated, and θ, which holds the current estimate of the parameter. For simplicity, the rows and columns of these matrices are labeled from 0 to p rather than from 1 to $p + 1$. In addition, a single vector of length p, denoted by $c = (c_1, \ldots, c_p)$, is needed as a temporary workspace to hold the values of y_{ij}^* given by (5.36). The iteration begins by setting T equal to T_{obs}, which we assume has already been computed. The expectations of y_{ij} and $y_{ij}y_{ik}$ that contribute to T_{mis} are then calculated and added into T, one missingness pattern at a time. In order to calculate these expectations within a missingness pattern s, the θ-matrix must be put into the required $\text{SWP}[\mathcal{O}(s)]$ condition; for this, we use the convenient book-keeping device that a diagonal element θ_{jj} is negative if and only if θ has been swept on position j. Finally, after the expected sufficient statistics are fully accumulated into T, the new parameter estimate is calculated and stored in θ in preparation for the next iteration.

For efficiency, the code in Figure 5.2 does not calculate the off-diagonal elements of T more than once. If θ and T are stored as two-dimensional arrays, then only the upper-triangular portions should be used, and T_{jk} or θ_{jk} should be interpreted as the (j, k)th element if $j \leq k$ or the (k, j)th element if $j > k$. Memory requirements can be reduced by retaining only the upper-triangular parts of T and θ in packed storage. To reduce the impact of rounding errors, T, θ, and c should be stored in double precision. Rounding errors can also be reduced by centering and scaling the columns of Y at the outset; for example, we could transform the observed data in each column of Y to have mean zero and unit variance before running EM. If the data are centered and scaled, however, we should remember that θ will be expressed on this transformed scale, and for interpretability we may need to transform the estimate of θ back to the original scale at the end of the program.

Starting values

EM requires a starting value $\theta^{(0)} = (\mu^{(0)}, \Sigma^{(0)})$ for the first iteration. Any starting value may be used provided that $\Sigma^{(0)}$ is positive definite, but in practice it helps to choose a value that is likely to be close to the mode. Several choices for starting values are described by Little and Rubin (1987). The mean vector and covariance matrix calculated only from the completely observed rows of Y may work well, provided that there are at least $p + 1$ such rows. Another easy method is to use the observed data from each variable to supply starting values for the means and variances, and set the initial correlations to zero; if the columns of Y have been centered and scaled at the outset to have mean 0 and variance 1, then this corresponds to taking $\mu^{(0)} = (0, 0, \ldots, 0)^T$ and $\Sigma^{(0)} = I$.

Unless the fractions of missing information for some components of θ are very high, the choice of starting value is usually not crucial; when the missing information is low to moderate, the first few iterations of EM tend to bring θ to the vicinity of the mode from any sensible starting value. When writing a program for general use, it is helpful to give the user the option of supplying a starting value, because restarting EM from a variety of locations helps to diagnose unusual features of the observed-data likelihood, such as ridges and multiple modes.

Estimates on the boundary

It sometimes happens, particularly with sparse datasets, that the observed-data likelihood function increases without limit as θ approaches the boundary of the parameter space (i.e. as Σ approaches a singular matrix). When this occurs, the EM algorithm may behave in a variety of ways. In some problems, the elements of θ stabilize and EM appears to converge to a solution on the boundary. In other problems, the program halts due to numeric overflow or attempted division by zero. In yet other problems, the sweeps required for the E-step become numerically unstable as the iterates approach the boundary, and substantial rounding errors are introduced. We have found that these rounding errors sometimes 'deflect' θ away from the boundary, causing a sudden large drop in likelihood from one iteration to the next. The iterates may approach the boundary for a number of steps, deflect away, approach again, and deflect away again in a recurring fashion. If the elements of θ do not appear to have converged after a large number of iterations, then it is advisable to monitor both the loglikelihood (Section 5.3.5) and some aspect of Σ (e.g. the determinant, or the ratio of the largest eigenvalue to the smallest) to determine whether the iterates are approaching the boundary.

When an ML estimate falls on the boundary, it is often helpful to apply a ridge prior and use EM to find the posterior mode as described below.

5.3.4 EM for posterior modes

This EM algorithm can be easily altered to compute a mode of the observed-data posterior distribution rather than an MLE. As discussed in Section 3.2.3, the E-step is no different; only the M-step needs to be modified. The exact form of this modification will depend on the prior distribution applied to θ.

Priors for incomplete data

At this point, it is worthwhile to consider what prior distributions may be appropriate for an incomplete dataset. Because a prior distribution by definition reflects one's state of knowledge about θ before any data are observed, the fact that some data are missing should from a strictly Bayesian viewpoint have no effect whatsoever on the choice of a prior. To the Bayesian purist, any prior that is appropriate for complete data will be equally appropriate for incomplete data. Most statisticians would agree, however, that choosing a prior distribution (including its analytic form) purely by introspection can be difficult, and in practice most priors are chosen at least partly for computational convenience. The normal inverted-Wishart family of prior distributions, described in Sections 5.2.2 and 5.2.3, is computationally convenient for the EM and data augmentation algorithms in this chapter. In general, this family is not conjugate when data are incomplete; the observed-data posterior $P(\theta \mid Y_{obs})$ under a normal inverted-Wishart prior is tractable only in special cases. Yet EM and data augmentation are both easy to implement under this family of priors, because the simplicity of these algorithms depends upon the tractability of the complete-data problem.

When prior information about θ is scanty, we suggest that the customary diffuse prior for complete data,

$$\pi(\theta) \propto |\Sigma|^{-\left(\frac{p+1}{2}\right)},$$

may also be reasonable when some data are missing. Recall from Section 5.2.3 that one important justification for this prior with complete data is that Bayesian and frequentist inferences about μ coincide. This result does not immediately generalize to incomplete data, but limited experience suggests that Bayesian inferences under this prior may also be approximately valid from a frequentist point of view. Little (1988) reports that in the case of bivariate datasets with missing values on one variable generated by an ignorable mechanism, this prior leads to Bayesian inferences about μ that are well-calibrated; the HPD regions tend to have frequency coverage close to the nominal levels. Because this prior treats the variables $Y_1, Y_2, \ldots, Y_p$ in a symmetric fashion, we conjecture that similar results may hold for more complicated multivariate scenarios as well.

When data are sparse and certain aspects of Σ are poorly estimated, we suggested in Section 5.2.3 that a useful prior for complete data was the limiting form of the normal inverted-Wishart with $\tau = 0$, $m = \epsilon$ for some $\epsilon > 0$, and $\Lambda^{-1} = \epsilon \operatorname{Diag} S$, where S is the complete-data sample covariance matrix. With incomplete data S cannot be calculated, but a useful substitute is the matrix with diagonal elements equal to the sample variances among the observed values in each column of Y. This prior effectively smooths the variances in Σ toward the observed-data variances and the correlations toward zero. If the observed data in each column of Y have been scaled at the outset of the program to have unit variances, then this prior will simply take $\Lambda^{-1} = \epsilon I$.

Modifications to the M-step

The joint mode of the normal inverted-Wishart distribution,

$$\mu \mid \Sigma \quad \sim \quad N(\mu_0, \tau^{-1}\Sigma),$$
$$\Sigma \quad \sim \quad W^{-1}(m, \Lambda),$$

is achieved at μ_0 and $(m + p + 2)^{-1}\Lambda^{-1}$ for μ and Σ, respectively (Section 5.2.2). Thus the complete-data posterior mode for $\theta = (\mu, \Sigma)$ under the normal inverted-Wishart prior with hyperparameters $(\tau, m, \mu_0, \Lambda)$, denoted by $\tilde{\theta} = (\tilde{\mu}, \tilde{\Sigma})$, is

$$\tilde{\mu} = \mu_0' \quad \text{and} \quad \tilde{\Sigma} = \frac{1}{m' + p + 2} \, (\Lambda')^{-1},$$

where μ_0', m' and Λ' are the updated versions of the hyperparameters given in Section 5.2.2. By reverse-sweeping the mode on position 0 and equating the result to a matrix of modified sufficient statistics,

$$\text{RSW}[0] \begin{bmatrix} -1 & \tilde{\mu}^T \\ \tilde{\mu} & \tilde{\Sigma} \end{bmatrix} = \begin{bmatrix} 1 & \tilde{\mu}^T \\ \tilde{\mu} & \tilde{\Sigma} + \tilde{\mu}\tilde{\mu}^T \end{bmatrix} = n^{-1} \begin{bmatrix} n & \tilde{T}_1^T \\ \tilde{T}_1 & \tilde{T}_2 \end{bmatrix},$$

the mode can be computed as if it were an ML estimate based on $\tilde{T}_1$ and $\tilde{T}_2$ rather than T_1 and T_2. Solving for $\tilde{T}_1$ and $\tilde{T}_2$ and substituting expressions for the updated hyperparameters gives

$$\tilde{T}_1 = \left(\frac{n}{n+\tau}\right) T_1 + \left(\frac{\tau}{n+\tau}\right) n\mu_0$$

and

$$\tilde{T}_2 = \frac{n}{n+m+p+2} \left(T_2 - \frac{1}{n} T_1 T_1^T + \Lambda^{-1} + A \right) + \frac{1}{n} \tilde{T}_1 \tilde{T}_1^T$$

as the modified sufficient statistics, where

$$A = \frac{\tau}{n(\tau+n)} (T_1 - n\mu_0)(T_1 - n\mu_0)^T.$$

To modify the EM algorithm shown in Figure 5.2 to compute a posterior mode rather than an MLE, we need only to replace the expected sufficient statistics T_1 and T_2 in the workspace T by the modified versions $\tilde{T}_1$ and $\tilde{T}_2$ immediately before executing the final step $\theta := \text{SWP}[0]\, n^{-1}T$.

5.3.5 Calculating the observed-data loglikelihood

One of the great advantages of the EM algorithm is that it never requires calculation of the observed-data loglikelihood function or its derivatives. The observed-data likelihood for this problem, discussed in Example 3 of Section 2.3.2, or its logarithm $l(\theta \mid Y_{obs})$, would be very tedious to differentiate or maximize by gradient-based methods. Evaluation of $l(\theta \mid Y_{obs})$ at a specific value of θ, however, is not overwhelmingly difficult; the computations required for a single evaluation are comparable to those needed for a single iteration of EM.

It follows from (2.10) that the observed data-loglikelihood function may be written as

$$\sum_{s=1}^{S} \sum_{i \in \mathcal{I}(s)} \left\{ -\tfrac{1}{2} \log|\Sigma_s^*| - \tfrac{1}{2} (y_{i(obs)} - \mu_s^*)^T \Sigma_s^{*-1} (y_{i(obs)} - \mu_s^*) \right\},$$

where $y_{i(obs)}$ denotes the observed part of y_i, and μ_s^* and Σ_s^* denote the subvector of μ and the submatrix of Σ, respectively, that pertain to the variables that are observed in pattern s. An equivalent but computationally more convenient expression is

$$l(\theta \mid Y_{obs}) = \sum_{s=1}^{S} \left\{ -\tfrac{n_s}{2} \log|\Sigma_s^*| - \tfrac{1}{2} \operatorname{tr} \Sigma_s^{*-1} M_s \right\}, \qquad (5.38)$$

where n_s is the number of observations in missingness pattern s and

$$M_s = \sum_{i \in \mathcal{I}(s)} (y_{i(obs)} - \mu_s^*)(y_{i(obs)} - \mu_s^*)^T.$$

```
d := 0
l := 0
for j := 1 to p do c_j := θ_0j
for s := 1 to S do
    for j := 1 to p do
        if r_sj = 1 and θ_jj > 0 then
            d := d + log θ_jj
            θ := SWP[j] θ
        else if r_sj = 0 and θ_jj < 0 then
            θ := RSW[j] θ
            d := d − log θ_jj
        end if
    end do
    M := 0
    for i ∈ I(s), j, k ∈ O(s) and j ≤ k do
        M_jk := M_jk + (y_ij − c_j)(y_ik − c_k)
    end do
    t := 0
    for j, k ∈ O(s) do t := t − θ_jk M_jk
    l := l − (n_s d + t)/2
end do
```

Figure 5.3. *Calculation of observed-data loglikelihood function.*

Pseudocode for calculating $l(\theta \,|\, Y_{obs})$ is shown in Figure 5.3. This algorithm requires a $p \times p$ matrix workspace M to hold values of M_s, and a $p \times 1$ vector c for temporary storage of μ. The constants d and t hold $\log|\Sigma_s^*|$ and $\operatorname{tr}\Sigma_s^{*-1}M_s$, respectively, and after execution the loglikelihood value is contained in l. This program modifies the parameter matrix θ; if necessary, however, the single line

$$\theta := \mathrm{RSW}[O(S)]\,\theta$$

may be added at the end of the program, which will return θ to its original state except for rounding errors.

Notice that the algorithm for evaluating $l(\theta \,|\, Y_{obs})$ bears a strong resemblance to a single step of EM. An obvious question to ask is whether the two sets of code can be combined, so that an evaluation of the loglikelihood is efficiently woven into EM itself. This is certainly possible, but subject to the following caveats. First, the loglikelihood would have to be evaluated at the parameter estimate from the *previous* iteration; that is, we would have to evaluate $l(\theta^{(t)} \,|\, Y_{obs})$ as we computed $\theta^{(t+1)}$. Second, notice that a loglikelihood evaluation requires accumulation of the *observed* parts of the complete-data sufficient statistics, rather than the expected values of the missing parts. Recall that the EM code in Figure 5.2 assumes that T_{obs}, the portion of the expected value of T that does not change over the iterations, has already been computed and stored at the outset of the program. Evaluation of the observed-data loglikelihood, however, requires access to the individual matrices $T_{obs}(s)$ for $s = 1, 2, \ldots, S$, which could be very cumbersome to store. If, as in Figure 5.3, the matrices $T_{obs}(s)$ are not stored but effectively recomputed at each iteration, then the proportionate reductions in computing time achieved by combining the two algorithms over running them separately would not be overwhelming.

When EM is used to find a posterior mode rather than an MLE, the function that is guaranteed to be non-decreasing at each iteration is no longer the observed-data likelihood but the observed-data posterior density. The logarithm of the observed-data posterior density is

$$\log P(\theta \mid Y_{obs}) = l(\theta \mid Y_{obs}) + \log \pi(\theta),$$

where unnecessary normalizing constants have been omitted. Thus the log-posterior density may be evaluated by adding $\log \pi(\theta)$ to the result of the algorithm in Figure 5.3. Under a normal inverted-Wishart prior with hyperparameters $(\tau, m, \mu_0, \Lambda)$, this additional term is

$$\log \pi(\theta) = -\tfrac{m+p+2}{2} \log |\Sigma| - \tfrac{1}{2} \operatorname{tr} \Sigma^{-1} M_0,$$

where

$$M_0 = \Lambda^{-1} + \tau(\mu - \mu_0)(\mu - \mu_0)^T,$$

and unnecessary constants have again been omitted.

5.3.6 Example: serum-cholesterol levels of heart-attack patients

Ryan and Joiner (1994, Table 9.1) report serum-cholesterol levels for $n = 28$ patients treated for heart attacks at a Pennsylvania medical center. For all patients in the sample, cholesterol levels were measured 2 days and 4 days after the attack. For 19 of the 28 patients, an additional measurement was taken 14 days after the attack. The data are displayed in Table 5.1 (a), with readings at 2, 4 and 14 days denoted by Y_1, Y_2 and Y_3, respectively.

Regarding the complete data as a random sample from a trivariate normal distribution, we applied EM to find the observed-data

Table 5.1. *EM algorithm applied to cholesterol levels for heart-attack patients measured 2, 4 and 14 days after attack*

(a) Observed data

Y_1	Y_2	Y_3
270	218	156
236	234	—
210	214	242
142	116	—
280	200	—
272	276	256
160	146	142
220	182	216
226	238	248
242	288	—
186	190	168
266	236	236
206	244	—
318	258	200
294	240	264
282	294	—
234	220	264
224	200	—
276	220	188
282	186	182
360	352	294
310	202	214
280	218	—
278	248	198
288	278	—
288	248	256
244	270	280
236	242	204

Source: Ryan and Joiner (1994)

(b) Iterations of EM

t	$\mu_3^{(t)}$	$\sigma_3^{(t)}$	$\rho_{13}^{(t)}$	$\rho_{23}^{(t)}$
0	200.000	50.0000	0.000000	0.000000
1	222.236	44.1831	0.403571	0.743661
2	222.237	44.1836	0.403566	0.743667
3	222.237	44.1839	0.403564	0.743669
4	222.237	44.1840	0.403563	0.743670
5	222.237	44.1840	0.403563	0.743671
6	222.237	44.1841	0.403563	0.743671
∞	222.237	44.1841	0.403563	0.743671

(c) Elementwise rates of convergence

t	$\hat{\lambda}_1^{(t)}$	$\hat{\lambda}_2^{(t)}$	$\hat{\lambda}_3^{(t)}$	$\hat{\lambda}_4^{(t)}$
0	—	—	—	—
1	0.000	0.000	0.000	0.000
2	0.469	0.468	0.476	0.456
3	0.468	0.467	0.474	0.458
4	0.468	0.466	0.472	0.460
5	0.468	0.466	0.471	0.462
6	0.467	0.466	0.470	0.463

ML estimates of the nine parameters in $\theta = (\mu, \Sigma)$ (ML estimates for this dataset could also be calculated noniteratively; see Section 6.5). Denote the elements of μ and Σ by μ_j and σ_{jk}, respectively, for $j, k = 1, 2, 3$, and let $\rho_{jk} = \sigma_{jk}(\sigma_{jj}\sigma_{kk})^{-1/2}$ denote the correlations. From starting values chosen based on a crude guess, $\mu^{(0)} = (200, 200, 200)^T$ and $\Sigma^{(0)} = (50)^2 I$, convergence within four significant digits to

$$\hat{\mu} = \begin{bmatrix} 253.9 \\ 230.6 \\ 222.2 \end{bmatrix}, \quad \hat{\Sigma} = \begin{bmatrix} 2195 & 1455 & 835.4 \\ & 2127 & 1515 \\ & & 1952 \end{bmatrix}$$

was achieved in just three iterations. Because no data are missing for Y_1 or Y_2, the five parameters $(\mu_1, \mu_2, \sigma_{11}, \sigma_{22}, \rho_{12})$ converge in a single step regardless of the starting value. Iterates of the four remaining parameters, expressed as μ_3, $\sigma_3 = \sqrt{\sigma_{33}}$, ρ_{13} and ρ_{23}, are displayed to six significant digits in Table 5.1 (b).

For estimation of θ, the iterations beyond $t = 4$ are superfluous because precision beyond three or four digits is rarely necessary. As discussed in Section 3.3.4, however, these additional iterations can be used to estimate elementwise rates of convergence, which are typically equal to the largest fraction of missing information. Elementwise rates of convergence for the four parameters that do not converge in one step, estimated using (3.27), are displayed in Table 5.1 (c). These estimates, which are all close to 47%, do not measure the individual rates of missing information for the four parameters μ_3, σ_3, ρ_{13} and ρ_{23}; rather, they pertain to the function of θ for which the rate of missing information is highest.

Notice that the 47% rate of missing information is somewhat higher than the $9/28 = 32\%$ rate of missing observations for Y_3. Because we know that the parameters pertaining to the joint distribution of (Y_1, Y_2) have no missing information, the 47% rate must pertain to some function of the parameters of the regression of Y_3 on Y_1 and Y_2. It is instructive to consider why the largest rate of missing information exceeds the rate of missing observations for Y_3. A hint is provided by the scatterplot of Y_1 versus Y_2 displayed in Figure 5.4 (a). The cases having missing values for Y_3 tend to be slightly farther, on average, from the center of the (Y_1, Y_2) distribution than do the cases for which Y_3 is observed. Because they are farther from the center, they exert more influence on the estimates of the regression parameters. A well known measure of influence in linear regression models is provided by the *leverage values*, the diagonal elements of the hat matrix (e.g. Draper and Smith, 1981).

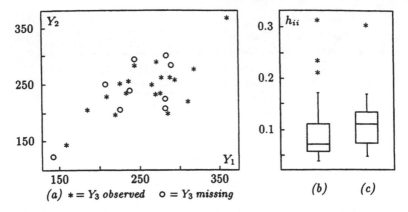

(a) * = Y_3 observed   o = Y_3 missing   (b)   (c)

Figure 5.4. (a) Scatterplot of Y_1 versus Y_2 for all cases, and boxplots of leverage values h_{ii} for cases having (b) Y_3 observed and (c) Y_3 missing.

The hat matrix for linear regression is defined to be

$$H = X(X^T X)^{-1} X^T,$$

where X is the matrix of predictor variables, in this case a 28×3 matrix containing the observed values of Y_1 and Y_2 and the column vector $\mathbf{1} = (1, 1, \ldots,)^T$. Boxplots of the diagonal elements h_{ii} of H for the cases having Y_3 observed and the cases having Y_3 missing are shown in Figures 5.4 (b) and (c), respectively. The incomplete cases tend to have slightly higher values of h_{ii} and thus exert greater influence on an average, per-case basis over the estimates of the regression parameters.

The parameters of greatest interest in this problem appear to be functions of μ, such as comparisons or contrasts among μ_1, μ_2 and μ_3. Although the rate of missing observations for Y_3 is 32%, we might conjecture that the rate of missing information for μ_3 or a contrast involving μ_3 is substantially lower, because of the high correlations between Y_3 and the completely observed variables Y_1 and Y_2. The rate of missing information for μ_3, a contrast involving μ_3 or any other function of θ may be estimated in a straightforward manner by multiple imputation; see Section 6.2.1.

5.3.7 Example: changes in heart rate due to marijuana use

Weil et al. (1968) describe a pilot study to investigate the clinical and psychological effects of marijuana use in human subjects. Nine

Table 5.2. *Change in heart rate recorded 15 and 90 minutes after marijuana use, measured in beats per minute above baseline*

Subject	15 minutes			90 minutes		
	Placebo	Low	High	Placebo	Low	High
1	16	20	16	20	−6	−4
2	12	24	12	−6	4	−8
3	8	8	26	−4	4	8
4	20	8	—	—	20	−4
5	8	4	−8	—	22	−8
6	10	20	28	−20	−4	−4
7	4	28	24	12	8	18
8	−8	20	24	−3	8	−24
9	—	20	24	8	12	—
mean	8.8	16.9	18.2	1.0	7.6	−3.2

Source: Weil *et al.* (1968)

healthy male subjects, all of whom claimed never to have used marijuana before, received doses in the form of cigarettes of uniform size. Each subject received each of the three treatments (low dose, high dose and placebo) and the order of treatments within subjects was balanced in a replicated 3×3 Latin square. Changes in heart rate for the $n = 9$ subjects measured 15 and 90 minutes after the smoking session are displayed in Table 5.2. Because the article does not specify the order in which the treatments were given to the individual subjects, we will ignore this feature of the data and proceed as if the order effects are negligible.

At first glance, it appears that missing data are only a minor problem here; only 5 of the 54 data values are missing. Yet, the EM algorithm converges very slowly. Depending on the starting values and convergence criterion, several hundred iterations may be needed to obtain convergence. The elementwise rates of convergence indicate that the largest fraction of missing information is approximately 97%. Moreover, the ML estimate of θ lies on the boundary of the parameter space. The ML estimates of the means, standard deviations and correlations are displayed in Table 5.3, along with the eigenvalues of the estimated correlation matrix. The smallest eigenvalue is zero to three decimal places, indicating that the estimated covariance matrix is singular or nearly so.

Why do so few missing values create such difficulty in this ex-

Table 5.3. *ML estimates of means, standard deviations and correlations for the columns of Table 5.2, with eigenvalues of the estimated correlation matrix*

(a) Means

7.38	16.90	14.00	10.60	7.56	−2.58

(b) Standard deviations

8.47	7.72	15.90	21.50	8.98	11.50

(c) Correlation matrix

1.000	−0.301	−0.565	0.385	−0.083	0.211
	1.000	0.620	−0.545	−0.558	0.150
		1.000	−0.860	−0.707	0.199
			1.000	0.705	0.024
				1.000	−0.059
					1.000

(d) Eigenvalues

3.186	1.262	0.890	0.498	0.165	0.000

ample? There are two primary reasons. First, the incomplete cases appear to be very influential. A comparison of the ML estimates of the means in Table 5.3 (a) with the means of the observed data in the columns of Table 5.2 is quite revealing. The large discrepancy for the fourth column (10.6 versus 1.0) demonstrates that a disproportionate amount of information about the mean for that column is provided by subjects 4 and 5. Further examination of Table 5.2 reveals that these two subjects have rather extreme values in some of the other columns, which gives them high leverage. When these two subjects are deleted, EM converges rapidly and the estimated largest fraction of missing information drops to 45%.

A second reason why this example is problematic is that the complete-data estimation problem is poorly conditioned. The number of subjects $n = 9$ is not much greater than the number of variables $p = 6$. When n and p are nearly equal, it becomes likely that certain linear combinations of the columns of Y will show little or no variability, particularly when the columns are correlated. The multivariate normal model for this example has 27 parameters, too many to be estimated well from a dataset of this size even with complete data. Although certain aspects of θ are poorly estimated, however, we can still make reasonable inferences about the parameters of interest; see Section 5.4.4.

5.4 Data augmentation

5.4.1 The I-step

Data augmentation for incomplete multivariate normal data is remarkably similar to the EM algorithm. The deterministic E- and M-steps are replaced by stochastic I- and P-steps, respectively, where the I-step simulates

$$Y_{mis}^{(t+1)} \sim P(Y_{mis} \mid Y_{obs}, \theta^{(t)}),$$

and the P-step simulates

$$\theta^{(t+1)} \sim P(\theta \mid Y_{obs}, Y_{mis}^{(t+1)}).$$

Because the rows $y_1, y_2, \ldots, y_n$ of Y are conditionally independent given θ, the I-step is carried out by drawing

$$y_{i(mis)}^{(t+1)} \sim P(y_{i(mis)} \mid y_{i(obs)}, \theta^{(t)})$$

independently for $i = 1, 2, \ldots, n$. As discussed in Section 5.3.2, if row i is in missingness pattern s then the conditional distribution of $y_{i(mis)}$ given $y_{i(obs)}$ and θ is multivariate normal with means

$$E(y_{ij} \mid Y_{obs}, \theta) = a_{0j} + \sum_{k \in \mathcal{O}(s)} a_{kj} y_{ik} \qquad (5.39)$$

and covariances

$$\text{Cov}(y_{ij}, y_{ik} \mid Y_{obs}, \theta) = a_{jk} \qquad (5.40)$$

for $j, k \in \mathcal{M}(s)$, where a_{jk} denotes an element of the matrix

$$A = \text{SWP}[\mathcal{O}(s)]\, \theta. \qquad (5.41)$$

Thus the I-step of data augmentation involves nothing more than the independent simulation of random normal vectors for each row of the data matrix, with means and covariances given by (5.39) and (5.40).

A convenient way to simulate random normal vectors within the I-step is to create a *Cholesky factorization* routine that operates

$$\boxed{\begin{array}{l} \textbf{for } i \in \mathcal{S} \textbf{ do} \\[4pt] \quad a_{ii} := \left(a_{ii} - \sum_{k \in \mathcal{S}, k < i} a_{ki}^2 \right)^{1/2} \\[6pt] \quad \textbf{for } j \in \mathcal{S},\, j > i \textbf{ do} \\[4pt] \qquad a_{ij} := a_{ii}^{-1} \left(a_{ij} - \sum_{k \in \mathcal{S}, k < i} a_{ki} a_{kj} \right) \\[6pt] \quad \textbf{end do} \\[2pt] \textbf{end do} \end{array}}$$

Figure 5.5. *Calculation of* $A := \text{Chol}_{\mathcal{S}} A$.

on square submatrices of (5.41). The Cholesky factor of a positive definite matrix A, denoted by

$$C = \text{Chol}\, A,$$

is an upper-triangular matrix of the same dimension of A having the property that $C^T C = A$. To simulate a random vector z from $N(b, A)$, we may take

$$z = b + (\text{Chol}\, A)^T z_0,$$

where z_0 is a vector of the same length as z containing independent standard normal variates. A typical Cholesky factorization routine operates on the upper-triangular portion of a symmetric matrix, overwriting it with its Cholesky factor. To draw from the distribution of $y_{i(mis)}$ given $y_{i(obs)}$ and θ, however, we need to calculate the Cholesky factor of only the square submatrix of (5.41) corresponding to the rows and columns in $\mathcal{M}(s)$. For a set $\mathcal{S}$ of row labels of a matrix A, let us use

$$A := \text{Chol}_{\mathcal{S}} A \tag{5.42}$$

to indicate the operation that overwrites (the upper triangular portion of) the square submatrix $\{a_{jk} : j, k \in \mathcal{S}\}$ with its Cholesky factor, while leaving the remaining elements of A unchanged. A simple algorithm for this operation, adapted from pseudocode given by Thisted (1988, p. 83), is shown in Figure 5.5.

Once the Cholesky factorization is available, the I-step becomes a simple matter of cycling through the missingness patterns $s = 1, \dots, S$, calculating

$$\text{Chol}_{\mathcal{M}(s)}\, \text{SWP}[\mathcal{O}(s)]\, \theta$$

for each s, and simulating $y_{i(mis)}$ for each $i \in \mathcal{I}(s)$. An implementation of the I-step is shown in Figure 5.6. The code simulates the

```
C   T := T_obs
    for s := 1 to S do
        for j := 1 to p do
            if r_sj = 1 and θ_jj > 0 then θ := SWP[j] θ
            if r_sj = 0 and θ_jj < 0 then θ := RSW[j] θ
            end do
        C := Chol_M(s) θ
        for i ∈ I(s) do
            for j ∈ M(s) do
                y_ij := θ_0j
                for k ∈ O(s) do y_ij := y_ij + θ_kj y_ik
                draw z_j ~ N(0,1)
                for k ∈ M(s) and k ≤ j do y_ij := y_ij + C_kj z_k
C               T_0j := T_0j + y_ij
C               for k ∈ O(s) do T_kj := T_kj + y_ij y_ik
C               for k ∈ M(s) and k ≤ j do T_kj := T_kj + y_ij y_ik
                end do
            end do
        end do
    end do
```

Figure 5.6. *I-step for incomplete multivariate normal data.*

missing values in Y_{mis} and stores them in the appropriate elements of Y. In addition, the code contains four lines preceded by the single character 'C' which accumulate the simulated complete-data sufficient statistics and store them in a $(p+1) \times (p+1)$ matrix workspace T. If the I-step is to be followed by a P-step, then these sufficient statistics will be needed to describe the complete-data posterior distribution of θ. If the I-step will not be followed by a P-step (e.g. if it is the final step of a chain for producing an imputation of Y_{mis}) then these four lines may be omitted. The code in Figure 5.5 requires two temporary workspaces: a $p \times p$ matrix C for storing Cholesky factors, and a $p \times 1$ vector z for holding simulated $N(0,1)$ variates.

5.4.2 The P-step

Under the prior distributions discussed in Sections 5.2.2 and 5.2.3, the complete data posterior $P(\theta \mid Y_{obs}, Y_{mis})$ is a normal inverted-Wishart distribution. The P-step of data augmentation, therefore, is merely a simulation of the normal inverted-Wishart distribution,

$$\mu \mid \Sigma \;\; \sim \;\; N(\mu_0, \tau^{-1}\Sigma),$$
$$\Sigma \;\; \sim \;\; W^{-1}(m, \Lambda),$$

for some $(\tau, m, \mu_0, \Lambda)$ determined by the prior, the observed data Y_{obs} and the missing data $Y_{mis}^{(t)}$ imputed at the last I-step. The specific values of $(\tau, m, \mu_0, \Lambda)$ are calculated using the formulas for updating hyperparameters given in Section 5.2.2.

The most obvious way to generate $\Sigma \sim W^{-1}(m, \Lambda)$ is to take $\Sigma = (X^T X)^{-1}$, where X is an $m \times p$ random matrix whose rows are independent draws from $N(0, \Lambda)$. This method cannot be used for non-integer values of m, however, and may be cumbersome for large m because it requires mp random variates. More efficient methods for generating random Wishart matrices are available that require simulation of only $p(p + 1)/2$ random variates. One such method relies on a characterization of the Wishart distribution known as the *Bartlett decomposition* (e.g. Muirhead, 1982). If $A \sim W(m, I)$ where I is a $p \times p$ identity matrix and $m \geq p$, then we can write $A = B^T B$ where B is an upper-triangular matrix whose elements are independently distributed as

$$b_{jj} \;\; \sim \;\; \sqrt{\chi^2_{m-j+1}}, \quad j = 1, \ldots, p, \tag{5.43}$$
$$b_{jk} \;\; \sim \;\; N(0, 1), \quad j < k. \tag{5.44}$$

Suppose that we generate an upper-triangular matrix B according to (5.43)–(5.44), so that $B^T B \sim W(m, I)$, and take

$$M \;=\; (B^T)^{-1} C,$$

where C is the Cholesky factor of Λ^{-1} (i.e. $C^T C = \Lambda^{-1}$). Then $\Sigma = M^T M$ will be distributed as $W^{-1}(m, \Lambda)$, because

$$(M^T M)^{-1} \;=\; C^{-1} B^T B (C^T)^{-1}$$
$$\sim \;\; W(m, (C^T C)^{-1}).$$

(Here we have made use of the property that $D \sim W(n, \Gamma)$ implies $C^T D C \sim W(n, C^T \Gamma C)$, which follows immediately from the definition of the Wishart distribution.) Moreover, taking

$$\mu \;=\; \mu_0 + \tau^{-1/2} M^T z,$$

where $z \sim N(0, I)$ is a $p \times 1$ vector of independent standard normal variates, results in $\mu \mid \Sigma \sim N(\mu_0, \tau^{-1}\Sigma)$. This method requires the inversion of only the triangular matrix B^T, which can be accomplished via a simple backsolving operation. Note that with the exception of M, all matrices used here are either symmetric or triangular, so memory requirements can be reduced by retaining only their upper-triangular portions in packed storage.

5.4.3 Example: cholesterol levels of heart-attack patients

Recall the example of Section 5.3.6 in which cholesterol measurements were recorded for patients 2, 4 and 14 days after heart attack. The EM algorithm converged rapidly with an estimated largest fraction of missing information equal to 47%. We applied data augmentation to this example under the noninformative prior (5.18). Output analysis from preliminary runs suggested that the data augmentation algorithm also converged rapidly. For illustration, we ran a single chain for 1100 iterations starting from the ML estimate of θ, discarded the first 100 iterations, and estimated ACFs for a variety of scalar functions of θ over the remaining 1000 iterations. We deliberately chose functions of θ for which the rates of missing information were thought to be high, including:

1. μ_3 and $\sigma_3 = \sqrt{\sigma_{33}}$, the mean and standard deviation of Y_3, respectively;

2. the parameters of the linear regression of Y_3 on Y_1 and Y_2, including the slopes

$$
\begin{bmatrix} \beta_{31\cdot 12} \\ \beta_{32\cdot 12} \end{bmatrix}^T = \begin{bmatrix} \sigma_{31} & \sigma_{32} \end{bmatrix} \begin{bmatrix} \sigma_{11} & \sigma_{12} \\ \sigma_{21} & \sigma_{22} \end{bmatrix}^{-1},
$$

the intercept

$$
\beta_{30\cdot 12} = \mu_3 - \begin{bmatrix} \sigma_{31} & \sigma_{32} \end{bmatrix} \begin{bmatrix} \sigma_{11} & \sigma_{12} \\ \sigma_{21} & \sigma_{22} \end{bmatrix}^{-1} \begin{bmatrix} \mu_1 \\ \mu_2 \end{bmatrix},
$$

and the residual standard deviation $\sigma_{3\cdot 12} = \sqrt{\sigma_{33\cdot 12}}$, where

$$
\sigma_{33\cdot 12} = \sigma_{33} - \begin{bmatrix} \sigma_{31} & \sigma_{32} \end{bmatrix} \begin{bmatrix} \sigma_{11} & \sigma_{12} \\ \sigma_{21} & \sigma_{22} \end{bmatrix}^{-1} \begin{bmatrix} \sigma_{13} \\ \sigma_{23} \end{bmatrix};
$$

and

3. the worst linear function $\xi = \xi(\theta)$ estimated from the final iterations of EM, as described in Section 4.4.3. This is the inner product of θ and the estimated eigenvector corresponding to the largest eigenvalue of EM's asymptotic rate matrix. Because there are no missing values on Y_1 or Y_2, ξ is a weighted sum of μ_3, σ_{13}, σ_{23} and σ_{33}, where the weights are the perturbations from the ML estimates in the final iterations of EM.

Table 5.4. *Sample ACFs of selected scalar parameters estimated over iterations of data augmentation*

lag	μ_3	σ_3	$\beta_{30\cdot12}$	$\beta_{31\cdot12}$	$\beta_{32\cdot12}$	$\sigma_{3\cdot12}$	ξ
0	1.00	1.00	1.00	1.00	1.00	1.00	1.00
1	.18*	.31*	.37*	.33*	.44*	.35*	.25*
2	.04	.19*	.18*	.09*	.19*	.15*	.17*
3	.02	.07*	.10*	.08*	.10*	.05	.06
4	−.02	.09*	.05	.03	.06	.05	.08*
5	−.01	.11*	.02	−.01	.04	.05	.09*
6	−.01	.09*	.06	−.01	.06	.06	.07*
7	.04	.05*	.03	−.08*	.01	.03	.04
8	.01	.04	.02	−.10*	−.02	.05	.04
9	.03	.08*	.04	−.02	−.02	.04	.07*
10	.05	.04	.03	.02	−.02	.02	.04
11	−.06	.07	.01	.04	.03	−.03	.07
12	.01	.07*	.04	.06	.05	.02	.06
13	.02	.07	.00	−.01	.08	.04	.07
14	−.01	.08*	−.01	.00	.09*	.02	.09*
15	−.02	−.02	.04	.04	.04	.00	−.01
16	−.02	.02	.02	.02	.06	−.03	.02
17	.02	.01	−.03	.00	.07	−.04	.01
18	.00	−.02	−.02	−.01	.04	−.06	−.02
19	−.03	−.01	.04	.02	.01	−.05	−.01
20	.05	.00	.02	.05	.01	−.03	.01

* significantly different from zero at the 0.05 level

Sample ACFs for these functions of θ up to lag 20 are displayed in Table 5.4. Correlations that are significantly different from zero at the 0.05 level, as determined by Bartlett's formula (4.49), are marked with an asterisk. Because the series is so long and the serial dependence is not high, the standard errors are small and even very small correlations are deemed significant. Even for the worst functions examined, however, the correlations are effectively zero by lag 10, and definitely negligible by lag 20. Time-series plots of these functions showed no unusual features and resembled those of the rapidly-converging series displayed in Figure 4.2 (a) and (b). Based on this evidence, we feel safe in concluding that the algorithm effectively achieves stationarity by 20 iterations.

The parameters of greatest interest in this problem are functions of $\mu = (\mu_1, \mu_2, \mu_3)^T$. For illustration, we will focus attention on three quantities: μ_3, the average cholesterol level at 14 days;

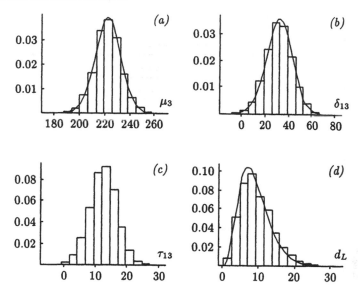

Figure 5.7. *Histograms of sample values of (a) μ_3, (b) δ_{13}, (c) τ_{13} and (d) d_L from 5000 consecutive iterations of data augmentation.*

$\delta_{13} = \mu_1 - \mu_3$, the average decrease in cholesterol level from day 2 to day 14; and $\tau_{13} = 100(\mu_1 - \mu_3)/\mu_1$, the relative percentage decrease in average cholesterol level from day 2 to day 14. To draw inferences about these quantities, we simulated another single chain of 5100 iterations starting from the ML estimate, discarded the first 100, and saved the 5000 remaining values of μ_3, δ_{13} and τ_{13}. Histograms of the sample values for these three quantities are shown in Figure 5.7 (a)–(c). Because μ_3 and δ_{13} are linear combinations of the elements of μ, obtaining Rao-Blackwellized estimates of the marginal densities of these quantities is straightforward. Under the prior (5.18), the complete-data posterior is given by (5.19)–(5.20). Using (5.17), it follows that the complete-data posterior density of a linear combination $\eta = a^T\mu$ is

$$P(\eta\,|\,Y_{obs}, Y_{mis}) \;=\; k\left[1 + \frac{(\eta - a^T\bar{y})^2}{(n-p)\sigma^2}\right]^{-(n-p+1)/2}, \qquad (5.45)$$

where $n = 28$ and $p = 3$ are the number of observations and variables, respectively; $\sigma^2 = (n-p)^{-1}a^T S a$; $\bar{y}$ and S are the sample mean vector (5.5) and covariance matrix (5.6) computed from

$Y = (Y_{obs}, Y_{mis})$; and

$$k = \frac{\Gamma\left(\frac{n-p+1}{2}\right)}{\Gamma\left(\frac{n-p}{2}\right)\sqrt{\pi(n-p)\sigma^2}} .$$

Rao-Blackwellized density estimates for $\mu_3 = (0, 0, 1)\mu$ and $\delta_{13} = (1, 0, -1)\mu$ estimated from the first 1000 iterations after the initial burn-in period are shown superimposed over the histograms in Figure 5.7 (a) and (b). Because τ_{13} is nonlinear its density is somewhat less easy to find, and Rao-Blackwellized estimates for this quantity are not shown.

In addition to μ_3, δ_{13} and τ_{13}, we also calculated and stored values of the likelihood-ratio statistic

$$d_L = d_L(\theta) = 2[l(\hat{\theta}|Y_{obs}) - l(\theta|Y_{obs})]$$

over the 5000 iterations, where $\hat{\theta}$ is the ML estimate. For large samples, the posterior distribution of d_L is approximately χ_d^2, where d is the dimension of θ (in this case, 9). A histogram of the sample values of d_L is displayed in Figure 5.7 (d) with the χ_9^2 density function superimposed over it, showing that the actual posterior matches the theoretical approximation quite closely.

Simulated posterior means for μ_3, δ_{13} and τ_{13} were found by averaging the 5000 iterates of each parameter. Simulated 95% posterior intervals were found by calculating the 2.5 and 97.5 percentiles of each sample using (4.8). To obtain a rough assessment of the random error in these estimates, a second chain was generated in an identical fashion with a different random-number generator seed. The simulated posterior means and 95% intervals (in parentheses) for the two replicate runs are shown below.

μ_3	δ_{13}	τ_{13}
222.2	31.8	12.4
(201.6, 244.0)	(8.9, 55.4)	(3.7, 20.9)
222.4	31.4	12.3
(201.7, 242.6)	(8.9, 53.3)	(3.7, 20.3)

Inferences about μ_3, δ_{13} and τ_{13} can also be conducted through multiple imputation. This will be demonstrated in Section 6.2.1.

5.4.4 Example: changes in heart rate due to marijuana use

Returning to the data in Table 5.2, let μ_j denote the population mean corresponding to column j, and let $\delta_{jk} = \mu_j - \mu_k$, $j, k = 1, \ldots, 6$. Following the original article be Weil *et al.* (1968), we will focus attention on the six treatment comparisons below.

15 minutes		90 minutes	
Low vs. Placebo	δ_{21}	Low vs. Placebo	δ_{54}
High vs. Placebo	δ_{31}	High vs. Placebo	δ_{64}
High vs. Low	δ_{32}	High vs. Low	δ_{65}

Data augmentation under the usual noninformative prior (5.18) does not work for this problem; the iterates of θ quickly wander to the boundary of the parameter space, causing numeric overflow. This pathological behavior suggests that the posterior is not proper. To stabilize the inference, we applied a ridge prior as described in Sections 5.2.3 and 5.3.4. After centering and scaling the columns of Y so that the observed data in each column have mean zero and unit variance, we set the hyperparameters of the normal inverted-Wishart prior to $\tau = 0$, $m = \epsilon$ and $\Lambda^{-1} = \epsilon I$ for $\epsilon = 0.5$. Under this weak prior, EM converges slowly but reliably to a posterior mode in the interior of the parameter space, with the largest fraction of missing information estimated at 95%.

The slow convergence of EM in this example suggests that data augmentation will also converge slowly, and output analysis from a preliminary run confirmed this. Using the same ridge prior, we simulated a single chain beginning at the posterior mode and monitored a variety of scalar summaries of θ. Time-series plots for δ_{21} and δ_{54} (on the original scale) from the first 100 iterations are shown in Figure 5.8 (a) and (b), respectively. The iterates of δ_{21} appear to approach stationarity quickly, whereas the series for δ_{54} shows long-range dependence. This is not surprising, because δ_{54} is a function of μ_4, and our earlier analysis led us to conjecture that the rate of missing information for μ_4 was very high. Sample ACFs for δ_{21} and δ_{54} estimated from 10 000 iterations are displayed in Figure 5.8 (c) and (d), respectively. Figure 5.8 (d) is typical of the ACFs for other slowly converging functions of θ. For all the functions we examined, the serial correlations effectively died out by lag 50.

The slow convergence in this example should lead us to use extra caution in designing the simulation experiment. Running independent chains from overdispersed starting values would be attractive,

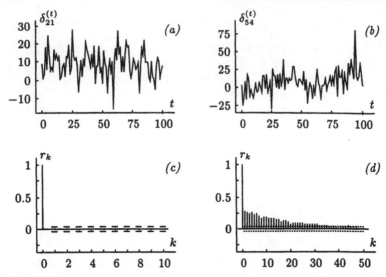

Figure 5.8. *Time-series plots of (a)* δ_{21} *and (b)* δ_{54} *over the first 100 iterations of data augmentation, and sample ACFs for (c)* δ_{21} *and (d)* δ_{54} *estimated from 10 000 iterations, with dashes indicating approximate 0.05-level critical values for testing* $\rho_k = \rho_{k+1} = \cdots = 0$.

but obtaining overdispersed starting values is not easy. Bootstrap resampling is unlikely to work well, because n is not much larger than p, so the distribution of $\hat{\theta}$ over bootstrap samples will probably bear little resemblance to the observed-data posterior. Sampling from the prior is not possible, because the prior is not a proper probability distribution. Because convergence to stationarity tends to be fastest when the starting value is near the center of the observed-data posterior, we decided to run ten independent chains of 5500 iterations each, starting each chain at the posterior mode. After discarding the first 500 values from each chain, the pth sample quantile for each contrast δ_{jk} was calculated for $p = 0.025$, 0.25, 0.5, 0.75 and 0.975 from the remaining 5000 values. Finally, the sample quantiles were averaged across the ten chains. For each of these averages, the variance of the quantiles across chains was used to estimate a standard error with nine degrees of freedom. The estimated quantiles for all six parameters are displayed in Figure 5.9. All of the simulated 95% posterior intervals cover zero, indicating that there is no strong evidence that any of the contrasts is different from zero. Standard errors for the simulated quantiles

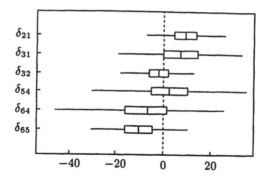

Figure 5.9. *Simulated posterior medians, quartiles and 95% equal-tailed intervals for six contrasts.*

ranged from 0.02 to 0.72, which is quite small relative to the width of the intervals displayed in Figure 5.9, so these simulation results are sharp enough for our purposes.

One could very well argue that the unrestricted multivariate normal model has too many parameters to be estimated from a dataset of this size, and that the unnecessarily large number of nuisance parameters hinders us from making clear inferences about the parameters of interest. Indeed, the long tails exhibited in the marginal posteriors of Figure 5.9, particularly for the two contrasts involving μ_4, suggest that some of the nuisance parameters are very poorly estimated, and we might do well to simplify the model. One possible simplification is to reduce the number of free parameters by applying a priori constraints to Σ. For example, we could require Σ to satisfy the condition of *compound symmetry* (i.e. equal diagonal elements and equal off-diagonal elements). Simulation algorithms for incomplete multivariate normal data with constrained covariance structure are possible, but they are beyond the scope of this book. A slightly different approach would be to specify fixed, additive effects for the rows and columns of the data matrix, and define the parameters of interest to be contrasts among the column effects (Chapter 9).

Yet another possibility is to perform a simple bivariate analysis for each contrast, making inferences about δ_{jk} using only the data in columns j and k. Under this bivariate approach, it is no longer possible to make joint inferences about the contrasts. Moreover, ignoring the data in columns other than j and k when making inferences about δ_{jk} may tend to introduce nonresponse biases;

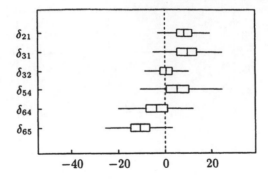

Figure 5.10. *Simulated posterior medians, quartiles and 95% equal-tailed intervals for six contrasts using a bivariate approach.*

the MAR assumption tends to be less plausible for the bivariate dataset than for the one with six variables. The decision whether to include additional variables in an analysis is not always an easy one, particularly for small datasets, and is an important topic worthy of further research.

Simulated posterior quantiles from a bivariate analysis are shown in Figure 5.10. For each contrast, data augmentation was applied to the bivariate dataset under the standard noninformative prior (5.18). Output analyses suggested that convergence to stationarity was rapid. For each contrast, 10 100 steps of a single Markov chain were simulated, beginning from the ML estimate. The first 100 values of the simulated contrast were discarded, and sample quantiles were calculated from the remaining 10 000. The distributions in Figure 5.10 are much narrower than those in Figure 5.9, and there is now a fair amount of evidence that the three contrasts δ_{21}, δ_{31} and δ_{65} are nonzero.

CHAPTER 6

More on the normal model

6.1 Introduction

In the last chapter, we introduced EM and data augmentation algorithms for the multivariate normal model. In this chapter, we illustrate how to effectively apply these algorithms with more real-data examples, and discuss modifications to the algorithms that can help to increase their efficiency.

Sections 6.2 and 6.3 present two examples of analysis by multiple imputation. The first, which was previously analyzed in Chapter 5 by parameter simulation, is straightforward and illustrates some of the basic properties of multiple-imputation point and interval estimates. The second is more complicated, involving categorical variables and inestimable parameters. By working through this second example, the reader will come to understand some of the complications and subtle issues that often arise with real data, and learn strategies for effectively dealing with these issues.

Real data often do not conform to normality, and it is important to know whether the multiple-imputation procedures advocated in this book are robust to departures from the modeling assumptions. Section 6.4 presents a simulation experiment to demonstrate the robustness of multiple imputation in a realistic setting.

When rates of missing information are high, EM and data augmentation tend to converge slowly. Section 6.5 presents a new class of simulation algorithms, called monotone data augmentation, that tend to converge quickly under certain types of missingness.

6.2 Multiple imputation: example 1

6.2.1 Cholesterol levels of heart-attack patients

Recall the example introduced in Section 5.3.6 in which serum cholesterol levels for heart-attack patients were recorded 2 days

(Y_1), 4 days (Y_2) and 14 days (Y_3) after attack. Nine of the $n = 28$ values of Y_3 were missing. In Section 5.4.3, we used data augmentation to simulate posterior distributions for three parameters of interest:

1. μ_3, the mean cholesterol level at 14 days;

2. $\delta_{13} = \mu_1 - \mu_3$, the average decrease in cholesterol level from day 2 to day 14; and

3. $\tau_{13} = 100(\mu_1 - \mu_3)/\mu_1$, the percentage decrease in cholesterol level from day 2 to day 14.

We now demonstrate how inferences for these same quantities can be conducted by multiple imputation.

6.2.2 Generating the imputations

Recall that proper multiple imputations are independent draws of Y_{mis} from the posterior predictive distribution of the missing data, $P(Y_{mis} \mid Y_{obs})$. The exploratory run of data augmentation revealed no discernible autocorrelations in scalar functions of θ beyond lag 10. Thus we can probably obtain acceptable imputations by (a) running data augmentation in a single chain starting from the MLE, and taking every tenth iterate of Y_{mis} as an imputation; or (b) running independent, parallel chains of ten iterations each starting from the MLE, and taking the final value of Y_{mis} from each chain as an imputation.

Because of the small size of this dataset, however, iterations are computationally inexpensive, and we can easily afford to increase the number of steps. To illustrate a conservative approach, we generated $m = 5$ multiple imputations by simulating five independent chains of 50 steps each. Independent starting values for the chains were obtained by running EM on independent bootstrap samples of size $n/2 = 14$ (Section 4.4.2). These starting values are probably overdispersed relative to the observed-data posterior $P(\theta \mid Y_{obs})$, so that in the unlikely event that stationarity has not been achieved by 50 steps, the resulting inferences will tend to be conservative. The $m = 5$ sets of imputed values for Y_3, rounded to integers, are displayed in Table 6.1.

6.2.3 Complete-data point and variance estimates

Multiple imputation requires that for each estimand Q we specify a complete-data point estimate $\hat{Q}$ and a complete-data variance

Table 6.1. *Cholesterol levels for heart-attack patients measured 2, 4 and 14 days after attack, with* $m = 5$ *multiple imputations*

Observed data			Imputed values for Y_3				
Y_1	Y_2	Y_3	1	2	3	4	5
270	218	156					
236	234	—	186	259	200	259	227
210	214	242					
142	116	—	238	50	116	133	197
280	200	—	187	190	186	222	169
272	276	256					
160	146	142					
220	182	216					
226	238	248					
242	288	—	243	264	295	234	215
186	190	168					
266	236	236					
206	244	—	264	169	295	197	246
318	258	200					
294	240	264					
282	294	—	254	257	303	230	302
234	220	264					
224	200	—	166	217	201	188	190
276	220	188					
282	186	182					
360	352	294					
310	202	214					
280	218	—	242	201	231	217	187
278	248	198					
288	278	—	209	319	259	235	228
288	248	256					
244	270	280					
236	242	204					

Source of observed data: Ryan and Joiner (1994)

estimate U. It also requires a sample size large enough for the approximation

$$\frac{\hat{Q} - Q}{\sqrt{U}} \sim N(0, 1) \tag{6.1}$$

to work well with complete data. Let

$$\bar{y}_j = \frac{1}{n} \sum_{i=1}^{n} y_{ij} \quad \text{and} \quad S_{jk} = \frac{1}{n-1} \sum_{i=1}^{n} (y_{ij} - \bar{y}_j)(y_{ik} - \bar{y}_k)$$

for $j, k = 1, 2, 3$ denote the complete-data sample means and covariances. For μ_3, the obvious complete-data estimates are $\hat{Q} = \bar{y}_3$ and $U = S_{33}/n$. For $\delta_{13} = \mu_1 - \mu_3$, the obvious choices are

$$\begin{aligned} \hat{Q} &= \bar{y}_1 - \bar{y}_3, \\ U &= (S_{11} - 2S_{13} + S_{33})/n. \end{aligned}$$

Asymptotic normality of $\bar{y}_3$ and $\bar{y}_1 - \bar{y}_3$ is guaranteed by the Central Limit Theorem, and a sample of size $n = 28$ should be large enough for the normal approximations to work well.

For the nonlinear parameter $\tau_{13} = 100(\mu_1 - \mu_3)/\mu_1$, a first-order Taylor expansion of the function $(\bar{y}_1 - \bar{y}_3)/\bar{y}_1$ about (μ_1, μ_3),

$$\frac{\bar{y}_1 - \bar{y}_3}{\bar{y}_1} - \frac{\mu_1 - \mu_3}{\mu_1} \approx \frac{\mu_3}{\mu_1^2}(\bar{y}_1 - \mu_1) - \frac{1}{\mu_1}(\bar{y}_3 - \mu_3),$$

suggests that the complete-data point estimate

$$\hat{Q} = 100(\bar{y}_1 - \bar{y}_3)/\bar{y}_1$$

will be approximately unbiased for τ_{13}, with approximate variance

$$V(\hat{Q}) \approx \frac{100^2}{n} \left[\left(\frac{\mu_3^2}{\mu_1^4}\right) \sigma_{11} - 2\left(\frac{\mu_3}{\mu_1^3}\right) \sigma_{13} + \left(\frac{1}{\mu_1^2}\right) \sigma_{33} \right].$$

A reasonable complete-data variance estimate is thus

$$U = \frac{100^2}{n} \left[\left(\frac{\bar{y}_3^2}{\bar{y}_1^4}\right) S_{11} - 2\left(\frac{\bar{y}_3}{\bar{y}_1^3}\right) S_{13} + \left(\frac{1}{\bar{y}_1^2}\right) S_{33} \right].$$

A handy rule-of-thumb used by survey statisticians is that a ratio of sample means will be approximately unbiased and normally distributed if the coefficient of variation (the standard deviation divided by the mean) of the denominator is 10% or less (e.g. Cochran, 1977, p. 166). The observed values of Y_1 in Table 6.1 have a mean and standard deviation of 253.9 and 47.7, respectively, so the estimated coefficient of variation for $\bar{y}_1$ is $(47.7/\sqrt{28})/253.9 = 0.036$, suggesting that the normal approximation should work well.

Table 6.2. *Complete-data point estimates and standard errors for μ_3, δ_{13} and τ_{13} from $m = 5$ multiply-imputed datasets*

	μ_3		δ_{13}		τ_{13}	
t	$\hat{Q}^{(t)}$	$\sqrt{U^{(t)}}$	$\hat{Q}^{(t)}$	$\sqrt{U^{(t)}}$	$\hat{Q}^{(t)}$	$\sqrt{U^{(t)}}$
1	221.3	7.56	32.61	10.21	12.84	3.72
2	219.1	10.35	34.86	9.34	13.73	3.53
3	224.8	9.31	29.14	9.97	11.48	3.73
4	218.7	7.69	35.25	8.39	13.88	3.03
5	220.3	7.82	33.61	9.83	13.23	3.58

Following the notation of Section 4.3.2, let $\hat{Q}^{(t)}$ and $U^{(t)}$ denote the complete-data point and variance estimates from the tth imputed dataset. Point and variance estimates for μ_1, δ_{13} and τ_{13} over the five imputations are displayed in Table 6.2.

6.2.4 Combining the estimates

Combining the complete-data point and interval estimates is a straightforward application of the formulas in Section 4.3.2 for inference with a scalar estimand. The overall estimates $\bar{Q}$, standard errors $\sqrt{T}$, degrees of freedom ν for the t-approximation and 95% interval estimates are displayed in Table 6.3. The values of ν are large, suggesting that the total variance estimates T are stable even though they are based on only $m = 5$ imputations. The point and interval estimates in Table 6.3 differ somewhat from those obtained by parameter simulation in Section 5.4.3, but the differences are mild relative to the sizes of the standard errors.

Table 6.3 also displays two diagnostics described in Section 4.3.2: the relative increase in variance due to nonresponse r, and the estimated fraction of missing information $\hat{\lambda}$. Although 32% of the Y_3 values are missing, the estimated rates of missing information for μ_3, δ_{13} and τ_{13} are under 10%, due undoubtedly to the correlations between Y_3 and the two variables that are never missing.

6.2.5 Alternative choices for the number of imputations

For this analysis we chose $m = 5$ imputations, because we knew that the fractions of missing information would not be severe. Recall that if the fraction of missing information for a parameter is λ, the relative efficiency of an estimate based on m imputations to one

Table 6.3. *Results of multiple-imputation inference for* μ_1, δ_{13} *and* τ_{13}

	$\bar{Q}$	$\sqrt{T}$	ν	95% interval	$100r$	$100\hat{\lambda}$
μ_3	220.8	9.02	517	(203.1, 238.6)	9.6	9.1
δ_{13}	33.09	9.94	760	(13.59, 52.60)	7.8	7.5
τ_{13}	13.03	3.68	595	(5.80, 20.26)	8.9	8.5

based on an infinite number is approximately $(1+\lambda/m)^{-1}$ (Section 4.3.1). From EM we learned that the worst fraction of missing information for this problem was about 47% (Section 5.3.6). Thus in the worst case, $m = 5$ would lead to a point estimate that is about $(1 + 0.47/5)^{-1} = 91\%$ as efficient as one with $m = \infty$. In fact, the estimated fractions of missing information for the parameters of interest were about 10%, so the estimates from $m = 5$ imputations appear to be about $(1 + 0.1/5)^{-1} = 98\%$ efficient.

To those unaccustomed to multiple imputation, basing any conclusion on a Monte Carlo simulation with only $m = 5$ draws might seem risky. A critic might argue that with only five imputations, one or more 'bad' (i.e. highly unusual) imputations could exert an undue influence on the results. To illustrate the effect of increasing the size of m, we generated an additional 95 imputations in the manner described above, for a total of 100 imputations. We then calculated point and interval estimates based on $m = 3$, 5, 10, 20 and 100. For $m = 3$ we used the first 3 imputations; for $m = 5$ we used the first 5 imputations; and so on. Finally, to get a rough idea of the amount of random variation in the estimates, we replicated the entire experiment, generating another 100 imputations from a different random-number generator seed and calculating another set of estimates for $m = 3$, 5, 10, 20 and 100.

The point and interval estimates for the various values of m are displayed graphically in Figure 6.1. For comparison, Figure 6.1 also displays the results of the two parameter-simulation runs of length 5000 described in Section 5.4.3. The multiple-imputation (MI) intervals for $m = 3$ and $m = 5$ appear to have more random variation than the parameter-simulation (PS) intervals. By $m = 10$, however, the MI intervals appear to remarkably stable, and there is little random variation (relative to the widths of the intervals) in any of the results for $m = 10$, 20 or 100.

The variability for $m = 3$ and $m = 5$ does not mean that these

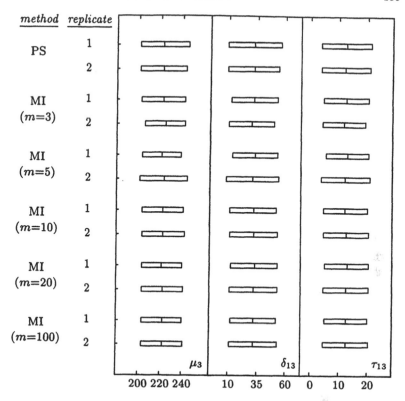

Figure 6.1. *Point and 95% interval estimates for* μ_3, δ_{13} *and* τ_{13} *from parameter simulation (PS) and multiple imputation (MI).*

intervals are unreliable. The intervals explicitly include simulation error as a component of uncertainty, and over repeated application they should still cover the true values of the parameters at least 95% of the time. To reduce random variation, one might consider increasing m, particularly if generating and storing imputations is not expensive. Based on Figure 6.1, however, there appears to be little reason to use more than $m = 10$ imputations for this problem.

Advantages of multiple imputation over parameter simulation

The PS estimates based on 5000 iterates of θ appear to be about as stable as MI estimates based on only $m = 10$ imputations of Y_{mis}. Notice, however, that the latter required only one-tenth as much

Table 6.4. *Estimated fractions of missing information from m=3, 5, 10, 20 and 100 imputations*

m	replicate	Parameter		
		μ_3	δ_{13}	τ_{13}
3	1	.13	.11	.12
3	2	.11	.09	.11
5	1	.09	.07	.08
5	2	.33	.29	.32
10	1	.11	.09	.10
10	2	.17	.15	.16
20	1	.15	.13	.14
20	2	.19	.16	.18
100	1	.16	.13	.14
100	2	.18	.15	.17

computation (500 steps of data augmentation versus 5000) and 0.6% as much storage ($10 \times 9 = 90$ locations to hold imputations of Y_{mis}, versus $5000 \times 3 = 15\,000$ to hold values of μ_3, δ_{13} and τ_{13}).

A further advantage of MI is that it provides an estimated fraction of missing information for each estimand. For small m, however, these estimates can be noisy. To illustrate, estimated fractions of missing information for μ_3, δ_{13} and τ_{13} based on $m = 3, 5, 10, 20,$ and 100 imputations (both replicates) are shown in Table 6.4. For small m the estimates vary substantially between replicates. This is to be expected, because they depend on the between-imputation components of variance which are estimated with only $m - 1$ degrees of freedom. Recall that our initial estimates of λ based on $m = 5$ imputations were all under 10% (Table 6.3); after increasing the value of m to 100, the estimates rose to 13–18%. Additional replications (not shown) demonstrate that even for $m = 100$, the estimates $\hat{\lambda}$ still have standard errors of approximately 0.02. Thus for small values of m, $\hat{\lambda}$ should be used only as a rough guide.

6.3 Multiple imputation: example 2

6.3.1 Predicting achievement in foreign language study.

Raymond (1987) describes data that were collected to investigate the usefulness of a newly developed instrument, the Foreign Lan-

Table 6.5. *Variables in foreign language achievement study, with number of missing values*

Variable	Description	Missing
LAN	foreign language studied (1=French, 2=Spanish, 3=German, 4=Russian)	0
AGE	age group (1=less than 20, 2=20–21, 3=22–23, 4=24–25, 5=26+)	11
PRI	Number of prior foreign language courses (1=none, 2=1, 3=2, 4=3, 5=4+)	11
SEX	1=male, 2=female	1
FLAS	score on foreign language attitude scale	0
MLAT	Modern Language Aptitude Test, fourth subtest score	49
SATV	Scholastic Aptitude Test, verbal score	34
SATM	Scholastic Aptitude Test, math score	34
ENG	score on Penn State English placement exam	37
HGPA	high school grade point average	1
CGPA	current college grade point average	34
GRD	final grade in foreign language course (4=A, 3=B, 2=C, 1=D, 0=F)	47

guage Attitude Scale (FLAS), for predicting success in the study of foreign languages. In particular, the investigators wanted to determine whether the FLAS had substantial predictive ability beyond that already provided by other well-established instruments such as the Modern Language Aptitude Test (MLAT). Twelve variables were collected for a sample of $n = 279$ students enrolled in foreign language courses at The Pennsylvania State University in the early 1980s (Raymond and Roberts, 1983). Descriptions of the variables, along with the number of missing values for each one, appear in Table 6.5. The raw data, kindly provided by Dr. Mark Raymond, are reproduced in Appendix A.

In this example, only 8% of all the values in the 279×12 data matrix are missing, and missingness rates per variable range from 0% to 18%. Only 62% of the cases (174 out of 279) have complete data for all twelve variables, however, so the case-deletion methods used by most statistical software packages would discard over one-

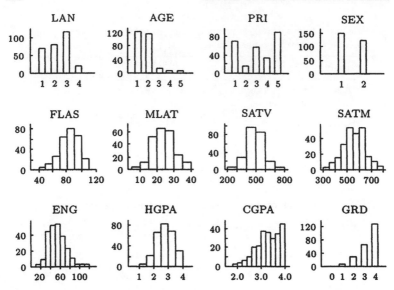

Figure 6.2. *Histograms of observed data for variables in foreign language achievement study.*

third of the entire dataset. Imputing for the missing values makes more efficient use of the available data.

6.3.2 Applying the normal model

Histograms of the observed values for each variable are displayed in Figure 6.2. Although these data clearly do not follow a multivariate normal distribution, we will still use the normal model for imputation. For the dichotomous and ordinal variables, we will impute under an assumption of normality and round off the continuous imputes to the nearest category. Examination of Figure 6.2 suggests that this strategy might not work well for AGE, PRI or GRD, because these variables are far from being symmetric and unimodal.

To make the variables AGE, PRI and GRD less troublesome, we recoded them by collapsing some adjacent categories. (In Chapter 9, when we are able to explicitly model mixed continuous and categorical data, we will analyze these data again without recoding.) An overwhelming majority of students received final grades of A or B; very few received C or below; the data provide relatively little information to characterize the C-or-below group, so we recoded

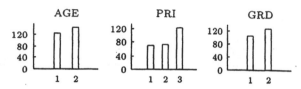

Figure 6.3. *Histograms of observed data for AGE, PRI and GRD after recoding.*

Table 6.6. *Definitions for AGE, PRI and GRD after recoding*

Variable	Description	Missing
AGE	age group (1=less than 20, 2=20+)	11
PRI	Number of prior foreign language courses (1=none, 2=1-2, 3=3+)	11
GRD	final grade in foreign language course (2=A, 1=B or lower)	47

final grade as a simple dichotomy (A, B or below). Similarly, the three highest age groups had very few students in them, so age was collapsed to a dichotomy as well (less than 20, 20+). Prior experience was reduced from five categories to three. Histograms of the recoded versions of AGE, PRI, and GRD and the revised definitions of these variables appear in Figure 6.3 and Table 6.6, respectively.

Notice that the variable LAN is nominal and should not be handled as a normal variable; the four language groups have no intrinsic ordering. To address this issue, LAN was replaced by a set of three dummy variables to distinguish among the four language groups: $LAN_2 = 1$ if Spanish and 0 otherwise, $LAN_3 = 1$ if German and 0 otherwise, and $LAN_4 = 1$ if Russian and 0 otherwise. Including LAN_2, LAN_3 and LAN_4 effectively treats the eleven remaining variables as multivariate normal within each of the four language groups, with a separate mean vector for each group and a common covariance matrix. The multivariate normal model clearly misspecifies the marginal distribution of the dummy variables, but this misspecification is of no consequence because the dummies are completely observed and do not need to be imputed (Section 2.6.2).

Finally, it is important to remember that a normal distribution has support on the whole real line, but the continuous variables in this dataset have a limited range of possible values. For example,

SAT scores may not exceed 800, and grade point averages may not exceed 4.0. Imputing under normality might occasionally result in an imputed value that is out of range. To handle this problem, we included a consistency check in our imputation routine. After performing the final I-step of data augmentation to create an imputation of Y_{mis}, each row of the imputed dataset was examined to see whether any of the imputed values were out of range; if so, the missing data for that row were re-drawn until the necessary constraints were satisfied. The final values of Y_{mis} created by this procedure approximate proper multiple imputations under a truncated multivariate normal model.

6.3.3 Exploring the observed-data likelihood and posterior

When LAN is replaced by three dummy variables, the dataset has $p = 14$ variables. The EM algorithm applied to these 14 variables converged rapidly; the parameter estimates stabilized to four significant digits after only ten iterations. When EM converges so quickly, estimating the largest fraction of missing information from the iterations can be difficult, because the estimated elementwise rates of convergence (3.27) tend to become numerically unstable after only a few iterations. Moreover, the iterations at which instability begins vary from component to component. The multivariate normal model for 14 variables has 119 parameters. With so many parameters, it is not easy to estimate the fraction of missing information by visually inspecting the elementwise rates. In situations like this it is helpful to apply graphical techniques.

To estimate the worst fraction of missing information, we first calculated elementwise rates (3.27) for each of the 119 parameters over the first 20 iterations of EM. After trimming away any values outside the interval $(0,1)$, we formed boxplots of the remaining values for each parameter, displaying them side-by-side. Boxplots for 50 randomly selected elements of μ and Σ are shown in Figure 6.4. Although a large number of outliers are present, all of the boxplots tend to be centered around 0.4. The median of the values in Figure 6.4 is 0.42, so a reasonable estimate of the worst fraction of missing information is 42%.

Inestimability of parameters

The moderate rates of missing information and the rapid convergence of EM might lead one to believe that the observed-data

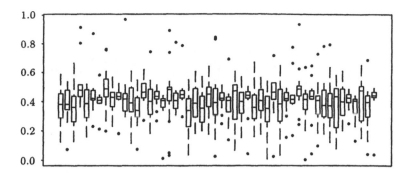

Figure 6.4. *Boxplots of estimated elementwise rates of convergence for 50 randomly selected parameters.*

likelihood function for this problem is well behaved. It turns out, however, that the likelihood is pathological. We performed a long exploratory run of data augmentation under the usual noninformative prior (5.18) and constructed time-series plots for selected elements of μ and Σ. For most parameters, the algorithm appeared to achieve stationarity very quickly. For a few parameters, however, the simulated values drifted into implausible regions of the parameter space. Time series plots for the means of the two variables with the highest rates of missingness, MLAT and GRD, are shown in Figure 6.5. Figure 6.5 (a) is typical of the plots for most parameters, with no discernible trends. Figure 6.5 (b), however, shows extreme long-range dependence. The mean of the dichotomous variable GRD is known to lie between 1 and 2, but by the 900th iteration the series has drifted above 2. This unusual behavior suggests that one or more components of θ are nearly or entirely inestimable from the observed data.

Additional runs of EM confirmed the presence of inestimable parameters. Using various simulated values of θ from the data-augmentation series as starting values, we re-ran EM and found that in each case it converged to a different stationary value. Moreover, when we evaluated the observed-data loglikelihood function at these stationary values, the loglikelihood was exactly the same in each case. Thus it appears that the stationary values are not distinct modes, but form a ridge of constant likelihood. The pathological behavior in Figure 6.5 (b) arises because the observed-data posterior distribution is not proper; although the I- and P-steps of data augmentation are both well defined, the algorithm is not

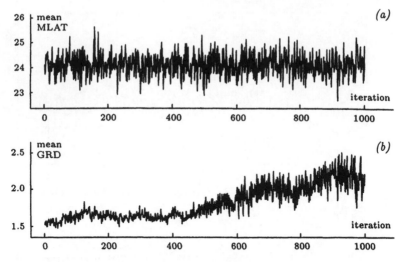

Figure 6.5. *Time series plots of (a) mean MLAT and (b) mean GRD over 1000 iterations of data augmentation.*

Table 6.7. *Cross-tabulation of LAN with GRD*

	LAN = 1	LAN = 2	LAN = 3	LAN = 4
GRD = 1	36	34	36	0
GRD = 2	27	31	68	0
GRD missing	4	13	10	20

converging to any stationary distribution (Section 3.5.2).

With a little exploration it is easy to detect the source of difficulty. Figure 6.5 (b) suggests that the inestimable part of θ pertains to the distribution of GRD. A cross-tabulation of GRD with LAN, shown in Table 6.7, reveals that GRD is missing for all cases with LAN = 4. Because no values of GRD are available for any students enrolled in Russian courses, it is impossible to estimate the parameters of the conditional distribution of GRD given LAN = 4 from this dataset.

6.3.4 Overcoming the problem of inestimability

One way to solve the problem of inestimability is to simply exclude the Russian language group and the variable LAN_4 from the analysis. Because GRD is missing for all 20 of these cases, they contribute little or no information about the main question of scientific interest, which pertains to the quality of FLAS as a predictor of GRD. Another way to handle the problem is to introduce a small amount of information about the inestimable portions of θ through a mildly informative prior distribution. Although excluding the Russian language group is certainly reasonable, we will adopt the latter approach to illustrate the use of an informative prior distribution.

After centering and scaling the observed data for each variable to have mean 0 and variance 1, we applied the ridge prior described in Section 5.2.3 with $\tau = 0$, $m = \epsilon$, and $\Lambda^{-1} = \epsilon I$ for $\epsilon = 3$. This prior adds the equivalent of three degrees of freedom to the estimation of Σ and smooths the estimated correlation matrix toward I. With a sample size of $n = 279$ the degree of smoothing is slight, and the effect on those portions of θ that are already well estimated is almost negligible. For portions of θ that are poorly estimated, however, this prior smooths the estimates toward a model of mutual independence among all variables. Inferences under this prior will thus tend to be conservative in the sense that we will be less likely to conclude that associations among variables are present when in fact they are not.

Under this prior, EM was found to converge reliably from a variety of starting values to a single posterior mode. The convergence was slower than before, requiring about 30 iterations, and the largest fraction of missing information was estimated at 92%. It may seem somewhat counterintuitive that the introduction of prior information appears to *raise* the worst fraction of missing information rather than lower it. This fraction, however, pertains only to those directions or functions of θ for which the function being maximized (i.e. the observed-data likelihood or posterior) is not flat. The elementwise rates estimate the largest eigenvalue of the asymptotic rate matrix that is less than one (Section 3.3.2). A ridge in the function produces one or more eigenvalues equal to one, and thus the inestimable functions of θ do not contribute to the estimated worst fraction of missing information when EM is used to maximize the likelihood. When an informative prior is introduced, however, the posterior is no longer precisely flat in any direction, and every function of θ then contributes to the estimated worst fraction of missing information.

Under the informative prior, data augmentation also appears to converge reliably. Starting at the mode, we ran a single chain for 1000 iterations and monitored a variety of functions of θ. Sample

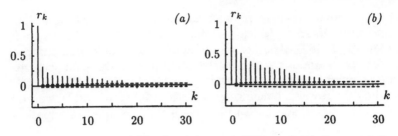

Figure 6.6. *Sample ACFs for (a) mean GRD and (b) the worst linear function of θ, estimated from 1000 iterations of data augmentation, with dashed lines indicating approximate critical values for testing $\rho_k = \rho_{k+1} = \cdots = 0$.*

ACFs for two functions are shown in Figure 6.6. The mean of GRD, which behaved pathologically under the noninformative prior, now shows no appreciable dependence after lag 20. The worst linear function of θ, as estimated by the trajectory of EM in the vicinity of the posterior mode (Section 4.4.3), appears to achieve stationarity in about 25 steps.

6.3.5 Analysis by multiple imputation

Following the preliminary run, we created $m = 20$ multiple imputations of the missing data by running 20 independent chains for 100 steps each. Starting values for the chains were obtained by finding posterior modes from independent bootstrap samples of 140 subjects each.

Inferences for logistic-regression coefficients

Because the response variable GRD was collapsed to a dichotomy, we decided to measure the predictive ability of FLAS and the other variables by logistic regression (e.g. McCullagh and Nelder, 1989). Let π_i denote the probability of GRD $= 2$ for subject i. We examined the model

$$\log \frac{\pi_i}{1 - \pi_i} = x_i^T \beta, \qquad (6.2)$$

where x_i is a vector of covariates for subject i and β a vector of unknown coefficients. Covariates in x_i included a term for the intercept; three dummy indicators for language (LAN_2, LAN_3 and LAN_4); an indicator for age ($\text{AGE}_2 = 1$ if 20+ and 0 otherwise); an indicator for sex ($\text{SEX}_2 = 1$ if female and 0 otherwise); linear and quadratic contrasts for PRI ($\text{PRI}_L = -1, 0, 1$ and $\text{PRI}_Q =$

Table 6.8. *Multiple-imputation inferences for logistic-regression coefficients, full model*

variable	$\bar{Q}$	$\sqrt{T}$	$\bar{Q}/\sqrt{T}$	ν	p	$100r$	$100\hat{\lambda}$
intercept	−15.5	3.07	−5.07	181	0.00	48	33
LAN$_2$	0.312	0.518	0.60	629	0.55	21	18
LAN$_3$	1.12	0.453	2.48	1187	0.01	15	13
LAN$_4$	−0.110	4.13	−0.03	79	0.98	96	50
AGE$_2$	1.40	0.457	3.07	227	0.00	41	30
PRI$_L$	0.350	0.261	1.34	249	0.18	38	28
PRI$_Q$	−0.165	0.150	−1.10	357	0.27	30	23
SEX$_2$	0.861	0.443	1.94	440	0.05	26	21
FLAS	0.0386	0.0166	2.33	161	0.02	52	35
MLAT	0.114	0.0480	2.37	201	0.02	44	31
SATV	−0.0033	0.0033	−1.01	301	0.32	34	26
SATM	0.0004	0.0026	0.13	1034	0.89	16	14
ENG	0.0110	0.0238	0.46	164	0.65	52	35
HGPA	2.27	0.439	5.18	884	0.00	17	15
CGPA	0.809	0.588	1.38	132	0.17	61	39

$1, -2, 1$ for PRI $= 1, 2, 3$, respectively); and the variables FLAS, MLAT, SATV, SATM, ENG, HGPA and CGPA. For each of the 20 imputed datasets, we computed ML estimates and asymptotic standard errors for the elements of β, and then combined the 20 sets using the formulas for multiple-imputation inference for scalar estimands (Section 4.3.2).

The results of the analysis are summarized in Table 6.8. For each coefficient, Table 6.8 displays the point estimate $\bar{Q}$ and standard error $\sqrt{T}$, the t-statistic $\bar{Q}/\sqrt{T}$, the degrees of freedom ν for the Student's t-approximation, and the p-value for testing the hypothesis $Q = 0$ against a two-sided alternative. Also shown are the relative increase in variance due to nonresponse r and the estimated fraction of missing information $\hat{\lambda}$. The p-value for FLAS (0.021) suggests that this variable is useful for predicting GRD. Increasing FLAS by ten points multiplies the odds $\pi_i/(1 - \pi_i)$ by an estimated factor $e^{10 \times 0.0386} = 1.47$; in other words, every ten-point increase in FLAS makes a student 47% more likely (on the odds scale) to receive a grade of A, if other covariates are held constant. The most powerful predictor of final grade appears to be high-school GPA; a one-unit increase in HGPA causes the predicted odds to be multiplied by $e^{2.27} = 9.68$. The only significant language effect is the coefficient of LAN_3, which distinguishes between the German and French groups; a student taking German appears to be about $e^{1.12} = 3.06$ times as likely to receive an A as a student taking French. Notice that LAN_4, which contrasts Russian with French, has a non-significant effect ($p = 0.979$) and a high fraction of missing information (50%). This is to be expected, because essentially all information about this parameter comes from the prior distribution which tends to pull the estimated coefficient toward zero.

Joint inferences for groups of coefficients

The inferences in Table 6.8 pertain to the logistic-regression coefficients individually. To make joint inferences about groups of coefficients, we need the methods for multidimensional estimands presented in Section 4.3.3. Of the three methods described there, we will demonstrate the procedure of Meng and Rubin (1992b) for combining likelihood-ratio test statistics.

With complete data, the loglikelihood function for the logistic model (6.2) may be written as

$$l(\beta \,|\, Y_{obs}, Y_{mis}) = \sum_{i=1}^{n} \left[z_i \log \frac{e^{x_i^T \beta}}{1 + e^{x_i^T \beta}} + (1 - z_i) \log \frac{1}{1 + e^{x_i^T \beta}} \right],$$

where $z_i = 1$ if individual i has $GRD = 2$, and $z_i = 0$ otherwise (e.g. McCullagh and Nelder, 1989). Suppose we want to test whether the coefficients for a group of variables (say, LAN_2 and LAN_4) are simultaneously zero. The usual likelihood-ratio test with complete data requires us to fit (a) the full model with all variables, and (b) the reduced model with all variables except LAN_2 and LAN_4. Denote the ML estimates of β under the full and reduced models by $\hat{\beta}$ and $\tilde{\beta}$, respectively. For notational convenience, we assume that $\hat{\beta}$ and $\tilde{\beta}$ are of the same length, with the elements of $\tilde{\beta}$ corresponding to the omitted variables set to zero. The likelihood-ratio test statistic is

$$d_L(\hat{\beta}, \tilde{\beta} \,|\, Y_{obs}, Y_{mis}) = 2[\,l(\hat{\beta} \,|\, Y_{obs}, Y_{mis}) - l(\tilde{\beta} \,|\, Y_{obs}, Y_{mis})\,],$$

which, under the reduced model, is approximately distributed as χ_2^2 because the reduced model differs from the full model by two parameters.

The method of Meng and Rubin (1992b) requires two passes through the imputed data. Let $\hat{\beta}^{(t)}$ and $\tilde{\beta}^{(t)}$ denote the ML estimates for the full and reduced models, respectively, fit to the tth

Table 6.9. *Multiple-imputation likelihood-ratio tests for eliminating groups of variables from the regression model*

variables omitted	D_3	k	ν_3	p	$100r_3$	$100\hat{\lambda}$
(a) LAN_2, LAN_4	−0.02	2	59	1.000	341	77
(b) SATV, SATM, ENG	0.40	3	941	0.750	30	23
(c) PRI_L, PRI_Q	1.62	2	461	0.200	36	26

imputed dataset. In the first pass, we calculate the likelihood-ratio statistic for each imputed dataset and find their average,

$$\bar{d}_L = \frac{1}{m} \sum_{t=1}^{m} d_L(\hat{\beta}^{(t)}, \tilde{\beta}^{(t)} \,|\, Y_{obs}, Y_{mis}^{(t)}).$$

In the second pass, we calculate the average of the likelihood-ratio test statistics with $\hat{\beta}^{(t)}$ and $\tilde{\beta}^{(t)}$ replaced by their averages,

$$\tilde{d}_L = \frac{1}{m} \sum_{t=1}^{m} d_L(m^{-1}\sum_{t=1}^{m}\hat{\beta}^{(t)}, m^{-1}\sum_{t=1}^{m}\tilde{\beta}^{(t)} \,|\, Y_{obs}, Y_{mis}^{(t)}).$$

The test statistic D_3 and p-value are then found by (4.44)–(4.46).

Using this technique, we tested three groups of variables and removed them from the model in turn after confirming that their p-values were high. The three groups were (a) the language indicators LAN_2 and LAN_4; (b) the test scores SATV, SATM and ENG; and (c) the linear and quadratic contrasts for PRI. Results from each test are shown in Table 6.9, including the test statistic D_3, the degrees of freedom k and ν_3 for the F-approximation, the p-value, the relative increase in variance due to nonresponse r_3, and the fraction of missing information $\hat{\lambda}$ calculated as $\hat{\lambda} = r_3/(1-r_3)$. Notice that D_3 for omitting LAN_2 and LAN_4 is slightly less than zero. With complete data, a likelihood-ratio test statistic cannot be negative. With Meng and Rubin's method, however, negative values do sometimes occur, particularly when the estimates of the coefficients in question are close to zero and their fractions of missing information are high. Multiple-imputation inferences for the coefficients of the final regression model are shown in Table 6.10.

6.4 A simulation study

We have claimed that it is often sensible to use a normal model to create multiple imputations even when the observed data are some-

Table 6.10. *Multiple-imputation inferences for logistic-regression co-efficients, final model*

variable	$\bar{Q}$	$\sqrt{T}$	$\bar{Q}/\sqrt{T}$	ν	p	$100r$	$100\hat{\lambda}$
intercept	−15.0	2.53	−5.91	160	0.00	53	35
LAN$_3$	0.874	0.401	2.18	235	0.03	40	29
AGE$_2$	1.30	0.434	3.01	197	0.00	28	32
SEX$_2$	0.891	0.405	2.20	398	0.03	28	22
FLAS	0.0351	0.0153	2.29	167	0.02	51	34
MLAT	0.0963	0.0399	2.41	269	0.02	36	27
HGPA	1.99	0.375	5.31	1417	0.00	13	12
CGPA	0.904	0.536	1.68	136	0.09	60	38

what nonnormal. A growing body of evidence supports this claim. The simulation results of Rubin and Schenker (1986), also reported by Rubin (1987, Chap. 4), demonstrate that for estimating the mean of a univariate population, imputations based on a normal model result in interval estimates with excellent repeated-sampling properties. Even for populations that are skewed or heavy-tailed, the actual coverage of multiple-imputation intervals is very close to the nominal coverage, except when the fraction of missing information is high (in excess of 50%). A recent simulation study in the context of a large national health survey produced encouraging results for a wide variety of linear and nonlinear estimators under plausible non-normal populations (Schafer *et al.*, 1996). The study was designed to mimic the specific features of a health examination survey conducted by the U.S. National Center for Health Statistics, including a complex sampling plan with unequal selection probabilities and multiple phases of data collection. Results of that simulation, which involved a mixed model for continuous and categorical variables, will be discussed in Chapter 9. Here we present a miniature version of the simulation to convey the essential result: model-based multiple imputation tends to work well for a wide variety of estimands, and is robust to moderate departures from the data model.

6.4.1 Simulation procedures

Data for this simulation, provided by the National Center for Health Statistics (NCHS), were drawn from Phase 1 of the Third National Health and Nutrition Examination Survey (NHANES III) (NCHS,

Table 6.11. *Variables in the simulation study*

Variable	Description
AGE	age group (1=20–39, 2=40–59, 3=60+)
BMI	body mass index (kg/m²)
HYP	hypertensive (1=no, 2=yes)
CHL	total serum cholesterol (mg/dL)

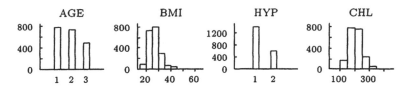

Figure 6.7. *Histograms of AGE, BMI, HYP and CHL in the population.*

1994). The data were collected by interviews and medical examinations in mobile examination centers. Because many of the sampled persons did not show up for examination, missingness rates for key exam variables exceeded 30%. To keep matters simple, this study is restricted to adult males (age 20+) and four variables. Definitions of the variables are given in Table 6.11.

An artificial population of 2000 subjects was created by drawing a simple random sample without replacement of all the adult males in the survey who had complete data for all four variables. Histograms for the variables in this population are shown in Figure 6.7. Because the survey used disproportionate sampling in certain racial, ethnic and age categories, and because we have omitted cases with missing data, these 2000 subjects are not representative of any population of substantive interest; the data and results presented here should not be regarded as estimates for any meaningful segment of the U.S. population. This study is meant only to illustrate the properties of model-based multiple imputation when applied to a population of real data that do not conform to simplistic modeling assumptions.

Sampling and response mechanism

From the population of 2000 subjects, simple random samples of size $n = 100$ were drawn without replacement. After a sample was drawn, a random pattern of missingness was imposed on BMI,

Table 6.12. *Probabilities for response patterns by AGE, with observed and missing variables denoted by × and ?, respectively*

	pattern							
BMI	×	?	×	?	×	?	×	?
HYP	×	×	?	?	×	×	?	?
CHL	×	×	×	×	?	?	?	?

	probability							
AGE=1	.725	.037	.031	.008	.053	.002	.004	.142
AGE=2	.737	.034	.036	.014	.029	.007	.003	.141
AGE=3	.650	.037	.039	.063	.034	.007	.004	.166

HYP and CHL for each sampled person according to his age. The probabilities for the $2^3 = 8$ possible response patterns by age were estimated from all adult males in the NHANES III sample, and are shown in Table 6.12. Because the response probabilities depend only on AGE, which is always observed, this mechanism is ignorable. The mechanism creates missingness rates of approximately 20% for each of the three variables BMI, HYP and CHL over repetitions of the sampling procedure.

Imputation

After imposing a pattern of missingness, the 'missing' values were then imputed $m = 5$ times under a multivariate normal model. AGE was entered into the model as two dummy variables: $AGE_2 = 1$ for AGE = 2 and 0 otherwise; and $AGE_3 = 1$ for AGE = 3 and 0 otherwise. BMI, HYP and CHL were entered without recoding or transformation. The imputations were created by running five independent chains of data augmentation under the standard non-informative prior (5.18). Each chain was started at the ML estimate and allowed to run for 20 cycles. The final value of Y_{mis} from each chain was taken as an imputation, and the continuous imputes for HYP were rounded off to the nearest category.

6.4.2 Complete-data inferences

After imputing five times, five sets of complete-data point and variance estimates were calculated for a variety of scalar estimands, and the results were combined in the usual way (Section 4.3.2).

Eighteen different estimands were examined, including population means, proportions, quantiles, a correlation coefficient and an odds ratio. Methods of complete-data inference for means and proportions are well known. If μ is the mean of a population, and $\bar{y}$ and S^2 are the sample mean and variance, respectively, from a simple random sample of size n, then the standard point and variance estimates are $\bar{y}$ and S^2/n. Similarly, if p is a population proportion and $\hat{p}$ is a sample proportion, the point and variance estimates are $\hat{p}$ and $\hat{p}(1 - \hat{p})/n$. Complete-data inferences for quantiles, correlations and odds ratios are described below.

Quantiles

The following approximate method for quantiles was described by Woodruff (1952). Suppose that Q is the pth quantile of a distribution function F, and $\hat{Q}$ is an estimate of Q based on a simple random sample of size n. Then

$$Q_1 \leq Q \leq Q_2$$

will be true if and only if

$$F(Q_1) \leq p \leq F(Q_2),$$

because F and F^{-1} are strictly increasing. Rather than finding an interval estimate for Q directly, we instead construct an interval estimate for the proportion of the population that lies below Q, and then translate the endpoints of this interval into quantiles. For example, an approximate 95% interval for p ranges from

$$p_1 = p - 2\sqrt{\frac{p(1-p)}{n}} \quad \text{to} \quad p_2 = p + 2\sqrt{\frac{p(1-p)}{n}}.$$

If we set Q_1 and Q_2 equal to the p_1th and p_2th sample quantiles, respectively, then the approximate 95% confidence interval for Q ranges from Q_1 to Q_2. This interval is not necessarily symmetric about $\hat{Q}$. It is well known, however that under mild smoothness conditions for F the sample quantiles are asymptotically normally distributed (e.g Serfling, 1980), and for large samples we can take $(Q_2 - Q_1)/4$ as an estimated standard deviation for $\hat{Q}$ (Francisco and Fuller, 1991).

Correlation coefficients

Suppose that r is a correlation coefficient from a simple random sample of n units, and ρ is the corresponding population value.

The familiar transformation due to Fisher (1921),

$$z(r) = \tanh^{-1}(r) = \tfrac{1}{2} \log \frac{1+r}{1-r},$$

makes $z(r)$ approximately normally distributed about $z(\rho)$ with variance $1/(n-3)$. This result is derived under an assumption of bivariate normality. An interval estimate for ρ can be calculated by first finding an interval for $z(\rho)$ using the normal approximation, and then applying the inverse transformation $z^{-1}(\cdot) = \tanh(\cdot)$ to the endpoints. Because $z(r) \approx r$ for values of r near zero (they agree to two decimal places for $|r| < 0.24$), the approximation $V(r) \approx 1/(n-3)$ is also acceptable in the vicinity of $r = 0$.

Odds ratios

Suppose that Y_1 and Y_2 are two binary variables taking values 1 and 2. In a simple random sample of size n, let x_{ij} be the number of sample units for which $Y_1 = i$ and $Y_2 = j$, $i, j = 1, 2$. The population odds ratio, defined as

$$\omega = \frac{P(Y_1 = 1 | Y_2 = 1)/P(Y_1 = 2 | Y_2 = 1)}{P(Y_1 = 1 | Y_2 = 2)/P(Y_1 = 2 | Y_2 = 2)},$$

is estimated by $\hat{\omega} = (x_{11} x_{22})/(x_{12} x_{21})$. In large samples, the log-odds ratio $\hat{\beta} = \log \hat{\omega}$ is approximately normally distributed about $\beta = \log \omega$, and a large-sample variance estimate for β is $x_{11}^{-1} + x_{12}^{-1} + x_{21}^{-1} + x_{22}^{-1}$ (e.g. Agresti, 1990). An interval estimate for ω can be obtained by first finding an interval for β using the normal approximation, and then taking antilogs of the endpoints.

6.4.3 Results

The entire simulation procedure of drawing a sample, imposing patterns of missingness, creating five imputations and calculating point and interval estimates was carried out 1000 times. The results are summarized in Table 6.13. For each of the eighteen estimands, this table shows the true estimand Q (i.e. the population value), the multiple-imputation point estimates $\bar{Q}$, the endpoints of the nominal 95% interval estimates (low and high) and the estimated fraction of missing information $\hat{\lambda}$ averaged over 1000 iterations. In addition, the table reports the simulated actual coverage (cvg.), the number of intervals out of 1000 that covered the true estimand. The average simulated coverage across all eighteen estimands is 952.7, indicating that the procedure is well calibrated. Some of the

Table 6.13. *Summary of simulation results for eighteen estimands*

Estimand	Q	$\bar{Q}$	low	high	cvg.	$100\hat{\lambda}$
Mean BMI						
overall	26.6	26.6	25.5	27.7	956	25
AGE = 1	25.7	25.7	24.0	27.4	941	22
AGE = 2	27.7	27.7	25.9	29.5	942	22
AGE = 3	26.3	26.3	24.1	28.5	961	34
Mean CHL						
overall	206	207	197	216	956	22
AGE = 1	192	192	177	206	960	25
AGE = 2	219	220*	204	235	949	20
AGE = 3	210	211	191	230	956	24
Proportion HYP = 2						
overall	.294	.299*	.197	.402	959	22
AGE = 1	.107	.117*	.000	.235	951	26
AGE = 2	.323	.329*	.156	.502	941	20
AGE = 3	.545	.540	.304	.776	927	27
Percentiles						
BMI (50%)	26.0	26.1*	24.8	27.4	951	24
BMI (90%)	32.7	32.8*	30.1	35.5	960	19
CHL (50%)	202	204*	192	216	961	20
CHL (90%)	262	264*	241	287	960	19
Correlation						
BMI and CHL	.171	.174	−.064	.393	940	29
Odds ratio						
BMI > 27.8 by HYP	1.64	1.81	.614	5.47	977	27

* denotes a point estimate with statistically significant bias

multiple-imputation point estimates, those denoted by an asterisk, have a statistically significant bias; for these, the average of the 1000 values of $\bar{Q}$ was significantly different from Q at the 0.05 level as judged by an ordinary t-test. But the biases are minor when compared to the average width of the 95% interval estimates, and thus are of little consequence.

Multiple imputation performs well in this example even though the normality assumption of the imputation model is clearly violated: the distributions of BMI and CHL are skewed to the right, and CHL is binary. In practice, one would probably transform BMI

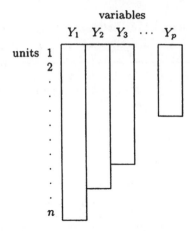

Figure 6.8. *Monotone missingness pattern.*

and CHL (e.g. to the log scale) before applying the normal model, in which case the performance should be even better.

6.5 Fast algorithms based on factored likelihoods

6.5.1 Monotone missingness patterns

This section presents a class of simulation algorithms for incomplete multivariate normal data which, in certain cases, will achieve stationarity more rapidly than ordinary data augmentation. These algorithms are based on the observation, first made by Li (1988), that we do not really need to fill in the entire set of missing data Y_{mis} at each I-step. The function of the I-step is to impute enough of the missing values to make the P-step into a tractable, complete-data posterior simulation. Under the multivariate normal model, however, the P-step can be made tractable by filling in only enough of the missing values to complete a *monotone pattern*.

The missingness pattern for a data matrix is said to be monotone if, whenever an element y_{ij} is missing, y_{ik} is also missing for all $k > j$ (Rubin, 1974; Little and Rubin, 1987). A monotone pattern is shown in Figure 6.8. Monotone patterns often arise in repeated-measures or longitudinal datasets, because if a subject drops out of the study in a given time period, then his or her data will typically be missing in all subsequent time periods. Sometimes a non-monotone dataset can be made monotone or nearly so by reordering the variables according to their missingness rates. Let n_j

denote the number of rows of the data matrix for which Y_j is observed. If the pattern is monotone, then $n_p \leq n_{p-1} \leq \cdots \leq n_1 = n$. We will assume that the rows of the monotone dataset have been sorted as in Figure 6.8, so that Y_j (and hence $Y_1, \ldots, Y_{j-1}$ as well) is observed for rows $1, \ldots, n_j$ and missing for rows $n_j + 1, \ldots, n$.

Factoring the observed-data likelihood

When the observed data Y_{obs} are monotone, the observed-data likelihood function can be expressed in a very convenient form. Let $\phi = (\phi_1, \phi_2, \ldots, \phi_p)$, where ϕ_1 denotes the parameters of the marginal distribution of variable Y_1, ϕ_2 the parameters of the conditional distribution of Y_2 given Y_1, ϕ_3 the parameters of the conditional distribution of Y_3 given Y_1 and Y_2, and so on. In other words, ϕ_j contains the intercept, slopes and residual variance from the normal linear regression of Y_j on $Y_1, \ldots, Y_{j-1}$. It is easy to show that $\phi = \phi(\theta)$ is a one-to-one function of the usual parameters $\theta = (\mu, \Sigma)$. Moreover, if no prior restrictions are imposed upon θ, then the components $\phi_1, \ldots, \phi_p$ are distinct in the sense that the parameter space of ϕ is the cross-product of the individual parameter spaces for $\phi_1, \ldots, \phi_p$. Expressions for $\phi_1, \ldots, \phi_p$ in terms of $\theta = (\mu, \Sigma)$ can be found by partitioning μ and Σ and applying the formulas given in Section 5.2.4.

When Y_{obs} is monotone, the observed-data likelihood function for ϕ factors neatly into independent likelihoods for $\phi_1, \ldots, \phi_p$. To see this, notice that the joint density of the variables $Y_1, \ldots, Y_p$ can be factored as

$$
\begin{aligned}
P(Y_1, \ldots, Y_p | \phi) &= P(Y_1 | \phi_1) \, P(Y_2 | Y_1, \phi_2) \\
&\quad \cdots P(Y_p | Y_1, \ldots, Y_{p-1}, \phi_p),
\end{aligned}
$$

which allows us to write the complete-data likelihood as

$$
\begin{aligned}
L(\phi | Y) &= \prod_{i=1}^{n} P(y_{i1}, \ldots, y_{ip} | \phi) \\
&= \prod_{i=1}^{n} \prod_{j=1}^{p} P(y_{ij} | y_{i1}, \ldots, y_{i,j-1}, \phi_j) \\
&= \prod_{j=1}^{p} \prod_{i=1}^{n} P(y_{ij} | y_{i1}, \ldots, y_{i,j-1}, \phi_j). \quad (6.3)
\end{aligned}
$$

The inner product in (6.3),

$$\prod_{i=1}^{n} P(y_{ij} \mid y_{i1}, \dots, y_{i,j-1}, \phi_j),$$

can also be written

$$\prod_{i=1}^{n_j} P(y_{ij} \mid y_{i1}, \dots, y_{i,j-1}, \phi_j) \prod_{i=n_j+1}^{n} P(y_{ij} \mid y_{i1}, \dots, y_{i,j-1}, \phi_j). \quad (6.4)$$

The observed-data likelihood $L(\phi \mid Y_{obs})$ is by definition the integral of (6.3) over Y_{mis}. But notice that the first product in (6.4) does not involve Y_{mis} because variable Y_j is observed in rows $1, \dots, n_j$, whereas the second product integrates to unity because Y_j is missing in rows $n_j + 1, \dots, n$. It follows that

$$L(\phi \mid Y_{obs}) = \prod_{j=1}^{p} L(\phi_j \mid Y_{obs}), \quad (6.5)$$

where

$$L(\phi_j \mid Y_{obs}) = \prod_{i=1}^{n_j} P(y_{ij} \mid y_{i1}, \dots, y_{i,j-1}, \phi_j). \quad (6.6)$$

Under the multivariate normal model, (6.6) is simply the likelihood for the normal linear regression of Y_j on $Y_1, \dots, Y_{j-1}$, based on the rows $1, \dots, n_j$ of the data matrix. Thus the factorization (6.5) effectively reduces the problem of inference about ϕ to a sequence of complete-data regressions over subsets of the rows of the data matrix.

6.5.2 Computing alternative parameterizations

When the data are monotone, the observed-data likelihood has a convenient form when expressed in terms of $\phi = (\phi_1, \dots, \phi_p)$. The parameters of the multivariate normal, however, are usually expressed in terms of $\theta = (\mu, \Sigma)$, a vector of means and a covariance matrix. To make use of the convenient form of the likelihood, we will need to switch back and forth between the two parameterizations.

A numerical procedure for computing $\phi = \phi(\theta)$ or $\theta = \phi^{-1}(\phi)$ can be formulated in terms of the sweep operator (Section 5.2.4). For convenience, we introduce a slight generalization of sweep which gives a compact notation to the process of sweeping a square submatrix of a larger matrix. Let G be a $p \times p$ symmetric matrix with elements g_{ij}, and let A be a subset of the p columns (and rows) of G. The generalized sweep operator SWP_A performs the usual sweep computations on the rows and columns of G in the set A but leaves the rest of G unchanged. Formally, $\text{SWP}_A[k]$ for some $k \in A$ operates on G by replacing it with another $p \times p$ matrix H,

$$H = \text{SWP}_A[k]\, G,$$

where the elements of H are given by

$$h_{kk} = -1/g_{kk},$$

$$h_{jk} = h_{kj} = \begin{cases} g_{jk}/g_{kk} & j \in A, \ j \neq k, \\ g_{jk} & j \notin A, \end{cases}$$

$$h_{jl} = h_{lj} = \begin{cases} g_{jl} - g_{jk}g_{kl}/g_{kk} & j \in A, \ l \in A, \ j \neq k, \ l \neq k, \\ g_{jl} & j \notin A \text{ or } l \notin A. \end{cases}$$

This operation will be referred to as *sweeping submatrix A of G on position k*. Similarly, the corresponding reverse sweep operator RSW_A applies the usual reverse-sweep computations to the rows and columns of G in set A, while leaving the rest of G unchanged. Formally, $\text{RSW}_A[k]$ for some $k \in A$ operates on G by replacing it with another $p \times p$ matrix H,

$$H = \text{RSW}_A[k]\, G,$$

where the elements of H are given by

$$h_{kk} = -1/g_{kk},$$

$$h_{jk} = h_{kj} = \begin{cases} -g_{jk}/g_{kk} & j \in A, \ j \neq k, \\ g_{jk} & j \notin A, \end{cases}$$

$$h_{jl} = h_{lj} = \begin{cases} g_{jl} - g_{jk}g_{kl}/g_{kk} & j \in A, \ l \in A, \ j \neq k, \ l \neq k, \\ g_{jl} & j \notin A \text{ or } l \notin A. \end{cases}$$

When the sweep or reverse sweep operators are written without a subscripting set, as in $\text{SWP}[k]$ or $\text{RSW}[k]$, it will be understood that the operation is being applied to the entire matrix.

We are now ready to give a compact notation to the process of computing ϕ from θ and vice-versa. Let

$$\phi_j = (\beta_j^T, \gamma_j)^T \tag{6.7}$$

where β_j is the $j \times 1$ vector of coefficients (including the intercept) from the linear regression of Y_j on $Y_1, Y_2, \ldots, Y_{j-1}$ and γ_j is the residual variance, so that

$$Y_j | Y_1, \ldots, Y_{j-1}, \phi_j \sim N((1, Y_1, \ldots, Y_{j-1}) \beta_j, \gamma_j). \qquad (6.8)$$

Let μ_j denote the jth element of μ and σ_{jk} the (j, k)th element of Σ, and define

$$\theta_j = (\mu_j, \sigma_{1j}, \sigma_{2j}, \ldots, \sigma_{jj})^T, \qquad (6.9)$$

so that $\theta = (\theta_1, \theta_2, \ldots, \theta_p)$. As in Section 5.2.4, let us express θ as a symmetric $(p+1) \times (p+1)$ matrix,

$$\theta = \begin{bmatrix} -1 & \mu^T \\ \mu & \Sigma \end{bmatrix} = \begin{bmatrix} \boxed{-1} & \boxed{\theta_1} & \boxed{\theta_2} & \boxed{\theta_3} & \cdots \\ & & & & \end{bmatrix},$$

where the lower portion of the matrix is not shown to avoid redundancy. Finally, let the row and column labels for this matrix run from 0 to p, so that θ_j appear in column j. To convert θ to

$$\phi = \begin{bmatrix} \boxed{-1} & \boxed{\phi_1} & \boxed{\phi_2} & \boxed{\phi_3} & \cdots \\ & & & & \end{bmatrix},$$

note that sweeping θ on positions $1, 2, \ldots, j - 1$ produces a new matrix whose jth column is ϕ_j. Therefore, if we sweep the full θ matrix on positions $1, 2, \ldots, p - 1$, then ϕ_p appears in the pth column. If we then reverse-sweep all but the last row and column on position $p - 1$, then ϕ_{p-1} appears in column $p - 1$. Reverse-sweeping all but the last two rows and columns on position $p - 2$ makes ϕ_{p-2} appears in column $p - 2$, and so on.

This procedure can be expressed very concisely in pseudocode. Let $A_j = \{0, 1, \ldots, j\}$ for $j = 1, 2, \ldots, p$. The following two lines will overwrite a θ matrix, replacing it with $\phi = \phi(\theta)$.

```
for j:=1 to p-1 do θ:=SWP[j] θ
for j:=p-1 down to 1 do θ:=RSW_{A_j}[j] θ
```

The transformation from ϕ back to θ is simply a reversal of these steps. The following two lines will overwrite a ϕ matrix, replacing it with $\theta = \phi^{-1}(\phi)$.

$$\text{for } j := 1 \text{ to } p-1 \text{ do } \phi := \text{SWP}_{A_j}[j]\,\phi$$
$$\text{for } j := p-1 \text{ down to } 1 \text{ do } \phi := \text{RSW}[j]\,\phi$$

6.5.3 Noniterative inference for monotone data

Maximum-likelihood estimation

When Y_{obs} has a monotone pattern, the factorization of the likelihood in terms of $\phi = (\phi_1, \ldots, \phi_p)$,

$$L(\phi \,|\, Y_{obs}) = \prod_{j=1}^{p} L(\phi_j \,|\, Y_{obs}),$$

enables us to calculate ML estimates without iteration (Little and Rubin, 1987, Chapter 6). Because the parameters $\phi_1, \ldots, \phi_p$ are distinct, maximizing $L(\phi \,|\, Y_{obs})$ is equivalent to maximizing each factor $L(\phi_j \,|\, Y_{obs})$ separately for $j = 1, \ldots, p$. The ML estimate of ϕ is $\hat{\phi} = (\hat{\phi}_1, \ldots, \hat{\phi}_p)$, where $\hat{\phi}_j$ is the maximizer of $L(\phi_j \,|\, Y_{obs})$.

The maximization of each factor $L(\phi_j \,|\, Y_{obs})$ is accomplished by ordinary least-squares regression of Y_j on $Y_1, \ldots, Y_{j-1}$, using rows $1, \ldots, n_j$ of the data matrix. Let z_j denote the observed data in column j,

$$z_j = (y_{1j}, y_{2j}, \ldots, y_{n_j, j})^T, \tag{6.10}$$

and X_j the upper-left $n_j \times (j-1)$ submatrix augmented by a column of ones,

$$X_j = \begin{bmatrix} 1 & y_{11} & y_{12} & \cdots & y_{1,j-1} \\ 1 & y_{21} & y_{22} & \cdots & y_{2,j-1} \\ \vdots & \vdots & \vdots & & \vdots \\ 1 & y_{n_j,1} & y_{n_j,2} & \cdots & y_{n_j,j-1} \end{bmatrix}. \tag{6.11}$$

By (6.8), the conditional distribution of z_j given X_j and ϕ_j is

$$z_j \,|\, X_j, \phi_j \sim N(X_j \beta_j, \gamma_j I),$$

so the likelihood for ϕ_j is

$$L(\phi_j \,|\, Y_{obs}) \propto \gamma_j^{-n_j/2} \exp\left\{ -\frac{1}{2\gamma_j} (z_j - X_j \beta_j)^T (z_j - X_j \beta_j) \right\}.$$

Using well-known properties of the normal linear regression model, the ML estimate of $\phi_j = (\beta_j^T, \gamma_j)^T$ is given by

$$\hat{\beta}_j = (X_j^T X_j)^{-1} X_j^T z_j, \tag{6.12}$$

$$\hat{\gamma}_j = n_j^{-1} \hat{\epsilon}_j^T \hat{\epsilon}_j, \qquad (6.13)$$

where $\hat{\epsilon}_j = z_j - X_j \hat{\beta}_j$ (e.g. Draper and Smith, 1981). Notice that $\hat{\gamma}_j$, the ML estimate of the residual variance, is biased because its denominator is n_j rather than $n_j - j$. Calculating (6.12)–(6.13) for $j = 1, 2, \ldots, p$ yields $\hat{\phi}$, the ML estimate of ϕ. Because ML estimates are invariant under transformations of the parameter, the ML estimate for θ can be calculated as $\hat{\theta} = \phi^{-1}(\hat{\phi})$.

Bayesian inference

Similarly, when Y_{obs} has a monotone pattern, we can also conduct Bayesian inferences without iteration provided that the prior distribution has a certain form. If we apply a prior density to ϕ that factors into independent densities,

$$\pi(\phi) = \pi_1(\phi_1) \, \pi_2(\phi_2) \, \cdots \, \pi_p(\phi_p), \qquad (6.14)$$

then it is obvious that the posterior distribution $P(\phi \mid Y_{obs})$ will also factor into independent posteriors for $\phi_1, \ldots, \phi_p$, a structure that Rubin (1987) calls *monotone distinct*. Bayesian inferences for ϕ can then be carried out as a sequence of independent inferences based on the posteriors

$$P(\phi_j \mid Y_{obs}) \propto L(\phi_j \mid Y_{obs}) \, \pi_j(\phi_j)$$

for $j = 1, \ldots, p$. For example, we can simulate a value of ϕ from $P(\phi \mid Y_{obs})$ by drawing ϕ_j from $P(\phi_j \mid Y_{obs})$ independently for $j = 1, \ldots, p$. A simulated value of θ from $P(\theta \mid Y_{obs})$ can then be obtained by applying the back-transformation $\theta = \phi^{-1}(\phi)$ to the simulated value of ϕ.

The noninformative prior most commonly used for multivariate normal data,

$$\pi(\theta) \propto |\Sigma|^{-\left(\frac{p+1}{2}\right)}, \qquad (6.15)$$

can be factored as in (6.14). To avoid confusion, let us refer to the density (6.15) as $\pi_\theta(\theta)$, and the corresponding density for ϕ induced by (6.15) as $\pi_\phi(\phi)$. The relationship between π_θ and π_ϕ is

$$\pi_\phi(\phi) = \pi_\theta(\phi^{-1}(\phi)) \, \|J\|^{-1}, \qquad (6.16)$$

where $\theta = \phi^{-1}(\phi)$ is the inverse of the transformation $\phi = \phi(\theta)$, J is the Jacobian or first-derivative matrix of the transformation $\phi = \phi(\theta)$ and $\|J\|$ is the absolute value of the determinant of J.

By a well known property of determinants, $|\Sigma|$ can be written as

$$\left| \begin{array}{cc} \Sigma_{11} & \Sigma_{12} \\ \Sigma_{21} & \Sigma_{22} \end{array} \right| = |\Sigma_{11}| \, |\Sigma_{22} - \Sigma_{21}\Sigma_{11}^{-1}\Sigma_{12}|$$

for square submatrices Σ_{11} and Σ_{22}. But $\Sigma_{22} - \Sigma_{21}\Sigma_{11}^{-1}\Sigma_{12}$ is the residual covariance matrix from the regression of the variables corresponding to Σ_{22} on the variables corresponding to Σ_{11} (Section 5.2.4). Taking $\Sigma_{22} = \sigma_{pp}$, the determinant of Σ becomes

$$|\Sigma| = |\Sigma_{11}| \, \gamma_p, \tag{6.17}$$

where Σ_{11} is Σ without the last row and column. Applying (6.17) recursively to Σ_{11} leads to

$$|\Sigma| = \prod_{j=1}^{p} \gamma_j. \tag{6.18}$$

To find $\pi_\phi(\phi)$, we also need to evaluate $||J||$. In Section 5.4.2, we derived the determinant of the Jacobian that arises when we condition on a subset of the variables $Y_1, \ldots, Y_p$. Suppose that we first transform θ to the intermediate parameter (ξ_{p-1}, ϕ_p), where ξ_{p-1} represents the portions of μ and Σ pertaining to the marginal distribution of $Y_1, \ldots, Y_{p-1}$, and ϕ_p pertains to the regression of Y_p on $Y_1, \ldots, Y_{p-1}$. From (5.28), the determinant of the Jacobian for going from θ to (ξ_{p-1}, ϕ_p) is $|\Sigma_{11}|^{-1}$, where Σ_{11} is the covariance matrix for $Y_1, \ldots, Y_{p-1}$. But $|\Sigma_{11}| = \gamma_1\gamma_2\cdots\gamma_{p-1}$, so the determinant of the Jacobian of this intermediate transformation is $(\gamma_1\gamma_2\cdots\gamma_{p-1})^{-1}$. If we then transform ξ_{p-1} to (ξ_{p-2}, ϕ_{p-1}), where ξ_{p-2} contains the portions of μ and Σ pertaining to $Y_1, \ldots, Y_{p-2}$ and ϕ_{p-1} pertains to the regression of Y_{p-1} on $Y_1, \ldots, Y_{p-2}$, the determinant of the Jacobian is $(\gamma_1\gamma_2\cdots\gamma_{p-2})^{-1}$. We can repeat this procedure until we have reached the final parameterization $\phi = (\phi_1, \ldots, \phi_p)$, and the determinant of the Jacobian for $\phi = \phi(\theta)$ will be the product of the determinants for each of the intermediate transformations. The result is

$$||J|| = \gamma_1^{-(p-1)}\gamma_2^{-(p-2)}\cdots\gamma_{p-1}^{-1}. \tag{6.19}$$

Substituting (6.19) and (6.18) into (6.16) gives

$$\pi_\phi(\phi) \propto \prod_{j=1}^{p} \gamma_j^{-\left(\frac{p+1}{2}-p+j\right)} \tag{6.20}$$

as the prior density for $\phi = \phi(\theta)$ induced by (6.15).

Now we show the posterior that results when this prior is combined with the observed-data likelihood from a monotone dataset. Consider the likelihood factor for ϕ_j,

$$L(\phi_j \,|\, Y_{obs}) \propto \gamma_j^{-n_j/2} \exp\left\{ -\frac{1}{2\gamma_j}(z_j - X_j\beta_j)^T(z_j - X_j\beta_j) \right\}.$$

With some algebraic manipulation, it can be shown that

$$(z_j - X_j\beta_j)^T(z_j - X_j\beta_j) = \hat{\epsilon}_j^T\hat{\epsilon}_j + (\beta_j - \hat{\beta}_j)^T X^T X (\beta_j - \hat{\beta}_j),$$

where $\hat{\beta}_j = (X^TX_j)^{-1}X_j^T z_j$ and $\hat{\epsilon}_j = X_j\hat{\beta}_j$. When $L(\phi_j \,|\, Y_{obs})$ is combined with the factor in (6.20) involving ϕ_j,

$$\pi_j(\phi_j) \propto \gamma_j^{-\left(\frac{p+1}{2} - p + j\right)},$$

the resulting posterior can be written as

$$P(\phi_j \,|\, Y_{obs}) \propto \gamma_j^{-j/2} \exp\left\{ -\frac{1}{2\gamma_j}(\beta_j - \hat{\beta}_j)^T X^T X (\beta_j - \hat{\beta}_j) \right\}$$

$$\times \gamma_j^{-((n_j - p + j - 1)/2) - 1} \exp\left\{ -\frac{1}{2\gamma_j}\hat{\epsilon}_j^T\hat{\epsilon}_j \right\},$$

which is the product of a multivariate normal and a scaled inverted-chisquare density,

$$\beta_j \,|\, \gamma_j, Y_{obs} \;\sim\; N(\hat{\beta}_j, \, \gamma_j(X^TX)^{-1}), \qquad (6.21)$$

$$\gamma_j \,|\, Y_{obs} \;\sim\; \hat{\epsilon}_j^T\hat{\epsilon}_j \, \chi^{-2}_{n_j - p + j - 1}. \qquad (6.22)$$

6.5.4 Monotone data augmentation

Thus far we have discussed methods of inference that are appropriate when the observed data Y_{obs} are monotone. It often happens in practice that a dataset is not precisely monotone, but would become monotone if a relatively small portion of the missing data were filled in. This situation often arises with double sampling, where investigators attempt to measure certain variables for all units in a sample, and then measure additional variables for only a subsample. If there were no missing values except for those missing by design, then the data would be perfectly monotone; in practice, however, there is usually some additional unplanned missingness which makes the overall pattern deviate slightly from monotonicity. Near-monotonicity also results in many longitudinal or panel studies, in which variables are measured for individuals on multiple occasions. Subjects who drop out of the study at a particular occasion or wave usually do not reappear in subsequent waves, so that if the variables are ordered by wave the overall pattern is nearly monotone.

When this situation arises, we can exploit the near-monotone pattern to devise simulation algorithms that are computationally more efficient than the data augmentation procedures described in Chapter 5. These new procedures, which we call *monotone data augmentation*, differ from ordinary data augmentation in that they fill in only enough of the missing data at each I-step to complete a monotone pattern. Suppose that we partition the missing data as $Y_{mis} = (Y_{mis^*}, Y_{mis^{**}})$, where Y_{mis^*} is some subset of the missing values which, if filled in, would result in (Y_{obs}, Y_{mis^*}) having a monotone pattern. Monotone data augmentation proceeds in the following two steps.

1. I-step: Given the current simulated value $\theta^{(t)}$ of the parameter, draw a value from the conditional predictive distribution of Y_{mis^*},

$$Y_{mis^*}^{(t+1)} \sim P(Y_{mis^*} | Y_{obs}, \theta^{(t)}). \tag{6.23}$$

2. P-step: Conditioning on $Y_{mis^*}^{(t+1)}$, draw a new value of θ from its posterior given the now-completed monotone pattern,

$$\theta^{(t+1)} \sim P(\theta | Y_{obs}, Y_{mis^*}^{(t+1)}). \tag{6.24}$$

In practice, the P-step will have to be carried out using the parameterization $\phi = (\phi_1, \ldots, \phi_p)$ that corresponds to the monotone pattern of (Y_{obs}, Y_{mis^*}). That is, we will have to draw

$$\phi^{(t+1)} = (\phi_1^{(t+1)}, \ldots, \phi_p^{(t+1)})$$

by drawing

$$\phi_j^{(t+1)} \sim P(\phi_j | Y_{obs}, Y_{mis^*}^{(t+1)})$$

independently for $j = 1, 2, \ldots, p$, and then calculate

$$\theta^{(t+1)} = \phi^{-1}(\phi^{(t+1)})$$

using the procedures for numerical transformation described earlier in this section.

Monotone data augmentation has two computational advantages over ordinary data augmentation. First, it requires fewer random number draws per iteration, i.e. it is typically faster to fill in Y_{mis^*} than the full Y_{mis}. Second, it will achieve approximate stationarity in fewer iterations. Liu, Wong and Kong (1994) show that 'collapsing' the data augmentation by drawing only a subset of the unknown quantities at each iteration leads to faster convergence

$$Y_1 \quad Y_2 \quad Y_3$$

1	1	1
0	1	1
1	0	1
0	0	1
1	1	0
0	1	0
1	0	0
0	0	0

Figure 6.9. *Possible missingness patterns for a three-variable dataset, with observed and missing variables denoted by 1 and 0, respectively.*

and smaller autocorrelations between successive iterates. With ordinary data augmentation, convergence is governed by the amount of information contained in Y_{mis} relative to Y_{obs} (Section 3.5.3). With monotone data augmentation, however, convergence is governed by the amount of information in Y_{mis^*} relative to Y_{obs}. When Y_{obs} is not far from monotone, Y_{mis^*} is relatively small; the distribution $P(\theta \mid Y_{obs}, Y_{mis^*})$ is then nearly independent of Y_{mis^*}, and only a few steps of monotone data augmentation will be needed to achieve approximate stationarity. In the extreme case where Y_{obs} is precisely monotone, Y_{mis^*} is empty and the algorithm reaches stationarity in one step.

Monotone data augmentation was first proposed by Li (1988) who demonstrated its use in simple bivariate examples. The algorithm presented here, which assumes multivariate normal data and the customary noninformative prior

$$\pi(\theta) \propto |\Sigma|^{-\left(\frac{p+1}{2}\right)},$$

has also been described by Liu (1993).

Choosing the monotone pattern to be completed

To identify a Y_{mis^*}, it helps to group the rows of the data matrix by their patterns of missingness. For example, the possible patterns of missingness for a three-variable dataset are shown in Figure 6.9. The missing values in the unshaded region constitute Y_{mis^*} and need to be filled in at every I-step; missing data in the shaded region constitute $Y_{mis^{**}}$ and do not need to be filled in.

In most cases, of course, there is no unique set of missing data Y_{mis^*} that will complete a monotone pattern. By simply reordering the columns $Y_1, Y_2, \ldots, Y_p$ of the data matrix, we can identify alternative sets of missing values that are candidates for Y_{mis^*}. For computational efficiency, it is advantageous to choose Y_{mis^*} to be 'small' in two senses. First, the actual number of missing values contained in Y_{mis^*} should be small, to reduce the number of random variates that need to be drawn at each I-step. Second, Y_{mis^*} should contain as little information as possible about the unknown parameters, to reduce the number of steps required to achieve approximate stationarity. These two objectives may sometimes conflict. In a normal dataset, for example, there may be a tradeoff between filling in a large number of relatively noninfluential observations and filling in a smaller number with high leverage. Finding a set Y_{mis^*} to maximize the efficiency of the algorithm is a difficult problem, as it involves questions about the convergence of Markov chain Monte Carlo algorithms that are not easy to answer at present. Moreover, finding such an optimal set may itself require substantial computation, offsetting the potential gains of a more efficient algorithm.

To choose Y_{mis^*}, we suggest the naive approach of simply ordering the columns of Y according to their fractions of missing observations. That is, choose Y_1 to be the variable with the fewest missing values, Y_2 the variable with the second fewest, and so on. This approach is attractive because it is computationally trivial. Moreover, it has the feature that if Y_{obs} is already monotone, it will find the monotone pattern and identify Y_{mis^*} to be empty.

6.5.5 Implementation of the algorithm

In discussing how to implement monotone data augmentation for the multivariate normal model, we will need to build on the bookkeeping notation of Chapter 5. Suppose that the rows of the data matrix have been grouped together according to their patterns of missingness as shown in Figure 6.10. Index the missingness patterns by $s = 1, 2, \ldots, S$. Let s_j denote the last pattern for which variable Y_j may need to be filled in to complete the overall monotone pattern, so that

$$S = s_1 \geq s_2 \geq \cdots \geq s_p.$$

Following Section 5.3.1, let

$$r_{sj} = \begin{cases} 1 & \text{if } Y_j \text{ is observed in pattern } s, \\ 0 & \text{if } Y_j \text{ is missing in pattern } s. \end{cases}$$

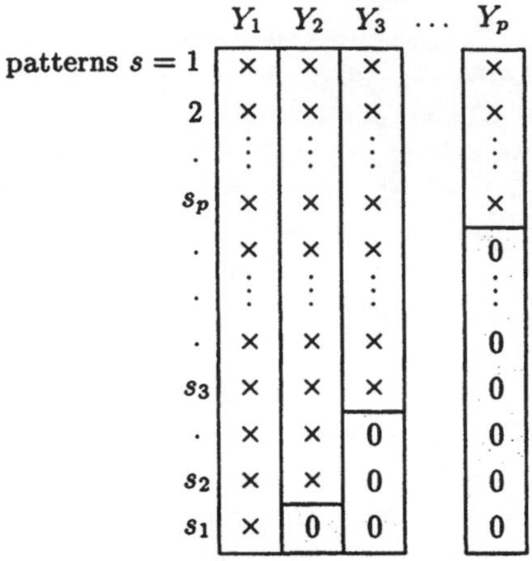

Figure 6.10. *Arrangement of missingness patterns for monotone data augmentation, with 0 denoting a variable that is missing and × denoting a variable that is either observed or missing.*

Let $\mathcal{O}(s)$ and $\mathcal{M}(s)$ denote the column labels corresponding to variables that are observed and missing, respectively, in pattern s,

$$\mathcal{O}(s) = \{j : r_{sj} = 1\},$$
$$\mathcal{M}(s) = \{j : r_{sj} = 0\}.$$

Also, let $\mathcal{M}^*(s)$ denote the subset of $\mathcal{M}(s)$ that must be filled in to complete the monotone pattern, and let $\mathcal{M}^{**}(s)$ be the remainder of $\mathcal{M}(s)$,

$$\mathcal{M}^*(s) = \{j : r_{sj} = 0 \text{ and } s_j \geq s\},$$
$$\mathcal{M}^{**}(s) = \{j : r_{sj} = 0 \text{ and } s_j < s\}.$$

For any s, $\mathcal{M}^*(s)$ lists the columns with missing values in the unshaded region of Figure 6.10, and $\mathcal{M}^{**}(s)$ lists the columns in the shaded region. Finally, let $\mathcal{I}(s)$ denote the subset of $\{1, 2, \ldots, n\}$ corresponding to the rows of the data matrix Y in pattern s.

The I- and P-steps

The I-step for monotone data augmentation is nearly identical to the I-step for ordinary data augmentation; the only difference is that rather than imputing all the missing values Y_{mis}, we need only impute the portion Y_{mis^*} to complete the monotone pattern. Consequently, the pseudocode for the I-step shown in Figure 5.6

can be used for monotone data augmentation with only one modification: replace every occurrence of $\mathcal{M}(s)$ with the potentially smaller set $\mathcal{M}^*(s)$. The four lines of code in Figure 5.6 preceded by the character 'C' are not needed and may be removed.

The P-step, however, is computationally more complicated than the P-step for ordinary data augmentation, because the posterior distributions of $\phi_1, \phi_2, \ldots, \phi_p$ depend on different sets of sufficient statistics. The posterior of ϕ_j, given by (6.21)–(6.22), depends on $\hat{\beta}_j$, $(X_j^T X_j)^{-1}$, and $\hat{\epsilon}_j^T \hat{\epsilon}_j$, which are obtained from the regression of Y_j on $Y_1, \ldots, Y_{j-1}$ over the rows of the data matrix in missingness patterns $s = 1, \ldots, s_j$. To perform this regression, we need to accumulate sums of squares and cross-products for variables $Y_1, \ldots, Y_j$ and patterns $s = 1, \ldots, s_j$.

As in Section 5.3.3, define $T(s)$ to be the $(p+1) \times (p+1)$ matrix of complete-data sufficient statistics from missingness pattern s,

$$
T(s) = \begin{bmatrix}
n_s & \sum y_{i1} & \sum y_{i2} & \cdots & \sum y_{ip} \\
 & \sum y_{i1}^2 & \sum y_{i1} y_{i2} & \cdots & \sum y_{i1} y_{ip} \\
 & & \sum y_{i2}^2 & \cdots & \sum y_{i2} y_{ip} \\
 & & & \ddots & \vdots \\
 & & & & \sum y_{ip}^2
\end{bmatrix},
$$

where all sums are taken over $i \in \mathcal{I}(s)$, and $n_s = \sum_{i \in \mathcal{I}(s)} 1$ is the sample size in pattern s. For simplicity, we will number the rows and columns of $T(s)$ from 0 to p rather than from 1 to $p+1$. Let $T_{mis}(s)$ and $T_{obs}(s)$ be matrices of the same size as $T(s)$ with elements defined as follows: the (j,k)th element of $T_{mis}(s)$ is equal to the (j,k)th element of $T(s)$ if $j \in \mathcal{M}(s)$ or $k \in \mathcal{M}(s)$, and zero otherwise; and $T_{obs}(s) = T(s) - T_{mis}(s)$. Notice that $T_{mis}(s)$ contains the sufficient statistics that depend on Y_{mis}, whereas $T_{obs}(s)$ contains the sufficient statistics that are functions only of Y_{obs}. Finally, let $T_{mis^*}(s)$ be a matrix identical to $T_{mis}(s)$, but with the following exception: the rows and columns corresponding to variables that are not needed to complete the monotone pattern are set to zero. That is, set the (j,k)th element of $T_{mis^*}(s)$ equal to zero if $j \in \mathcal{M}^{**}(s)$ or $k \in \mathcal{M}^{**}(s)$, otherwise set it equal to the (j,k)th element of $T_{mis}(s)$. Thus T_{mis^*} contains the sufficient statistics that depend on Y_{mis^*} but not on $Y_{mis^{**}}$.

Suppose that the unknown values in Y_{mis^*} have been filled in by an I-step so that $T_{mis^*}(s)$ can be calculated. If we let

$$T_j = \sum_{s=1}^{s_j} T_{obs}(s) + \sum_{s=1}^{s_j} T_{mis^*}(s),$$

then

$$T_j = \begin{bmatrix} X_j^T X_j & X_j^T z_j & 0 \\ z_j^T X_j & z_j^T z_j & 0 \\ 0 & 0 & 0 \end{bmatrix},$$

where z_j and X_j, given by (6.10) and (6.11), are the response vector and covariate matrix needed for the regression of Y_j on $Y_1, \ldots, Y_{j-1}$. If this matrix is swept on positions $0, 1, \ldots, j-1$, the result is

$$\begin{bmatrix} -(X_j^T X_j)^{-1} & (X_j^T X_j)^{-1} X_j^T z_j & 0 \\ z_j^T X_j (X_j^T X_j)^{-1} & z_j^T z_j - z_j^T X_j (X_j^T X_j)^{-1} X_j^T z_j & 0 \\ 0 & 0 & 0 \end{bmatrix}.$$

But notice that

$$(X_j^T X_j)^{-1} X_j^T z_j = \hat{\beta}_j$$

is the vector of estimated coefficients from ordinary least-squares regression of z_j on X_j. Moreover, it is straightforward to show that

$$z_j^T z_j - z_j^T X_j (X_j^T X_j)^{-1} X_j^T z_j = \hat{\epsilon}_j^T \hat{\epsilon}_j,$$

where $\hat{\epsilon}_j = z_j - X_j \hat{\beta}_j$ is the vector of estimated residuals. The quantities needed to describe the posterior distribution of ϕ_j, given the observed data Y_{obs} and imputed data in Y_{mis^*}, can thus be obtained by sweeping the matrix T_j. Note that all of the elements of T_j in rows and columns $j+1, \ldots, p$ are zero before and after sweeping. Superfluous arithmetic can be avoided by applying the generalized sweep operator (Section 6.5.2) to sweep only the nonzero portions of T. The regression computations become

$$\text{SWP}_{A_j}[0, \ldots, j-1] T_j = \begin{bmatrix} -(X_j^T X_j)^{-1} & \hat{\beta}_j & 0 \\ \hat{\beta}_j^T & \hat{\epsilon}_j^T \hat{\epsilon}_j & 0 \\ 0 & 0 & 0 \end{bmatrix},$$

where $A_j = \{0, 1, \ldots, j\}$.

An implementation of the P-step is shown in Figure 6.11. The components of ϕ are simulated in the reverse order $\phi_p, \phi_{p-1}, \ldots, \phi_1$ and placed in a $(p+1) \times (p+1)$ matrix as shown in Section 6.5.2. This implementation requires two matrix workspaces of the same

```
s_{p+1} := 0
T := 0
for j := p down to 1 do
    for s := s_{j+1} + 1 to s_j do T := T + T_{obs}(s) + T_{mis*}(s)
    if s_j > s_{j+1} then T := SWP_{A_j}[0, 1, ..., j - 1] T
    draw φ_{jj} ~ T_{jj}/χ²_{N_j-p+j-1}
    C := Chol_{A_{j-1}}(-φ_{jj}T)
    for k := 0 to j - 1 do
        draw v_k ~ N(0, 1)
        φ_{kj} := T_{kj}
        for l := 0 to k do φ_{kj} := φ_{kj} + C_{lk}v_l
    end do
    if j > 1 and s_{j-1} > s_j then
        T := RSWA_{A_{j-1}}[0, 1, ..., j - 1] T
    else if j > 1 and s_{j-1} = s_j then
        T := RSWA_{A_{j-1}}[j - 1] T
    end if
end do
```

Figure 6.11. *P-step for monotone data augmentation.*

size as ϕ: T, in which the sufficient statistics T_j are accumulated and swept; and C, which holds the Cholesky factors required for simulating the vectors of regression coefficients β_j. In addition, a vector workspace $v = (v_0, v_1, \ldots, v_{p-1})$ is needed for temporary storage of normal random variates. The quantity N_j, which appears in the degrees of freedom of the chisquare random variate, is

$$N_j = \sum_{s=1}^{s_j} n_s,$$

the total number of rows of the data matrix Y for which variable Y_j is either observed or imputed.

The algorithm of Figure 6.11 operates as follows. After the elements of T are initialized to zero, the sufficient statistics for $Y_1, \ldots, Y_p$ are accumulated in T over missingness patterns $1, \ldots, s_p$. The matrix T is swept on positions $0, \ldots, p - 1$, producing statistics from the regression of Y_p on $Y_1, \ldots, Y_{p-1}$. A random value of $\phi_p = (\gamma_p, \beta_p)$ is then drawn from its posterior distribution. If additional rows of Y will enter into the next regression, i.e. if $s_{p-1} > s_p$, then T is reverse-swept on positions $0, \ldots, p - 1$ to prepare for the accumulation of sufficient statistics over these additional rows.

Otherwise, T is reverse-swept only on position $p - 1$, yielding the results from the regression of Y_{p-1} on $Y_1, \ldots, Y_{p-2}$. Continuing in this fashion, the algorithm draws $\phi_{p-1}, \phi_{p-2}, \ldots, \phi_1$. Upon completion, the resulting value of ϕ should be transformed to the θ-scale (Section 6.5.2) to prepare for the next I-step.

The accumulation of sufficient statistics in line 4 of this algorithm may be rewritten as

$$T := T + \sum_{s=s_{j+1}+1}^{s_j} T_{obs}(s) + \sum_{s=s_{j+1}+1}^{s_j} T_{mis^*}(s). \qquad (6.25)$$

The first sum on the right-hand side of (6.25) depends only on the observed data Y_{obs} and does not need to be recalculated at each P-step. Calculating

$$B_j = \sum_{s=s_{j+1}+1}^{s_j} T_{obs}(s)$$

once at the outset of the program and storing it for future iterations can substantially reduce the amount of computation required at each P-step. Notice that we do not need to calculate and store B_j for every $j = 1, 2, \ldots, p$, but only for those values of j for which $s_{j+1} < s_j$. The second sum on the right-hand side of (6.25) depends on Y_{mis^*}, the missing values imputed at the I-step, so these terms will need to be recalculated at each P-step.

6.5.6 Uses and extensions

Like ordinary data augmentation, monotone data augmentation enables us to (a) simulate values of θ from the observed-data posterior $P(\theta \mid Y_{obs})$, and (b) create proper multiple imputations of Y_{mis}. The output stream is a sequence

$$(Y_{mis^*}^{(1)}, \theta^{(1)}), (Y_{mis^*}^{(2)}, \theta^{(2)}), \ldots, (Y_{mis^*}^{(t)}, \theta^{(t)}), \ldots$$

with $P(Y_{mis^*}, \theta \mid Y_{obs})$ as its stationary distribution. After a sufficient burn-in period, successive values of θ,

$$\theta^{(t)}, \theta^{(t+1)}, \theta^{(t+2)}, \ldots,$$

constitute a dependent sample from $P(\theta \mid Y_{obs})$ and may be summarized using any of the methods described in Chapter 4. Iterates of Y_{mis^*} that are sufficiently far apart in the output stream, say

$$Y_{mis^*}^{(t)}, Y_{mis^*}^{(t+k)}, Y_{mis^*}^{(t+2k)}, \ldots$$

for some large value of k, can be taken as proper multiple imputations of Y_{mis^*}.

In many applications, we will want proper multiple imputations of all the missing data in Y_{mis}, not just the missing data Y_{mis^*} needed to complete a monotone pattern. To obtain m proper multiple imputations of Y_{mis}, we should first generate m values of θ that are approximately independent, say

$$\theta^{(t)}, \theta^{(t+k)}, \ldots, \theta^{(t+mk)},$$

and then draw a value of Y_{mis} given each one,

$$
\begin{aligned}
Y_{mis}^{(1)} &\sim P(Y_{mis} \mid Y_{obs}, \theta^{(t)}), \\
Y_{mis}^{(2)} &\sim P(Y_{mis} \mid Y_{obs}, \theta^{(t+k)}), \\
&\vdots \\
Y_{mis}^{(m)} &\sim P(Y_{mis} \mid Y_{obs}, \theta^{(t+mk)}),
\end{aligned}
$$

using the I-step for ordinary data augmentation described in Chapter 5. Of course, to obtain independent values of θ we do not necessarily need to subsample every kth value from a single chain of monotone data augmentation; we can also run m independent chains of length k from a common starting value, or better still, from m independent starting values drawn from an overdispersed starting distribution (Section 4.4.2).

Alternative priors

The monotone data augmentation algorithm described above uses the customary noninformative prior distribution

$$\pi(\theta) \propto |\Sigma|^{-\left(\frac{p+1}{2}\right)}.$$

It is occasionally helpful to use other priors. For example, in sparse-data situations where some aspects of the covariance structure are poorly estimated, we may want to apply the ridge prior described in Section 5.2.3. A strategy for monotone data augmentation under an arbitrary inverted-Wishart prior distribution for Σ is outlined by Liu (1993). Liu's algorithm uses a clever factorization of the posterior distribution under monotone data, derived using an extension of the Bartlett decomposition (Section 5.4.2).

6.5.7 Example

Section 6.4 presented a small simulation study designed to mimic the types of data and missingness found in a national health examination survey. The response mechanism shown in Table 6.12, which was estimated from an actual survey, tends to produce samples that are nearly monotone. The most common missingness pattern, which occurs for about 70% of sampled individuals, has all four survey variables (AGE, BMI, HYP, CHL) observed. The next most common pattern, which occurs about 15% of the time, has AGE observed and the other three variables missing. If AGE is placed in the first column of the data matrix, then at least 85% of the sampled individuals will tend to conform to a monotone pattern. This is precisely the type of situation in which monotone data augmentation should outperform ordinary data augmentation.

To illustrate, a simple random sample of $n = 25$ individuals was drawn from the study population, and a random pattern of missingness was imposed on the sample according to the estimated mechanism. The simulated data and missingness patterns are shown in Table 6.14. Overall there are 27 missing values, but only three of them (one value of HYP and two of BMI) are needed to complete a monotone pattern.

As in the simulation study, we replaced AGE by two dummy indicators ($AGE_2 = 1$ for AGE $= 2$ and 0 otherwise; $AGE_3 = 1$ for AGE $= 3$ and 0 otherwise) and modeled the resulting five-variable dataset as multivariate normal. An exploratory run of the EM algorithm revealed that the worst fraction of missing information, as estimated from the elementwise rates of convergence, is about 66%. Runs of data augmentation and monotone data augmentation under the customary noninformative prior verified that monotone data augmentation does indeed converge faster. Sample autocorrelations for two functions of the parameter θ, calculated over 5000 iterations of each algorithm, are displayed in Figure 6.12. Figure 6.12 (a) shows ACFs for the correlation between BMI and CHL, and Figure 6.12 (b) shows ACFs for the worst linear function of θ, which was estimated from the trajectory of EM. With respect to these two parameters, data augmentation appears to be approximately stationary by lag $k = 4$, whereas monotone data augmentation seems nearly stationary at lag $k = 1$.

For a dataset of this size, iterations of either algorithm can be executed so quickly on modern computers that the advantage of monotone data augmentation is of little practical importance. In

Table 6.14. *Sample data from a health examination survey with simulated pattern of missingness (1=observed, 0=missing)*

(a) Observed data			
AGE	HYP	BMI	CHL
1	—	—	—
2	0	22.7	187
1	0	—	187
3	—	—	—
1	0	20.4	113
3	—	—	184
1	0	22.5	118
1	0	30.1	187
2	0	22.0	238
2	—	—	—
1	—	—	—
2	—	—	—
3	0	21.7	206
2	1	28.7	204
1	0	29.6	—
1	—	—	—
3	1	27.2	284
2	1	26.3	199
1	0	35.3	218
3	1	25.5	—
1	—	—	—
1	0	33.2	229
1	0	27.5	131
3	0	24.9	—
2	0	27.4	186

(b) Missingness patterns				
count	AGE	HYP	BMI	CHL
13	1	1	1	1
1	1	1	0	1
1	1	0	0	1
3	1	1	1	0
7	1	0	0	0

a large database, however, a four-fold reduction in the time required to produce a given number of multiple imputations can be a substantial improvement. Moreover, the gains tend to become even more dramatic as the rates of missing information increase. In studies that employ double sampling or matrix sampling, it is not uncommon for the rates of missing information for some parameters to be 90% or more. These high rates of missingness, due primarily to data that are missing by design, can make the convergence of ordinary data augmentation painfully slow. It is easy to envision scenarios where exploiting a near-monotone pattern that

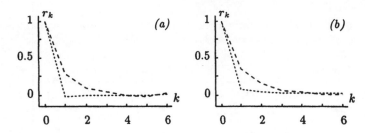

Figure 6.12. *Sample ACFs of series from ordinary data augmentation (dashed line) and monotone data augmentation (dotted line) for (a) the correlation between BMI and CHL, and (b) the worst linear function of the parameter.*

arises by design can reduce the computations by one or more orders of magnitude.

CHAPTER 7

Methods for categorical data

7.1 Introduction

The past three decades have seen enormous growth in the theory
and application of models for categorical data. Categorical-data
techniques such as logistic regression and loglinear modeling are
now commonplace in the social and biomedical sciences and nearly
every other major area of statistical application. For the most part,
however, principled methods for handling missing values in categorical data analysis have not been readily available.

We have already demonstrated that, under certain circumstances,
categorical variables can be handled quite reasonably by applying the multivariate normal distribution (Sections 6.3 and 6.4).
In other situations, however, it is desirable to use a model specifically designed for categorical data. This chapter develops techniques for parameter simulation and multiple imputation for incomplete categorical data under the saturated multinomial model.
The saturated multinomial is more general than the multivariate
normal in the sense that it allows for three-way and higher associations among the variables; the multivariate normal captures simple (two-way) associations only. When maintaining higher-order
associations among continuous variables is a priority, it may even
be worthwhile to categorize them and apply the methods of this
chapter rather than normal-based methods, even though the cate-
gorization may result in a slight loss of information.

The generality of the saturated multinomial model can also be
a drawback, however, because in many applications (particularly
as the number of variables grows) some of the higher-order associations may be poorly estimated. In these situations, it often helps
to simplify the model by selectively removing some of these complex associations. Elimination of higher-order associations will be
discussed within the framework of loglinear modeling, which will
be covered in Chapter 8.

Section 7.2 lays the groundwork for our categorical-data methods by reviewing fundamental properties of two multivariate distributions, the multinomial and the Dirichlet. Basic EM and data augmentation algorithms for the saturated multinomial model are developed in Section 7.3. Section 7.4 introduces a class of algorithms that tends to be more efficient when the missing values fall in a pattern that is nearly monotone.

7.2 The multinomial model and Dirichlet prior

7.2.1 The multinomial distribution

Let $Y_1, Y_2, \ldots, Y_p$ denote a set of categorical variables. For notational convenience, we will suppose that the levels of each variable are coded as positive integers, so that

$$Y_j \text{ takes possible values } 1, 2, \ldots, d_j$$

for $j = 1, 2, \ldots, p$. Throughout this chapter, we will regard the levels $1, 2, \ldots, d_j$ as nominal or unordered categories; we do not consider models that explicitly account for ordering, e.g. the models for ordinal variables discussed by Agresti (1984) and Clogg and Shihadeh (1994). Incomplete ordinal data can sometimes be handled, at least approximately, by pretending that they are normally distributed and applying the methods of Chapters 5–6. Alternatively, one can disregard the order of the levels and apply the methods described here. Disregarding the order results in some loss of information and may lead to models that are more complex (i.e. having more parameters) than necessary to describe the essential relationships among the variables. For developing models that are parsimonious and scientifically meaningful, it is usually desirable to retain the ordering of the levels, if possible. On the other hand, if the immediate goal is to create plausible multiple imputations of missing data for future analyses, then disregarding the order and applying the methods of this chapter may be a perfectly reasonable approach.

If values of $Y_1, Y_2, \ldots, Y_p$ are recorded for a sample of n units, then the complete data can be expressed as an $n \times p$ data matrix Y. If the sample units are independent and identically distributed (iid), then without loss of information we can reduce Y to a contingency table with D cells, where $D = \prod_{j=1}^{p} d_j$ is the number of distinct combinations of the levels of $Y_1, Y_2, \ldots, Y_p$. In practice, logical constraints among the variables may render some of these combinations impossible. For example, if Y_1 represents age (1=0–9 years, 2=10–19 years, ...) and Y_2 represents marital status (1=never married, 2=currently married, ...) then under most circumstances ($Y_1 = 1, Y_2 = 2$) should be regarded as an impossible event. Cells of the contingency table that are necessarily empty due to logical constraints are called *structural zeroes* (e.g. Agresti, 1990). Structural zeroes present only minor complications, most of which are notational. For now, we will proceed as if there are no structural zeroes.

Let us index the cells of the contingency table by the single subscript $d = 1, 2, \ldots, D$. Let x_d be the number of sample units that fall into cell d, and let

$$x = (x_1, x_2, \ldots, x_D)$$

denote the entire set of cell frequencies or counts. If the sample units are iid and the sample size $n = \sum_{d=1}^{D} x_d$ is regarded as fixed, then x has a multinomial distribution. We will write

$$x \mid \theta \sim M(n, \theta)$$

to indicate that x is multinomial with index n and parameter

$$\theta = (\theta_1, \theta_2, \ldots, \theta_D),$$

where θ_d is the probability that a unit falls into cell d. The probability distribution for x is given by

$$P(x \mid \theta) = \frac{n!}{x_1! \, x_2! \cdots x_D!} \, \theta_1^{x_1} \theta_2^{x_2} \cdots \theta_D^{x_D} \qquad (7.1)$$

for $\sum_{d=1}^{D} x_d = n$ and 0 otherwise. Because the total sample size n is fixed, one of the elements of x is redundant; we can replace x_D by $n - \sum_{d=1}^{D-1} x_d$ and regard (7.1) as the probability distribution for $(x_1, \ldots, x_{D-1})$.

Notice that the cell probabilities must satisfy $\sum_{d=1}^{D} \theta_d = 1$, so the multinomial model has only $D - 1$ free parameters; θ_D can be replaced by $1 - \sum_{d=1}^{D-1} \theta_d$. Alternatively, we can regard the full vector $\theta = (\theta_1, \ldots, \theta_D)$ as the unknown parameter, with the understanding that it must lie within the simplex

$$\Theta = \left\{ \theta : \theta_d \geq 0 \text{ for all } d \text{ and } \sum_{d=1}^{D} \theta_d = 1 \right\}, \qquad (7.2)$$

a $(D-1)$-dimensional subset of D-dimensional space. When $D = 3$, for example, Θ is the region encompassed by the triangle with vertices $(1, 0, 0)$, $(0, 1, 0)$ and $(0, 0, 1)$.

The simplex Θ is the natural parameter space for the multinomial, i.e. the set of all possible values of θ for which (7.1) is a valid probability model. Throughout this chapter, we allow θ to lie anywhere in Θ. Such a model is said to be *saturated*, because it includes the maximum number of free parameters $(D-1)$. The saturated model is very general; it allows for any kind of relationships to exist among the variables $Y_1, Y_2, \ldots, Y_p$. In many applications, however, such generality is undesirable because the information contained in the observed data may not be sufficient to estimate so many parameters adequately. Moreover, when the goal is to develop a model that is scientifically meaningful, models that are more parsimonious (i.e. having fewer parameters) than the saturated model may be easier to interpret. In Chapter 8, we will show how to reduce the number of free parameters by imposing loglinear constraints on the elements of θ.

When the multinomial vector x has only $D = 2$ cells, x_2 and θ_2 can be replaced by $n - x_1$ and $1 - \theta_1$, respectively, and (7.1) reduces to a binomial distribution,

$$P(x \mid n) = \frac{n!}{x_1! \, (n - x_1)!} \, \theta_1^{x_1} (1 - \theta_1)^{n - x_1}.$$

In this special case, we will sometimes use the notation

$$x_1 \mid \theta_1 \sim B(n, \theta_1)$$

as an alternative to

$$(x_1, n - x_1) \mid \theta \sim M(n, (\theta_1, n - \theta_1)).$$

The first two moments of the multinomial distribution are given by

$$\begin{aligned}
E(x_d \mid \theta) &= n \, \theta_d, \\
V(x_d \mid \theta) &= n \, \theta_d (1 - \theta_d), \\
\mathrm{Cov}(x_d, x_{d'} \mid \theta) &= -n \, \theta_d \theta_{d'}, \quad d' \neq d.
\end{aligned}$$

Further properties of the multinomial distribution can be found in texts on discrete data (e.g. Bishop, Fienberg and Holland, 1975; Agresti, 1990).

Maximum-likelihood estimation

The likelihood function for the multinomial parameter is

$$L(\theta \mid Y) \propto \prod_{d=1}^{D} \theta_d^{x_d} \, I_\Theta(\theta), \tag{7.3}$$

where $I_\Theta(\theta)$ is an indicator function equal to 1 if $\theta \in \Theta$ and 0 otherwise. Notice that we have written $L(\theta|Y)$ rather than $L(\theta|x)$. We are allowed to do this because all relevant information about θ in the data matrix Y is captured in the contingency table x; that is, we can reconstruct Y from x except for the order of the sample units, which under the iid assumption is statistically irrelevant. The loglikelihood is

$$l(\theta|Y) = \sum_{d=1}^{D} x_d \log \theta_d, \qquad (7.4)$$

defined over the simplex Θ. The multinomial is a regular exponential family distribution whose sufficient statistics are simply the cell counts $x = (x_1, \ldots, x_D)$. Therefore, complete-data ML estimates can be obtained simply by equating each observed cell count x_d to its expectation $E(x_d|\theta) = n\theta_d$, leading to the well-known result that the ML estimates for the cell probabilities are the observed proportions

$$\hat{\theta}_d = \frac{x_d}{n}, \quad d = 1, \ldots, D. \qquad (7.5)$$

7.2.2 Collapsing and partitioning the multinomial

The multinomial distribution has two convenient properties that enable us to factor the probability distribution $P(x|\theta)$ and the likelihood $L(\theta|Y)$. Suppose that we collapse two cells of the contingency table, say x_1 and x_2, adding the frequencies together to produce a new table $x^* = (z, x_3, \ldots, x_D)$ where $z = x_1 + x_2$. Then (a) the distribution of of x^* is multinomial,

$$x^* \mid \theta \sim M(n, \theta^*), \qquad (7.6)$$

where $\theta^* = (\xi, \theta_3, \ldots, \theta_D)$ and $\xi = \theta_1 + \theta_2$; and (b) the conditional distribution of (x_1, x_2) given z is also multinomial,

$$(x_1, x_2) \mid z, \theta \sim M(z, (\theta_1/\xi, \theta_2/\xi)). \qquad (7.7)$$

Property (a) is derived by summing the multinomial probabilities for all x-vectors consistent with $x_1 + x_2 = z$,

$$P(x^*|\theta) = \sum_{j=0}^{z} P(x_1 = j, x_2 = z - j, x_3, \ldots, x_D)$$

$$= \sum_{j=0}^{z} \frac{n!}{j!\,(z-j)!\,x_3! \cdots x_D!} \theta_1^j \theta_2^{z-j} \theta_3^{x_3} \cdots \theta_D^{x_D}$$

$$= \frac{n!}{z!\,x_3!\cdots x_D!}\, \theta_3^{x_3}\cdots\theta_D^{x_D} \sum_{j=0}^{z} \frac{z!}{j!\,(z-j)!}\, \theta_1^j\theta_2^{z-j},$$

and noting that

$$\sum_{j=0}^{z} \frac{z!}{j!\,(z-j)!}\, \theta_1^j\theta_2^{z-j} = (\theta_1+\theta_2)^z$$

by the Binomial Theorem. Property (b) can be deduced as follows. Notice that if we repeatedly apply Property (a) to collapse the table down to $x_1+x_2=z$ and $x_3+\cdots+x_D=n-z$, we obtain

$$(z,n-z)\mid\theta \sim M(n,\,(\xi,1-\xi)).$$

Moreover, if we collapse $x_3+\cdots+x_D=n-z$ but leave x_1 and x_2 intact, then

$$(x_1,x_2,n-z)\mid\theta \sim M(n,\,(\theta_1,\theta_2,1-\xi)).$$

The conditional distribution of (x_1,x_2) given z is by definition

$$P(x_1,x_2\mid z,\theta) = \frac{P(x_1,x_2,n-z\mid\theta)}{P(z,n-z\mid\theta)} \qquad (7.8)$$

for $x_1+x_2=z$ and 0 otherwise. Substituting expressions for the numerator and denominator, the right-hand side of (7.8) becomes

$$\left[\frac{n!}{x_1!\,x_2!\,(n-z)!}\, \theta_1^{x_1}\theta_2^{x_2}(1-\xi)^{n-z}\right]\left[\frac{n!}{z!\,(n-z)!}\, \xi^z(1-\xi)^{n-z}\right]^{-1}$$

which reduces to

$$P(x_1,x_2\mid z,\theta) = \frac{z!}{x_1!\,x_2!}\left(\frac{\theta_1}{\xi}\right)^{x_1}\left(\frac{\theta_2}{\xi}\right)^{x_2},$$

the desired result.

We have stated these results in terms of collapsing just two cells $(x_1+x_2=z)$, but they extend to arbitrary types of collapsing. Suppose that we partition the cell numbers $\{1,2,\ldots,D\}$ into subsets $A_1,A_2,\ldots,A_K$ that are mutually exclusive and collectively exhaustive. Denote the part of x corresponding to A_k by

$$x_{(k)} = \{x_d : d \in A_k\}.$$

The collection $\{x_{(1)},x_{(2)},\ldots,x_{(K)}\}$ of these parts will be called the *partitioned table*, and $x_{(k)}$ will be called the *kth part of x*. Denote the total frequency for the kth part by

$$z_k = \sum_{d\in A_k} x_d.$$

The collection $z = (z_1, z_2, \ldots, z_K)$ of these total frequencies will be called the *collapsed table*. Denote the probability that a sample unit falls into the kth part by

$$\xi_k = \sum_{d \in A_k} \theta_d, \qquad (7.9)$$

and the conditional probability that a sample unit falls into cell d given that it falls into the kth part by

$$\phi_{kd} = \theta_d / \xi_k \quad \text{for all } d \in A_k. \qquad (7.10)$$

Denote the collection of all such conditional probabilities for the kth part by

$$\phi_k = \{\phi_{kd} : d \in A_k\}.$$

Notice that ϕ_k is simply the kth part of θ, rescaled so that its elements sum to one. Under these conditions, it can be shown that (a) the marginal distribution of the collapsed table is multinomial,

$$z \mid \theta \sim M(n, \xi), \qquad (7.11)$$

where $\xi = (\xi_1, \xi_2, \ldots, \xi_K)$; and (b) the conditional distribution of the partitioned table given the collapsed table is a set of independent multinomials,

$$
\begin{aligned}
x_{(1)} \mid z, \theta &\sim M(z_1, \phi_1), \\
x_{(2)} \mid z, \theta &\sim M(z_2, \phi_2), \\
&\vdots \\
x_{(K)} \mid z, \theta &\sim M(z_K, \phi_K).
\end{aligned}
\qquad (7.12)
$$

A set of independent multinomial distributions over a partitioned contingency table is often called a *product multinomial*. For any collapsing scheme, we can thus factor the multinomial distribution into a multinomial for the frequencies in the collapsed table, whose parameters are obtained by summing or collapsing θ in the same manner that x was collapsed, and a product multinomial for the conditional distribution of the partitioned table given the collapsed table, whose parameters are obtained by partitioning θ and rescaling each part to sum to one.

Factoring the likelihood

It is easy to see that the parameters for the collapsed table and the partitioned table, which we denote collectively by

$$\psi = (\xi, \phi_1, \ldots, \phi_K),$$

are a one-to-one function of $\theta = (\theta_1, \ldots, \theta_d)$; the forward transformation $\psi = \psi(\theta)$ is defined by (7.9)–(7.10), and the back transformation $\theta = \psi^{-1}(\psi)$ is

$$\theta_d = \xi_k \phi_{kd} \quad \text{for all } d \in A_k, \tag{7.13}$$

$k = 1, 2, \ldots, K$. Moreover, the parameters for the collapsed table and each part of the partitioned table are mutually distinct; any values of $\xi, \phi_1, \ldots, \phi_K$ in their respective simplexes will produce a value of θ in its simplex Θ. It follows that the likelihood function for ψ can be factored into a sequence of independent multinomial likelihoods,

$$L(\psi|x) = L(\xi|z) \, L(\phi_1|x_{(1)}) \, \cdots \, L(\phi_K|x_{(K)}).$$

Likelihood-based inferences about each part of ψ can be carried out independently, and the results can then be combined to produce a valid overall inference. For example, ML estimates for each part $\xi, \phi_1, \ldots, \phi_K$ can be calculated independently; they are

$$\hat{\xi}_k = \frac{z_k}{n} \quad \text{and} \quad \hat{\phi}_{kd} = \frac{x_d}{z_k} \quad \text{for all } d \in A_k.$$

Applying the back transformation $\theta = \psi^{-1}(\psi)$ to these values gives $\hat{\theta}_d = x_d/n$, the ML estimates for θ. Bayesian inferences for each part can also proceed independently, provided that the prior distribution applied to ψ factors into independent priors for $\xi, \phi_1, \ldots, \phi_K$.

Non-multinomial sampling

This factorization of the multinomial likelihood has important implications for statistical inference. In many datasets, the distribution of one or more categorical variables is not random but fixed by design. Common examples of this include (a) treatment indicators in randomized experiments and (b) variables used to define strata in sample surveys. When the distribution of one or more variables is fixed by design, the cell frequencies $x = (x_1, x_2, \ldots, x_D)$ are not multinomial; rather, they follow a product-multinomial distribution. If we erroneously apply a multinomial model, however, we can still obtain valid likelihood-based or Bayesian inferences about the parameters of the non-fixed portion of the model. This result holds for incomplete data, provided that the missing values are confined to variables that are not fixed (Section 2.6.2). In addition, the multinomial likelihood may lead to valid conditional inferences in situations where the total sample size n is random (e.g. Poisson sampling) (Bishop, Fienberg and Holland, 1975; Agresti, 1990). Although we will speak almost exclusively of the multinomial model throughout this chapter and the next, the reader should be aware that the methods presented here can be reasonably applied in many non-multinomial situations.

7.2.3 The Dirichlet distribution

The simplest way to conduct Bayesian inference with a multinomial model is to choose a parametric family of prior distributions whose density has the same functional form as the likelihood (7.3). Suppose that $\theta = (\theta_1, \dots, \theta_D)$ is a vector of random variables with the property that $\theta_d \geq 0$ for $d = 1, \dots, D$ and $\sum_{d=1}^{D} \theta_d = 1$. Then θ is said to have a Dirichlet distribution with parameter $\alpha = (\alpha_1, \dots, \alpha_D)$ if its density is

$$P(\theta|\alpha) = \frac{\Gamma(\alpha_0)}{\Gamma(\alpha_1)\,\Gamma(\alpha_2)\cdots\Gamma(\alpha_D)}\,\theta_1^{\alpha_1-1}\theta_2^{\alpha_2-1}\cdots\theta_D^{\alpha_D-1} \quad (7.14)$$

over the simplex Θ, where $\alpha_0 = \sum_{d=1}^{D} \alpha_d$ and $\Gamma(\cdot)$ denotes the gamma function. As a shorthand for (7.14), we will write

$$\theta \mid \alpha \sim D(\alpha).$$

The right-hand side of (7.14) is a valid probability density provided that $\alpha_d > 0$ for $d = 1, \dots, D$.

When the Dirichlet is used as a prior distribution for the parameters of the multinomial, we will typically omit the normalizing constant and write the prior density as

$$\pi(\theta) \propto \theta_1^{\alpha_1-1}\theta_2^{\alpha_2-1}\cdots\theta_D^{\alpha_D-1}, \quad (7.15)$$

where $\alpha_1, \dots, \alpha_D$ are understood to be user-specified hyperparameters. Although this appears to be a joint density for D random variables, we must remember that one of the elements of θ is redundant. In taking expectations, for example, we would replace θ_D by $1 - \sum_{d=1}^{D-1} \theta_d$ and integrate with respect to $\theta_1, \dots, \theta_{D-1}$. In the special case of $D = 2$, $\theta_2 = 1 - \theta_1$ and the Dirichlet reduces to a beta distribution for θ_1. In this special case we may write

$$\theta_1 \mid \alpha \sim Beta(\alpha_1, \alpha_2)$$

as an alternative to

$$(\theta_1, \theta_2) \mid \alpha \sim D(\alpha).$$

(a)   *(b)*

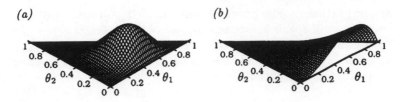

Figure 7.1. *Dirichlet densities for (a)* $\alpha = (5,3,4)$ *and (b)* $\alpha = (3,1,2)$, *plotted as functions of* θ_1 *and* θ_2.

Properties of the Dirichlet distribution

Here we state without proof some basic properties of the Dirichlet distribution. For a more detailed treatment, see Wilks (1962). The first two moments are given by

$$E(\theta_d) = \frac{\alpha_d}{\alpha_0},$$

$$V(\theta_d) = \frac{\alpha_d(\alpha_0 - \alpha_d)}{\alpha_0^2(\alpha_0 + 1)},$$

$$\mathrm{Cov}(\alpha_d, \alpha_{d'}) = -\frac{\alpha_d \alpha_{d'}}{\alpha_0^2(\alpha_0 + 1)}, \quad d' \neq d.$$

If the means α_d/α_0 are held constant but α_0 is allowed to increase, then the variances and covariances are of order $O(\alpha_0^{-1})$. For this reason, α_0 may be regarded as a precision parameter; as it increases, the distribution becomes more tightly concentrated about the mean.

The mode of the Dirichlet can be found by noting that its density is equivalent to the likelihood function from a multinomial contingency table $x = (x_1, \ldots, x_D)$ with $x_d = \alpha_d - 1$, $d = 1, \ldots, D$. This function is maximized at $\theta_d = x_d / \sum_{d'=1}^{D} x_{d'}$ provided that every x_d is nonnegative. Therefore, the mode of the Dirichlet density occurs at

$$\theta_d = \frac{\alpha_d - 1}{\alpha_0 - D} \quad d = 1, \ldots, D, \tag{7.16}$$

provided that every $\alpha_d \geq 1$.

Two examples of the Dirichlet density for $D = 3$ are shown in Figure 7.1. Because one of the elements of $\theta = (\theta_1, \theta_2, \theta_3)$ is redundant, the densities are plotted as functions of θ_1 and θ_2 over the triangular region $\theta_1 \geq 0$, $\theta_2 \geq 0$, $\theta_1 + \theta_2 \leq 1$. Figure 7.1 (a) shows the density for $\alpha = (5,3,4)$, and Figure 7.1 (b) shows the density for $\alpha = (3,1,2)$. Notice that in (a) the mode lies in the interior of the parameter space Θ, whereas in (b) the mode lies on the boundary. It is true in general that if every $\alpha_d > 1$, then the density has a unique mode in the interior of Θ. If every $\alpha_d = 1$, then the Dirichlet density is uniform over Θ. If one or more of the parameters α_d is equal to one but none are less than one, then the density is bounded and the mode occurs on the boundary. Finally, if $\alpha_d < 1$ for any d then the density function becomes infinite on the boundary. These properties suggest that if $\theta \sim D(\alpha)$ represents the current state of knowledge about θ, and if one or more elements of α are less than or equal to one, then the mode may not be a sensible point estimate for θ; a better estimate would be the mean.

Relationship to the gamma distribution

An important relationship exists between the Dirichlet distribution and the gamma distribution. A random variable v is said to have a *standard gamma distribution* with parameter $a > 0$ if its density is

$$P(v|a) = \frac{1}{\Gamma(a)} v^{a-1} e^{-v}$$

for $v > 0$, and we write

$$v \mid a \sim G(a).$$

The gamma distribution is usually presented as a two-parameter family, with one parameter determining the shape and the other determining the scale. The standard gamma distribution is obtained by setting the usual scale parameter to one. The mean and variance of the standard gamma are both equal to a. The standard gamma also has the following reproductive property: if $v_1 \sim G(a_1)$ and $v_2 \sim G(a_2)$ are independent, then $v_1 + v_2 \sim G(a_1 + a_2)$.

The Dirichlet distribution can be obtained from the standard gamma as follows. Suppose that $v_1, v_2, \ldots, v_D$ are independent standard gamma variates with parameters $\alpha_1, \alpha_2, \ldots, \alpha_D$, respectively. If we take

$$\theta_d = \frac{v_d}{\sum_{d'=1}^{D} v_{d'}}, \quad d = 1, 2, \ldots, D,$$

then $\theta = (\theta_1, \theta_2, \ldots, \theta_D)$ will have a Dirichlet distribution with parameter $\alpha = (\alpha_1, \alpha_2, \ldots, \alpha_D)$. This property enables us to simulate a Dirichlet random vector using a standard gamma variate generator. Methods for efficient generation of gamma random variates are reviewed by Kennedy and Gentle (1980).

Limitations of the Dirichlet prior

From a purely conceptual standpoint, the Dirichlet distribution is not the most attractive prior for cross-classified contingency tables. One of its drawbacks is that it treats the cells of the table in an unordered fashion, ignoring its cross-classified structure. We have adopted the Dirichlet prior mainly for computational convenience, because with complete data it leads to posterior distributions that are easily summarized. If the parameters of the data model are not well estimated by the data, and it becomes apparent that the choice of prior has a substantial impact on the results, then one should be wary of drawing firm conclusions from an analysis under a Dirichlet prior or, for that matter, any other type of prior.

7.2.4 Bayesian inference

It is easy to see what happens when a Dirichlet prior is applied to the parameters of the multinomial. Suppose that a contingency table $x = (x_1, \ldots, x_D)$ has a multinomial distribution with parameter $\theta = (\theta_1, \ldots, \theta_D)$, and the prior distribution for θ is Dirichlet with hyperparameter $\alpha = (\alpha_1, \ldots, \alpha_D)$,

$$x \mid \theta \;\sim\; M(n, \theta), \qquad (7.17)$$

$$\theta \;\sim\; D(\alpha). \qquad (7.18)$$

Multiplying the Dirichlet density (7.15) by the multinomial likelihood (7.3) produces

$$P(\theta | Y) \propto \theta_1^{\alpha_1 + x_1 - 1} \theta_2^{\alpha_2 + x_2 - 1} \cdots \theta_D^{\alpha_D + x_D - 1}, \qquad (7.19)$$

which is a Dirichlet density with parameters

$$
\begin{aligned}
\alpha' &= (\alpha_1', \alpha_2', \ldots, \alpha_D') \\
&= (\alpha_1 + x_1, \alpha_2 + x_2, \ldots, \alpha_D + x_D) \\
&= \alpha + x. \qquad (7.20)
\end{aligned}
$$

The posterior distribution of θ under (7.17)–(7.18) is thus

$$\theta \mid Y \sim D(\alpha').$$

The posterior mean is

$$E(\theta | Y) = \left(\frac{\alpha_1'}{\alpha_0'}, \; \frac{\alpha_2'}{\alpha_0'}, \; \ldots, \; \frac{\alpha_D'}{\alpha_0'} \right)$$

where $\alpha_0' = \sum_{d=1}^{D}(\alpha_d + x_d) = \alpha_0 + n$, and the posterior mode is

$$\text{mode}(\theta \mid Y) = \left(\frac{\alpha_1' - 1}{\alpha_0' - D}, \frac{\alpha_2' - 1}{\alpha_0' - D}, \ldots, \frac{\alpha_D' - 1}{\alpha_0' - D} \right)$$

provided that every $\alpha_d' \geq 1$.

The Dirichlet prior (7.17) is a proper probability distribution if $\alpha_1, \alpha_2, \ldots, \alpha_D$ are all positive. Notice, however, that for (7.19) to be proper, we only need the updated hyperparameters $\alpha_d' = \alpha_d + x_d$ to be positive. This means that we can adopt an improper prior density function such as

$$\pi(\theta) \propto \theta_1^{-1}\theta_2^{-1}\cdots\theta_D^{-1}, \qquad (7.21)$$

which is the limiting form of the $D(\alpha)$ density as α approaches $(0, 0, \ldots, 0)$, and still obtain a proper posterior if $\alpha_d + x_d > 0$ for every d. In a slight abuse of terminology, we will call (7.21) the Dirichlet density with $\alpha = (0, 0, \ldots, 0)$; it should be understood that this is not a density per se, but it leads to a proper Dirichlet posterior if there are no empty cells (i.e. if every $x_d \geq 1$).

7.2.5 Choosing the prior hyperparameters

Because of the rule (7.20) for updating the hyperparameters $\alpha = (\alpha_1, \ldots, \alpha_D)$, it is tempting to think of these as imaginary prior counts in the cells of the contingency table. This notion is certainly correct in a *relative* sense; increasing α_d by one has the same inferential effect as observing one additional sample unit in cell d. In an *absolute* sense, however, we hesitate to interpret α_d as the number of prior observations in cell d, because it is not necessarily true that $\alpha_d = 0$ represents no prior observations in cell d.

Noninformative priors

When little prior information is available about θ, it may be sensible to take $\alpha_1, \alpha_2, \ldots, \alpha_D$ equal to a common value—that is, to set $\alpha = (c, c, \ldots, c)$ for some constant c. However, there is no unique choice for c that clearly represents a state of ignorance about θ. Most statisticians would agree that without strong prior information, the ML estimate

$$\hat{\theta} = \left(\frac{x_1}{n}, \frac{x_2}{n}, \ldots, \frac{x_D}{n} \right) \qquad (7.22)$$

is a reasonable point estimate for θ. This is particularly true if $\hat{\theta}$ lies in the interior of the parameter space, i.e. if there are no empty cells. Notice that (7.22) is the posterior mean of θ under the improper prior with $c = 0$, assuming that there are no empty cells. But it is also the posterior mode under the uniform prior with $c = 1$. From the standpoint of estimating θ, one could thus argue that either (or neither!) of these priors is noninformative. Moreover, the Jeffreys invariance principle for choosing a noninformative prior (e.g. Box and Tiao, 1992) leads to the choice $c = 1/2$. Therefore, it seems reasonable to regard the whole range of values of c between zero and one as potentially noninformative.

With certain techniques or algorithms, there may be a natural choice for a noninformative prior. For example, with a mode-finding algorithm such as EM, the uniform prior ($c = 1$) will cause the procedure to converge to an ML estimate. In a general-purpose implementation of EM, therefore, it would be natural to adopt $c = 1$ as a default noninformative prior. In other situations, however, the choice is less clear. In data augmentation, for example, the parameters of interest are typically estimated by their simulated posterior means. Under the prior with $c = 0$, the posterior mean coincides with the ML estimate (at least in the complete-data case) for parameters that are linear functions of $\theta_1, \ldots, \theta_D$, but not for nonlinear parameters (e.g. odds ratios). Unlike ML estimates, posterior means are not invariant under nonlinear transformations. Therefore, we cannot really claim that $c = 0$ is a good default prior for a general-purpose data augmentation routine. The $c = 0$ prior is also unattractive because it is improper; the existence of a proper posterior under this prior is not guaranteed.

If the sample size is large relative to the number of parameters being estimated, the choice of prior will tend to have little impact on the final inferences. For the examples in this book, we will adopt the Jeffreys prior ($c = 1/2$) as a default noninformative prior for simulations where the sample size is large. This choice is admittedly somewhat arbitrary. If there is any doubt that the influence of the prior is minimal, one should always conduct a sensitivity analysis, applying a variety of alternative priors to see how the resulting inferences change. If the results vary dramatically over a range of plausible priors, then the only scientifically justifiable conclusion may be that no firm conclusions are possible.

Sparse tables and flattening priors

When the sample size n is not much larger than the number of cells D, a substantial number of cells may contain no observations.

A table $x = (x_1, \ldots, x_D)$ in which a high proportion of the frequencies x_d are zero is said to be *sparse*. It is well known that when common models for discrete data (e.g. loglinear or logistic models) are fit to sparse tables, the empty cells can lead to inestimable parameters and/or ML estimates on the boundary. For this reason, it has often been suggested that a small positive number such as 1/2 should be added to every cell of a sparse table prior to model fitting. The use of such a number, called a *flattening constant*, is reviewed by Clogg et al. (1991).

The effect of a flattening constant is to smooth the estimate of θ toward a uniform table in which all cell probabilities are equal. When $x = (x_1, \ldots, x_D)$ represents a cross-classification by discrete variables $Y_1, Y_2, \ldots, Y_p$, a uniform table has no relationships whatsoever among the variables. Adding a constant $\epsilon > 0$ to every cell thus tends to be conservative, in the sense that it makes us less likely to conclude that relationships among the variables exist when in fact they do not.

A prior distribution that smooths parameter estimates toward a uniform table will be called a *flattening prior*. Flattening priors can be helpful for ensuring that the mode of θ is unique and lies in the interior of the parameter space. For mode-finding algorithms, the prior with $\alpha = (c, c, \ldots, c)$ for some $c > 1$ is flattening; it adds the equivalent of $\epsilon = c - 1$ prior observations to every cell. Values of c less than one are not recommended for mode-finding algorithms because they are 'anti-flattening,' pushing the estimate of θ away from a uniform table. For simulations in which the results are summarized by posterior means, any prior with $c > 0$ has a flattening effect on the elements of θ, adding the equivalent of $\epsilon = c$ observations to every cell relative to the ML estimate. For odds ratios and other nonlinear parameters, however, the effect of these priors when c is near zero may hardly be flattening. For such parameters, priors with c close to zero may place too much mass near the boundary, causing inferences about nonlinear parameters to be unstable when the table is sparse. In sparse-data situations, it is always advisable to apply a variety of reasonable alternative priors and see how the results change.

When using a flattening prior, care should be taken not to over-smooth the data. Adding ϵ imaginary counts to every cell introduces information equivalent to $D\epsilon$ prior observations. In a very sparse table, adding, say, 1/2 to every cell may result in an effective prior sample size comparable to or greater than the actual sample size. In the absence of strong prior beliefs about θ, it is probably unwise to add prior information that amounts to more than about 10–20% of the actual sample size, so that the integrity of the observed data is not seriously compromised. If inferences about the parameters of interest cannot be stabilized by these modest amounts of prior information, then the model is probably too complex to be supported by the observed data. In such situations, it would be wise to simplify the model by eliminating unnecessary variables or by imposing loglinear constraints (Chapter 8).

Data-dependent priors

One obvious potential drawback of flattening priors is that when they are applied to cross-classified contingency tables, they smooth the data toward a model in which each variable Y_j has a uniform distribution over its levels $1, 2, \ldots, d_j$. In many contexts, it is more desirable to smooth toward a model of mutual independence among the variables but to leave the marginal distributions of the variables unaffected. This can be achieved by making the prior data-dependent.

Suppose that one of the variables (say Y_1) represents the response of greatest interest, and the other variables are potential predictors of Y_1. Clogg *et al.* (1991) advocate a strategy in which prior observations are divided among cells of the contingency table in such a way that the marginal distribution of Y_1 in the observed data is preserved. For example, suppose that Y_1 is dichotomous, with $Y_1 = 1$ and $Y_1 = 2$ observed for 30% and 70% of the sample units, respectively. After an appropriate total number of prior observations n_0 has been chosen, 30% of this total can be allocated to cells of the table corresponding to $Y_1 = 1$, with the remaining 70% going to cells corresponding to $Y_1 = 2$. This strategy, which has an empirical Bayes flavor, smooths the estimates of θ toward a null model in which none of the predictors has any effect on Y_1, but it does not affect the overall distribution of Y_1 itself.

This strategy can be extended to formulate a prior that simultaneously preserves the marginal distributions of all the variables in the dataset (Fienberg and Holland, 1970, 1973). Suppose that cell d of a frequency table corresponds to the event $Y_1 = y_1, Y_2 = y_2, \ldots, Y_p = y_p$. If $Y_1, Y_2, \ldots, Y_p$ are mutually independent, then the probability associated with this cell is

$$\theta_d = P(Y_1 = y_1)\, P(Y_2 = y_2) \cdots P(Y_p = y_p). \tag{7.23}$$

The probabilities on the right-hand side of (7.23) can be estimated by the observed proportions in the sample. Substituting these estimates into (7.23), and multiplying the resulting estimate of θ_d by the desired total number of prior observations n_0, gives the number of prior observations to be allocated to cell d. For mode-finding algorithms, the hyperparameter associated with cell d would be

$$\alpha_d = 1 + n_0 \prod_{j=1}^{p} \hat{P}(Y_j = y_j), \qquad (7.24)$$

where $\hat{P}(Y_j = y_j)$ is the observed proportion of sample units for which $Y_j = y_j$. For simulations,

$$\alpha_d = n_0 \prod_{j=1}^{p} \hat{P}(Y_j = y_j) \qquad (7.25)$$

is a more natural choice, at least when we are concerned with linear functions of the elements of θ. These data-dependent priors can be thought of as discrete-data versions of the ridge prior for the parameters of the multivariate normal (Section 5.2.3), which also smooths toward a model of mutual independence among variables.

If the marginal distribution of each Y_j is not far from uniform (i.e. if the levels $1, 2, \ldots, d_j$ occur with roughly the same frequency), then these data-dependent priors will have nearly the same effect as flattening priors. If some levels are relatively much rarer than others, however, then flattening priors may exert undue influence on these rarer categories, inflating their probabilities and distorting the inferences about certain functions of θ. When this is the case, data-dependent priors can be an attractive alternative to flattening priors, particularly when the data are sparse.

7.2.6 Collapsing and partitioning the Dirichlet

A Dirichlet random vector can be collapsed and partitioned in a manner analogous to that already described for the multinomial (Section 7.2.2), and the resulting vectors will have Dirichlet distributions. Let us first consider what happens when we collapse two elements. Suppose that $\theta = (\theta_1, \ldots, \theta_D)$ has a Dirichlet distribution with parameter $\alpha = (\alpha_1, \ldots, \alpha_D)$. If we form a new vector $\theta^* = (\xi, \theta_3, \ldots, \theta_D)$, where $\xi = \theta_1 + \theta_2$, then (a) the distribution of θ^* is Dirichlet with parameter $\alpha^* = (\beta, \alpha_3, \ldots, \alpha_D)$, where $\beta = \alpha_1 + \alpha_2$; and (b) the conditional distribution of $(\theta_1/\xi, \theta_2/\xi)$ given ξ is Dirichlet with parameter (α_1, α_2). Proofs of these properties are given by Wilks (1962); they can also be justified by appealing to the relationship between the Dirichlet and the standard gamma distribution (Section 7.2.3).

More generally, suppose that $\theta = (\theta_1, \ldots, \theta_D)$ represents the cell probabilities for a multinomial vector $x = (x_1, \ldots, x_D)$, and we apply the transformation described in Section 7.2.2 to θ, transforming it into the cell probabilities for the collapsed and partitioned versions of x. That is, suppose that $A_1, A_2, \ldots, A_K$ are mutually exclusive and collectively exhaustive subsets of $\{1, 2, \ldots, D\}$; let

$$x_{(k)} = \{x_d : d \in A_k\}$$

be the kth part of x; and let

$$z_k = \sum_{d \in A_k} x_d$$

be the total frequency for the kth part. The cell probabilities for the collapsed table $z = (z_1, z_2, \ldots, z_K)$ are $\xi = (\xi_1, \xi_2, \ldots, \xi_K)$, where

$$\xi_k = \sum_{d \in A_k} \theta_d,$$

and the conditional probability of falling into cell d given that we are already in the kth part of the table is

$$\phi_{kd} = \theta_d / \xi_k \quad \text{for all } d \in A_k.$$

If θ has a Dirichlet distribution with parameter $\alpha = (\alpha_1, \ldots, \alpha_D)$, then it can be shown that the distribution of ξ is Dirichlet,

$$\xi \mid \alpha \sim D(\beta),$$

where the parameters $\beta = (\beta_1, \ldots, \beta_K)$ are obtained by summing the elements of α in the same way the elements of θ were summed to obtain ξ,

$$\beta_k = \sum_{d \in A_k} \alpha_d.$$

Moreover, if $\phi_k = \{\phi_{kd} : d \in A_k\}$ is the set of conditional probabilities for the kth part of x, then the conditional distribution of $\phi = (\phi_1, \phi_2, \ldots, \phi_K)$ given ξ is a set of K independent Dirichlet distributions,

$$
\begin{aligned}
\phi_1 \mid \xi, \alpha &\sim D(\alpha_{(1)}), \\
\phi_2 \mid \xi, \alpha &\sim D(\alpha_{(2)}), \\
&\vdots \\
\phi_K \mid \xi, \alpha &\sim D(\alpha_{(K)}),
\end{aligned}
\tag{7.26}
$$

where $\alpha_{(k)} = \{\alpha_d : d \in A_k\}$ denotes the kth part of α.

These properties imply that if a Dirichlet prior is applied to the parameter θ of a multinomial contingency table x, then the prior distribution of $\psi = (\xi, \phi)$, which is a one-to-one function of θ, can be factored into independent Dirichlet distributions for $\xi, \phi_1, \ldots, \phi_K$. This ability of the Dirichlet distribution to be collapsed and partitioned makes it a very attractive prior for use in simulation algorithms, and provides the basis for a monotone data augmentation routine to be described in Section 7.4.

7.3 Basic algorithms for the saturated model

7.3.1 Characterizing an incomplete categorical dataset

This section presents EM and data augmentation algorithms for incomplete categorical datasets under the saturated multinomial model, which imposes no restrictions on the types of relationships that may exist among the variables $Y_1, Y_2, \ldots, Y_p$. These algorithms are conceptually simple, but the notation needed to describe them in a general setting is somewhat unwieldy. To characterize the information contained in an incomplete multivariate categorical dataset, we must extend our notation for contingency tables in several ways.

First, we must account for the fact that the complete-data contingency table $x = (x_1, x_2, \ldots, x_D)$ is actually a cross-classification by the levels of $Y_1, Y_2, \ldots, Y_p$, and as such can be regarded as a p-dimensional array. Suppose that variable Y_j takes possible values $1, 2, \ldots, d_j$. Let x_y, where $y = (y_1, y_2, \ldots, y_p)$, be the total number of units in the sample for which the event $Y_1 = y_1, Y_2 = y_2, \ldots, Y_p = y_p$ occurs, and let θ_y be the probability of this event for any unit. Here we are using y to represent a generic realization of $(Y_1, Y_2, \ldots, Y_p)$ for a single unit, i.e. a possible row of the $n \times p$ data matrix Y. We will denote the set of all possible values of y by $\mathcal{Y}$. Assuming for the moment that there are no structural zeroes, $\mathcal{Y}$ is the Cartesian cross-product of the sets $\{1, 2, \ldots, d_j\}$ for $j = 1, 2, \ldots, p$. When a cell count or probability appears with the vector subscript $y = (y_1, y_2, \ldots, y_p)$ it should be interpreted as an element of an array with dimensions $d_1 \times d_2 \times \cdots \times d_p$, but when it appears with the scalar subscript d it should be interpreted as the dth element of a vector of length $D = \prod_{j=1}^{p} d_j$. Depending on the context, we will sometimes think of the tables x and θ as vectors,

$$x = (x_1, x_2, \ldots, x_D), \quad \theta = (\theta_1, \theta_2, \ldots, \theta_D),$$

and at other times as p-dimensional arrays,

$$x = \{x_y : y \in \mathcal{Y}\}, \quad \theta = \{\theta_y : y \in \mathcal{Y}\}.$$

The distinction between the two forms is simply a matter of notational convenience, because it is always possible to turn an array into a vector by assigning a linear ordering to its cells.

Now we must extend the notation to allow for missing data. Let us assume that observations have been grouped according to their missingness patterns. Index the missingness patterns that appear in the dataset by $s = 1, 2, \ldots, S$, and define a set of binary response indicators

$$r_{sj} = \begin{cases} 1 & \text{if } Y_j \text{ is observed in pattern } s, \\ 0 & \text{if } Y_j \text{ is missing in pattern } s. \end{cases}$$

Let $x_y^{(s)}$ denote the number of sample units within missingness pattern s for which $(Y_1, Y_2, \ldots, Y_p) = y$, and let

$$x^{(s)} = \{x_y^{(s)} : y \in \mathcal{Y}\}$$

denote the full set of these counts for pattern s. If any variables are missing in pattern s, then $x^{(s)}$ is not observed; rather, we observe the counts for a lower dimensional table in which the sample units have been cross-classified only by the observed variables. Let $\mathcal{O}_s$ and $\mathcal{M}_s$ be functions that extract from $y = (y_1, y_2, \ldots, y_p)$ the elements corresponding to the variables that are observed and missing, respectively, in pattern s,

$$\begin{aligned} \mathcal{O}_s(y) &= \{y_j : r_{sj} = 1\}, \\ \mathcal{M}_s(y) &= \{y_j : r_{sj} = 0\}. \end{aligned}$$

Also, let O_s and M_s be, respectively, the sets of all possible values of $\mathcal{O}_s(y)$ and $\mathcal{M}_s(y)$. For example, suppose that in a dataset with $p = 4$ variables, missingness pattern s has Y_1 and Y_4 observed but Y_2 and Y_3 missing; then $\mathcal{O}_s(y) = (y_1, y_4)$, $\mathcal{M}_s(y) = (y_2, y_3)$,

$$\begin{aligned} O_s &= \{(y_1, y_4) : y_1 = 1, 2, \ldots, d_1; \ y_4 = 1, 2, \ldots, d_4\}, \\ M_s &= \{(y_2, y_3) : y_2 = 1, 2, \ldots, d_2; \ y_3 = 1, 2, \ldots, d_3\}. \end{aligned}$$

When the units within missingness pattern s are cross-classified only by their observed variables, the result is a table with counts that we shall denote by

$$z_{\mathcal{O}_s(y)}^{(s)} = \sum_{\mathcal{M}_s(y) \in M_s} x_y^{(s)} \quad \text{for all } \mathcal{O}_s(y) \in O_s. \tag{7.27}$$

The marginal probability that an observation falls within cell $\mathcal{O}_s(y)$ of this table will be called

$$\beta_{\mathcal{O}_s(y)} = \sum_{\mathcal{M}_s(y) \in M_s} \theta_y. \tag{7.28}$$

Observed-data likelihood

When $x = (x_1, x_2, \ldots, x_D)$ has a multinomial distribution with parameter $\theta = (\theta_1, \theta_2, \ldots, \theta_D)$, then the complete-data loglikelihood function for θ is

$$l(\theta|Y) = \sum_{d=1}^{D} x_d \log \theta_d$$

over the simplex Θ (Section 7.2.1). Equivalently, viewing x and θ as p-dimensional arrays, we can write the loglikelihood as

$$l(\theta|Y) = \sum_{y \in \mathcal{Y}} x_y \log \theta_y. \tag{7.29}$$

When some data are missing, the observed-data loglikelihood can be calculated as follows. For any missingness pattern s, the observed data are summarized by the table

$$z^{(s)} = \{z^{(s)}_{\mathcal{O}_s(y)} : \mathcal{O}_s(y) \in O_s\}. \tag{7.30}$$

Notice that $z^{(s)}$ is a collapsed version of the unobserved $x^{(s)}$. By our rules for collapsing multinomial tables (Section 7.2.2), it follows that the contribution of $z^{(s)}$ to the observed-data loglikelihood is equivalent to that of a multinomial distribution with index

$$n_s = \sum_{y \in \mathcal{Y}} x_y^{(s)}$$

and parameter

$$\beta^{(s)} = \{\beta_{\mathcal{O}_s(y)} : \mathcal{O}_s(y) \in O_s\}. \tag{7.31}$$

That is, the contribution of $z^{(s)}$ to the observed-data loglikelihood is

$$\sum_{\mathcal{O}_s(y) \in O_s} z^{(s)}_{\mathcal{O}_s(y)} \log \beta_{\mathcal{O}_s(y)}.$$

The observed-data loglikelihood is the sum of these contributions for missingness patterns $s = 1, 2, \ldots, S$,

$$l(\theta|Y_{obs}) = \sum_{s=1}^{S} \sum_{\mathcal{O}_s(y) \in O_s} z^{(s)}_{\mathcal{O}_s(y)} \log \beta_{\mathcal{O}_s(y)}. \tag{7.32}$$

Despite the concise appearance of (7.32), it is a rather compli-
cated function of the individual elements of θ. Evaluating $l(\theta \mid Y_{obs})$
at specific numerical values of θ is not difficult, but calculating analytic expressions for its first two derivatives can be tedious. For
this reason, it is inconvenient to maximize $l(\theta \mid Y_{obs})$ by gradient
methods. The EM algorithm is straightforward, however, because
it involves only the repeated maximization of the complete-data
loglikelihood (7.29).

7.3.2 The EM algorithm

EM for the saturated multinomial model was first described by
Chen and Fienberg (1974) in the special case of $p = 2$ variables, and
extended by Fuchs (1982) to arbitrary p. A description also appears
in Chapter 9 of Little and Rubin (1987). The algorithm, which was
already presented in Section 3.2.2 for two binary variables, is simple and intuitive. For each missingness pattern $s = 1, \ldots, S$, we
allocate the counts in the observed table $z^{(s)}$ to the cells of the full
p-way table $x^{(s)}$. This allocation is carried out in the proportions
implied by the current estimate of θ. When the allocation is complete, the proportions in the resulting table $x = x^{(1)} + x^{(2)} + \cdots x^{(S)}$
provide the updated estimate of θ.

Before running EM, the observed data for each missingness pattern should first be cross-classified according to the observed variables; that is, the data should be reduced to $z^{(1)}, \ldots, z^{(S)}$. Notice
that $z^{(1)}, \ldots, z^{(S)}$ can be regarded as arrays of varying dimensions;
the number of dimensions for $z^{(s)}$ is equal to the number of variables observed in pattern s. When implementing EM on a computer, however, storing $z^{(1)}, \ldots, z^{(S)}$ as multidimensional arrays
tends to be cumbersome and inefficient. As the number of variables p grows, the number of arrays S can increase very rapidly.
Moreover, these arrays can be very sparse; many of them may
contain only a few or perhaps even just one observation each. A
general-purpose computer program should be efficient in its use of
memory, and the data structures it creates should have predictable
size and shape. A more efficient way to store and manipulate the
counts in $z^{(1)}, \ldots, z^{(S)}$ is outlined in Appendix B.

The E- and M-steps

The complete-data loglikelihood (7.29) is a linear function of the
elements of $x = \{x_y : y \in \mathcal{Y}\}$, the unobserved p-dimensional table

that cross-classifies all sample units by their values of $Y_1, Y_2, \ldots, Y_p$. To perform the E-step, we must find the expectation of each count x_y given the observed data and an assumed value for θ. Notice that x can be expressed as $x = \sum_{s=1}^{S} x^{(s)}$, the sum of individual tables for missingness patterns $1, \ldots, S$. Moreover, the observed data $z^{(s)}$ for pattern s is a collapsed version of $x^{(s)}$, and by our rules for collapsing and partitioning (Section 7.2.2) it follows that the conditional distribution of $x^{(s)}$ given $z^{(s)}$ is product-multinomial. Let

$$x^{(s)}_{O_s(y)} = \{x^{(s)}_y : M_s(y) \in M_s\} \tag{7.33}$$

denote the portion of $x^{(s)}$ that is obtained by fixing $O_s(y)$ at a specific value but varying $M_s(y)$ over M_s; that is, $x^{(s)}_{O_s(y)}$ is simply the set of all cell counts in $x^{(s)}$ that contribute to the observed count $z^{(s)}_{O_s(y)}$. By the partitioning rules, $x^{(s)}_{O_s(y)}$ has, given $z^{(s)}_{O_s(y)}$, a multinomial distribution with index $z^{(s)}_{O_s(y)}$ and parameters

$$\gamma_{O_s(y)} = \{\theta_y/\beta_{O_s(y)} : M_s(y) \in M_s\}; \tag{7.34}$$

that is,

$$x^{(s)}_{O_s(y)} \mid z^{(s)}_{O_s(y)}, \theta \sim M(z^{(s)}_{O_s(y)}, \gamma_{O_s(y)}). \tag{7.35}$$

Notice that (7.34) is simply the portion of θ corresponding to $x^{(s)}_{O_s(y)}$, rescaled so that its elements sum to one. It follows that the conditional expectation of an element of $x^{(s)}$ is

$$E(x^{(s)}_y \mid z^{(s)}, \theta) = z^{(s)}_{O_s(y)} \theta_y/\beta_{O_s(y)}. \tag{7.36}$$

The E-step consists of calculating (7.36) for every $s = 1, \ldots, S$ and summing the results,

$$E(x_y \mid Y_{obs}, \theta) = \sum_{s=1}^{S} z^{(s)}_{O_s(y)} \theta_y/\beta_{O_s(y)}. \tag{7.37}$$

Once the E-step has been completed, the M-step is trivial. The complete-data loglikelihood (7.29) is maximized at $\theta_y = x_y/n$, so the M-step is simply to

$$\text{estimate } \theta_y \text{ by } E(x_y \mid Y_{obs}, \theta)/n \tag{7.38}$$

for all $y \in \mathcal{Y}$.

A pseudocode implementation of the E- and M-steps is shown in Figure 7.2. Given the observed counts $z^{(1)}, \ldots, z^{(S)}$ and the current value of θ, this code overwrites θ with its updated value. A temporary workspace x of the same size as θ is required for accumulating

```
for y ∈ 𝒴 do x_y := 0
for s := 1 to S do
    for 𝒪_s(y) ∈ O_s do
        if z^(s)_{𝒪_s(y)} ≠ 0 then
            if M_s = ∅ then
                x_y := x_y + z^(s)_{𝒪_s(y)}
            else
                sum := 0
                for ℳ_s(y) ∈ M_s do sum := sum + θ_y
                for ℳ_s(y) ∈ M_s do x_i := x_y + z^(s)_{𝒪_s(y)} θ_y/sum
                end if
            end if
        end do
    end do
for y ∈ 𝒴 do θ_y := x_y/n
```

Figure 7.2. *Single iteration of EM for the saturated multinomial model.*

the expected sufficient statistics. The algorithm cycles through the missingness patterns and checks to see whether the current pattern s has any missing variables (i.e. if $\mathcal{M}_s(y)$ is nonempty). If not, then the observed counts for pattern s are added into the elements of x; otherwise, the expectations (7.36) are calculated and added into x. After this is done for $s = 1, 2, \ldots, S$, the resulting elements of x are divided by n, which yields the updated value of θ.

Starting values and posterior modes

If the starting value of θ lies on the boundary of the parameter space Θ, i.e. if some of its elements are zero, then an inconsistency could arise in the initial E-step. It could happen that a nonzero count appears in one of the cells of the observed-data tables $z^{(1)}, \ldots, z^{(S)}$ for which the probability implied by the starting value of θ is zero. If this occurs, then the algorithm may halt due to attempted division by zero. To prevent such inconsistencies from arising, a starting value should be chosen in the interior of the parameter space. A good default starting value is a uniform table, in which all the elements of θ are equal.

The algorithm in Figure 7.2 calculates an ML estimate, but with a slight modification it can also be used to find a posterior mode under a Dirichlet prior. The E-step remains the same, but the M-step must be altered to maximize the complete-data posterior density rather than the complete-data likelihood. If the prior distribution of θ is Dirichlet with hyperparameter $\alpha = \{\alpha_y : y \in \mathcal{Y}\}$, then the last line in Figure 7.2 should be changed to

$$\text{for } y \in \mathcal{Y} \text{ do } \theta_y := (x_y + \alpha_y - 1)/(n + \alpha_0 - D), \qquad (7.39)$$

where $\alpha_0 = \sum_{y \in \mathcal{Y}} \alpha_y$ and D is the total number of cells in θ. Taking $\alpha_y = 1$ for all $y \in \mathcal{Y}$ results in a uniform prior, under which the posterior mode and the ML estimate coincide. Notice that if any $\alpha_y < 1$ and the corresponding cell count x_y is zero, then (7.39) will produce a negative estimate for θ_y. For computing posterior modes, priors with $\alpha_y < 1$ are not recommended.

Random zeroes and structural zeroes

When cells of the observed-data tables $z^{(1)}, \ldots, z^{(S)}$ are empty not because the events corresponding to those cells are impossible but merely as an artifact of chance, the cells are said to contain random zeroes. Random zeroes in $z^{(1)}, \ldots, z^{(S)}$ may have two undesirable effects. First, they may produce an ML estimate on the boundary of Θ. Such an estimate is conceptually unattractive, because it implies that some events in the discrete sample space have zero probability even though they have not been deemed impossible on a priori grounds. Second, random zeroes may render certain functions of θ inestimable, in which case the ML estimate will not be unique; the observed-data likelihood will be maximized along a ridge, and EM will converge to different stationary values depending on the starting value (Fuchs, 1982).

When random zeroes result in inestimable parameters or ML estimates on the boundary, the algorithm in Figure 7.2 does not experience any numerical difficulty; it still converges reliably from any starting value in the interior of Θ. The value to which it converges, however, may be a poor estimate for certain functions of θ. When this happens, it is often helpful to apply a Dirichlet prior distribution in which all the hyperparameters are greater than one, e.g. a flattening prior with $\alpha = (c, c, \ldots, c)$ for some $c > 1$, which adds the equivalent of $c - 1$ prior observations to each cell. Another good choice is a data-dependent prior that smooths the estimate toward a null model of independence (Section 7.2.5).

A cell that is empty because the corresponding event is logically impossible is said to contain a structural zero. Structural zeroes are qualitatively different from random zeroes and should not be handled in the same way. Because the probabilities associated with structural zeroes are known to be zero a priori, those cells should be omitted from the estimation procedure. In the algorithm of Figure 7.2, structural zeroes can be handled by providing a starting value for θ in which the elements corresponding to structural zeroes have been set to zero. If the initial value of θ_y is zero, then the first E-step will not allocate any portion of the observed counts in $z^{(1)}, \ldots, z^{(S)}$ to cell y, and the resulting expectation $E(x_y \,|\, Y_{obs}, \theta)$ will be zero. To ensure that the estimate of θ_y remains zero for all subsequent iterations, the last line of the algorithm should be revised to

$$\texttt{for } y \in \mathcal{Y}^* \texttt{ do } \theta_y := (x_y + \alpha_y - 1)/(n + \alpha_0^* - D^*), \qquad (7.40)$$

where $\mathcal{Y}^*$ is the set of all possible values of y excluding the structural zeroes, $\alpha_0^* = \sum_{y \in \mathcal{Y}^*} \alpha_y$ is the sum of the prior hyperparameters and D^* is the number of elements in $\mathcal{Y}^*$ (i.e. the total number of cells excluding structural zeroes).

Observed-data loglikelihood

The observed-data loglikelihood function $l(\theta \,|\, Y_{obs})$, given by (7.32), and the observed-data log-posterior density

$$\log P(\theta \,|\, Y_{obs}) = l(\theta \,|\, Y_{obs}) + \log \pi(\theta),$$

are not difficult to calculate for specific values of θ. Evaluating the loglikelihood or log-posterior density can be helpful for monitoring the progress of EM and data augmentation (Sections 3.3.4 and 4.4.3). Pseudocode for evaluating $l(\theta \,|\, Y_{obs})$ is shown in Figure 7.4. The loglikelihood at the current value of θ is calculated and stored in l. Notice that this code is very similar to the E-step and could easily be woven into EM.

7.3.3 Data augmentation

Data augmentation for the saturated multinomial model is quite similar to the EM algorithm described above. Recall that in data augmentation, we alternately draw from the predictive distribution of the missing data given the observed data and the parameters (the I-step) and from the complete-data posterior distribution of the parameters (the P-step). The observed data consist of the tables $z^{(s)}$ for missingness patterns $s = 1, \ldots, S$, and the missing data consist of the information needed to expand each $z^{(s)}$ into a full p-dimensional table $x^{(s)}$. The predictive distribution of $x^{(s)}$

```
l := 0
for s := 1 to S do
    for O_s(y) ∈ O_s do
        if z^(s)_{O_s(y)} ≠ 0 then
            if M_s = ∅ then
                l := l + z^(s)_{O_s(y)} log θ_y
            else
                sum := 0
                for M_s(y) ∈ M_s do sum := sum + θ_y
                l := l + z^(s)_{O_s(y)} log (sum)
            end if
        end if
    end do
end do
```

Figure 7.3. *Evaluation of the observed-data loglikelihood function.*

given $z^{(s)}$ and θ is the product multinomial given by (7.33)–(7.35). Therefore, the I-step consists of drawing each $x^{(s)}$ from its product multinomial distribution and summing them to obtain a simulated complete-data table $x = x^{(1)} + x^{(2)} + \cdots + x^{(S)}$. Under the Dirichlet prior $\theta \sim D(\alpha)$, the P-step is then just a simulation of θ from its complete-data posterior $D(\alpha + x)$.

In the pseudocode of Figure 7.2, the line

$$\text{for } M_s(y) \in M_s \text{ do } x_y := x_y + z^{(s)}_{O_s(y)} \theta_y / \text{sum} \qquad (7.41)$$

allocates an observed count $z^{(s)}_{O_s(y)}$ to the cells of the complete-data table in fixed proportions determined by the current value of θ. To convert this E-step into an I-step, the proportional allocation must be replaced by a random allocation; that is, we must replace (7.41) by a routine that will draw

$$x^{(s)}_{O_s(y)} \sim M(z^{(s)}_{O_s(y)}, \gamma_{O_s(y)})$$

and add the result into x. One method for simulating the multinomial counts, called *table sampling*, is to compare standard uniform $U(0, 1)$ random variates to cumulative sums of the probabilities in $\gamma_{O_s(y)}$. Pseudocode for table sampling is shown in Figure 7.4. Substituting this code for (7.41) will change the E-step into an I-step. Table sampling can be slow if the counts in the observed-data tables $z^{(s)}$ are large. A more efficient method for simulating multi-

```
        for m:= 1 to z^(s)_{O_s(y)} do
           draw u ~ U(0, 1)
           k:= 0
           for M_s(y) ∈ M_s do
              if k + θ_y/sum > u then
                 x_y := x_y + 1
                 goto 1
              else
                 k:= k + θ_y/sum
              end if
           end do
1          continue
        end do
```

Figure 7.4. *Table sampling for the data augmentation I-step.*

nomial draws in that situation, which relies on a Poisson variate generator, is described by Brown and Bromberg (1984).

To complete the conversion of the EM algorithm to data augmentation, the M-step (the final line of Figure 7.2) must be changed to a P-step; that is, the estimation of θ from the complete-data table x must be replaced by a random draw of θ from the Dirichlet posterior $D(\alpha + x)$. The Dirichlet is easily simulated using standard gamma variates (Section 7.2.3). If any structural zeroes are present, those cells should be omitted from the P-step and their probabilities should be set to zero. If random zeroes occur in $z^{(1)}, \ldots, z^{(S)}$ and the improper Dirichlet prior with $\alpha = (0, 0, \ldots, 0)$ is being used, then depending on the pattern of the zeroes the P-step could be undefined, because some elements of $\alpha + x$ could be zero. For this reason, the prior $\alpha = (0, 0, \ldots, 0)$ should be avoided whenever random zeroes are present. A proper prior, e.g. a flattening prior with $\alpha = (c, c, \ldots, c)$ for some positive value of c, should be used instead.

Imputation of unit-level missing data

The I- and P-steps of the data augmentation algorithm described above operate on the sufficient statistics stored in the workspace x. After enough steps have been taken to achieve approximate stationarity, x will contain a simulated draw from the posterior predictive distribution of the complete-data contingency table $P(x \mid Y_{obs})$. If the algorithm is being used for multiple imputation, however, it may be necessary at the end of the simulation run to impute the missing values at the unit level, i.e. to fill in the missing elements Y_{mis} of the $n \times p$ data matrix Y.

Figure 7.5 shows pseudocode for a modified I-step that imputes the missing elements of Y. Executing this code once at the end of a sufficiently long data augmentation run will result in a proper imputation of Y_{mis}, i.e. a simulated draw from $P(Y_{mis} \mid Y_{obs})$. In Figure 7.5, $y_{i(obs)}$ and $y_{i(mis)}$ denote the observed and missing portions, respectively, of the ith row of the data matrix Y, and $\mathcal{I}(s)$ denotes the rows of Y that exhibit missingness pattern s. The vector workspace $y = (y_1, y_2, \ldots, y_p)$ serves as a counter, indexing the cells of the p-dimensional contingency table. For any row i in missingness pattern s, the subvector $\mathcal{O}_s(y)$ of y is first set equal to the observed data in $y_{i(obs)}$, so that the remaining portion $\mathcal{M}_s(y)$ indexes all the cells of the contingency table into which observation i might fall. The missing values in $y_{i(mis)}$ are then drawn simultaneously by table sampling, comparing a single uniform variate u to the set of probabilities derived from θ that describe the conditional distribution of $y_{i(mis)}$ given $y_{i(obs)}$.

7.3.4 Example: victimization status from the National Crime Survey

Recall the data of Table 3.3 from the National Crime Survey, in which households were classified according to whether they had been victimized by crime in two six-month periods. In the sample of 756 households, 38 had victimization status missing for the first period, 42 had status missing for the second period and 115 had status missing for both periods. Using the EM algorithm and likelihood-ratio tests, we found very strong evidence that victimization status on the two occasions was related; the p-value for testing the hypothesis of independence was essentially zero. Moreover, we found fairly strong evidence that the rates of victimization in the two periods were not equal; the p-value for testing the hypothesis of marginal homogeneity/symmetry was 0.06 (Section 3.2.4).

Analysis by parameter simulation

Tests of independence and marginal homogeneity/symmetry can also be readily carried out by parameter simulation. To test a hypothesis by parameter simulation, we first select a function of the

```
for s:= 1 to S do
    if M_s ≠ ∅ then
        for i ∈ I(s) do
            O_s(y):= y_{i(obs)}
            sum:= 0
            for M_s(y) ∈ M_s do sum:= sum + θ_y
            draw u ~ U(0,1)
            k:= 0
            for M_s(y) ∈ M_s do
                if k + θ_y/sum > u then
                    y_{i(mis)}:= M_s(y)
                    goto 1
                else
                    k:= k + θ_y/sum
                end if
            end do
1           continue
        end do
    end if
end do
```

Figure 7.5. *I-step for imputing missing values at the unit level.*

cell probabilities θ that measures the degree to which θ departs from the null hypothesis, and simulate the posterior distribution of this quantity given the observed data. For independence, a natural quantity to examine is the odds ratio

$$\omega = \frac{\theta_{11}\,\theta_{22}}{\theta_{12}\,\theta_{21}}, \tag{7.42}$$

where θ_{ij} denotes the probability of $(Y_1 = i, Y_2 = j)$ for $i, j = 1, 2$. The proportion of simulated values of ω that are less than or equal to one can be taken as an approximate one-sided p-value for testing the hypothesis of independence ($\omega = 1$) against the alternative that households victimized in the first period were more likely to be victimized in the second period ($\omega > 1$). For marginal homogeneity/symmetry, we can examine the difference in victimization rates between the second period ($\theta_{+2} = \theta_{12} + \theta_{22}$) and the first period ($\theta_{2+} = \theta_{21} + \theta_{22}$),

$$\begin{aligned}
\delta &= \theta_{+2} - \theta_{2+} \\
&= \theta_{12} - \theta_{21}. \tag{7.43}
\end{aligned}$$

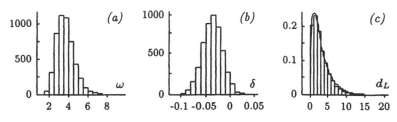

Figure 7.6. *Histograms of (a)* $\omega = (\theta_{11}\theta_{22})/(\theta_{12}\theta_{21})$ *and (b)* $\delta = \theta_{12} - \theta_{21}$ *over 5000 iterations of data augmentation, and of (c) the likelihood-ratio statistic* d_L *with the* χ_3^2 *density superimposed.*

The proportion of simulated values of δ that fall above zero is an approximate one-sided p-value for testing the hypothesis of no change ($\delta = 0$) against the alternative that the victimization rate has dropped ($\delta < 0$).

One interesting question is whether the 115 households for which both variables are missing should be included in the simulations. From an inferential standpoint it does not matter; under the ignorability assumption these sample units contribute nothing to the likelihood function for θ, so likelihood-based or Bayesian inferences for θ will be the same whether these units are included or not. From a computational standpoint, however, it is slightly better to omit them, because their presence needlessly increases the fractions of missing information and slows the convergence of data augmentation. In this particular example, the difference is barely noticeable. Without these 115 cases, the worst fraction of missing information as estimated from the iterations of EM (Section 3.3.4) is about 13%. Including these cases, it rises to 26%. Either way, data augmentation converges very quickly; in preliminary runs under the Jeffreys prior (all $\alpha_i = 1/2$), the autocorrelations in scalar functions of θ essentially died out after lag 2 or 3 even when the 115 cases were included.

Starting from the ML estimate of θ, we simulated 5000 steps of data augmentation under the Jeffreys prior following a burn-in period of 100 steps. Histograms of the simulated values of ω and δ are shown in Figure 7.6 (a) and (b), respectively. All 5000 values of ω were greater than one, so the simulated p-value for the test of independence is zero. Of the 5000 values of δ, 164 fell above zero, so the simulated p-value for testing $\delta = 0$ against the one-sided alternative $\delta < 0$ is 164/5000 = 0.033; the p-value against the two-sided alternative is $2 \times 0.033 = 0.066$.

Notice that these simulated p-values agree closely with those from the likelihood-ratio tests performed in Chapter 3. Because of the large sample size and the small number of parameters in this example, Bayesian and likelihood-based inferences are essentially identical. Further evidence that the large-sample properties are working well is provided by the posterior distribution of the likelihood-ratio statistic. The quantity

$$d_L = 2[\,l(\hat{\theta}|Y_{obs}) - l(\theta|Y_{obs})\,],$$

where $\hat{\theta}$ is the ML estimate, has (when regarded as a function of θ) a posterior distribution that is asymptotically chisquare with three degrees of freedom, because the multinomial model for this example has three free parameters. A histogram of the 5000 simulated values of d_L is shown in Figure 7.6 (c) with the χ_3^2 density function superimposed; the two are nearly indistinguishable.

By averaging the 5000 iterates of ω and δ, we obtain simulated posterior means

$$\hat{E}(\omega|Y_{obs}) = 3.67 \quad \text{and} \quad \hat{E}(\delta|Y_{obs}) = -0.036.$$

Comparing these to the ML estimates obtained in Section 3.2.2,

$$\hat{\omega} = 3.57 \quad \text{and} \quad \hat{\delta} = -0.037,$$

we find that the agreement is close. Simulated 95% posterior intervals for ω and δ based on sample quantiles of the 5000 iterates are (2.20, 5.77) and (−0.076, 0.001), respectively.

Analysis by multiple imputation

In this example, it is also straightforward to conduct inferences by multiple imputation. We generated a set of $m = 10$ imputations by running ten independent chains of data augmentation for 100 steps, starting each chain from the ML estimate. To speed convergence, the 115 households for which both variables were missing were omitted from the sample. At the final I-step of each chain, however, these households were restored to the sample so that their missing data could be imputed. Because these households contribute nothing to the observed-data likelihood, inferences will be essentially the same whether they are included or not. We decided to include them in the final I-steps so that the variation among the imputed datasets would more accurately reflect the real levels of missing-data uncertainty. The observed data and ten imputations of the complete-data table are shown in Table 7.1.

Table 7.1. *Victimization status for households in the National Crime Survey, with $m = 10$ multiple imputations*

(a) Observed data

Victimized in first period?	Victimized in second period?		
	No	Yes	Missing
No	392	55	33
Yes	76	38	9
Missing	31	7	115

Source: Kadane (1985, Table 1)

(b) Multiple imputations of the complete-data table

Responses	Imputation									
	1	2	3	4	5	6	7	8	9	10
no, no	522	540	525	539	528	532	517	539	522	517
no, yes	77	70	70	65	82	77	76	64	75	78
yes, no	106	99	106	96	99	96	113	105	102	108
yes, yes	51	47	55	56	47	51	50	48	57	53

As before, let us make inferences about the odds ratio $\omega = (\theta_{11}\theta_{22})/(\theta_{12}\theta_{21})$ and the difference $\delta = \theta_{12} - \theta_{21}$. The standard method for obtaining a point estimate and confidence interval for an odds ratio with complete data is given in Section 6.4.2. The obvious complete-data estimate of the difference δ is $\hat{\delta} = \hat{\theta}_{12} - \hat{\theta}_{21}$, where $\hat{\theta}_{12} = x_{12}/n$ and $\hat{\theta}_{21} = x_{21}/n$. In large samples $\hat{\delta}$ will be approximately normally distributed, and a consistent estimate of its variance is

$$\hat{V}(\hat{\delta}) = \frac{1}{n}\left[\hat{\theta}_{12}(1 - \hat{\theta}_{12}) + \hat{\theta}_{21}(1 - \hat{\theta}_{21}) + 2\hat{\theta}_{12}\hat{\theta}_{21}\right]$$

by elementary properties of the multinomial distribution (Section 7.2.1). Given these complete-data methods and the ten imputations in Table 7.1 (b), multiple-imputation point and interval estimates were obtained by Rubin's method for scalar estimands (Section 4.3.2). The resulting point estimates for ω and δ are 3.60 and -0.039, respectively, which agree closely with the ML estimates and the simulated posterior means. The resulting 95% interval estimates are $(2.15, 6.04)$ and $(-0.079, 0.001)$, which also agree well with the intervals obtained through parameter simulation. Estimated fractions of missing information for ω and δ are 35% and 26%, respectively.

7.3.5 Example: Protective Services Project for Older Persons

Fuchs (1982) analyzed data from the Protective Services Project for Older Persons, a longitudinal study designed to measure the impact of enriched social casework services on the well-being of elderly clients (Blenkner *et al.*, 1971). For 101 clients in the study, six dichotomous variables were recorded:

Variable	Levels	Code
Group membership	1 = experimental, 2 = control	G
Age	1 = under 75, 2 = 75+	A
Sex	1 = male, 2 = female	S
Survival status	1 = deceased, 2 = survived	D
Physical status	1 = poor, 2 = good	P
Mental status	1 = poor, 2 = good	M

For an additional 63 clients, values of physical and/or mental status were missing. The observed dataset, including complete and incomplete cases, is shown in Table 7.2.

Results from this project generated considerable controversy in the social work literature. Some (Fischer, 1973) argued that the enriched services seemed to be detrimental to the clients, because the mortality rate for the experimental group was actually higher than for the control group. Classifying the subjects by only G and D, both of which are observed for the entire sample, we obtain the marginal frequencies displayed in Table 7.3. The test for independence in this table, based on the well-known Pearson X^2 statistic, yields $X^2 = 5.03$ with one degree of freedom; the approximate p-value is 0.025, which provides fairly strong evidence that G and P are related. The estimated odds ratio is 2.04, suggesting that subjects in the experimental group were about twice as likely (on the odds scale) to die than subjects in the control group.

If subjects had been assigned to treatments in a random fashion, then Table 7.3 would indeed provide evidence that the services given to the experimental group were detrimental. If we examine the relationships between G and the other variables, however, we find that the treatment assignments were not random. Subjects in the experimental group tended to be older, and also tended to have poorer physical and mental status, than subjects in the

Table 7.2. *Data from the Protective Services Project for Older Persons*

			Male				Female			
			< 75		≥ 75		< 75		≥ 75	
Mental	*Physical*	*Survival*	E†	C†	E	C	E	C	E	C
(a) Fully categorized										
Poor	Poor	Deceased	0	2	5	3	0	0	2	1
		Survived	1	0	0	0	0	0	0	1
	Good	Deceased	0	0	2	2	1	1	1	0
		Survived	0	2	2	0	0	0	0	0
Good	Poor	Deceased	0	0	3	1	0	0	1	2
		Survived	3	1	1	2	0	1	1	0
	Good	Deceased	1	1	4	6	2	0	0	2
		Survived	5	10	6	8	3	5	2	4
(b) Missing physical status										
Poor	Missing	Deceased	0	0	0	0	0	0	0	0
		Survived	0	0	1	0	0	0	0	0
Good		Deceased	0	0	0	0	0	0	0	0
		Survived	0	0	0	0	0	0	0	0
(c) Missing mental status										
Missing	Poor	Deceased	2	0	5	3	1	1	2	0
		Survived	1	1	0	3	0	0	0	1
	Good	Deceased	1	0	0	0	0	0	1	2
		Survived	1	3	2	1	1	1	0	0
(d) Missing both physical and mental status										
Missing	Missing	Deceased	0	1	2	2	1	0	3	1
		Survived	2	8	1	2	1	1	2	2

†E denotes experimental; C denotes control. Source: Fuchs (1982)

Table 7.3. *Classification of subjects by G and D*

	Survived?	
Group	No	Yes
Experimental	40	36
Control	31	57

control group. It appears that the investigators tended to give the enriched services to clients who appeared to have the greatest need for them. The marginal association between G and D could thus be due, at least in part, to the fact that the subjects in the experimental group were simply more prone to die than the subjects in the control group, regardless of any services they received. Rather than examining the marginal association between G and D, we ought to focus on their conditional associations given the covariates A, S, P and M, to see whether G and D are still related after the possibly confounding effects of these covariates have been removed. That is, we should examine the odds ratios for G and D within the sixteen 2×2 tables that correspond to the unique combinations of the levels of A, S, P and M.

The complete-data contingency table has $2^6 = 64$ cells; with a sample size of $n = 164$, this results in an average of only 2.6 observations per cell. As noted by Fuchs (1982), the ML estimate of θ under the saturated model is not unique due to the pattern of random zeroes in the observed-data tables. Moreover, the suprema of the likelihood function lie on the boundary of the parameter space. To make EM converge to a unique mode in the interior, a Dirichlet prior was applied with $\alpha = (c, c, \ldots, c)$ for $c = 1.1$, which adds the equivalent of 6.4 prior observations and spreads them uniformly across the 64 cells. Then, taking this mode as a starting value, single chains of data augmentation were simulated under two alternative priors: $c = 0.1$ and $c = 1.5$. Each chain was run for 1000 steps following a burn-in period of 200 steps.

Boxplots of the simulated GD odds ratios for each of the sixteen $ASPM$ combinations are shown in Figure 7.7. The odds ratios are plotted on the natural log scale, with positive values indicating a positive association between enriched services $(G = 1)$ and death $(D = 1)$. Under the $c = 0.1$ prior, the simulated odds ratios show enormous variability; this prior assigns high probability to regions of the parameter space near the boundary, where odds ratios can approach 0 or $+\infty$. Under the stronger prior $c = 1.5$ the situation has improved, but the range of the simulated odds ratios is still implausibly wide. Notice that under either prior, all of the boxplots straddle the null value of zero, and there is no overwhelming tendency for the boxplots to be centered either to the left or to the right of zero. Thus there seems to be no strong evidence against the null hypothesis that G and D are unrelated.

To further sharpen the posterior distributions, we could increase the value of c even more. But this does not seem appropriate,

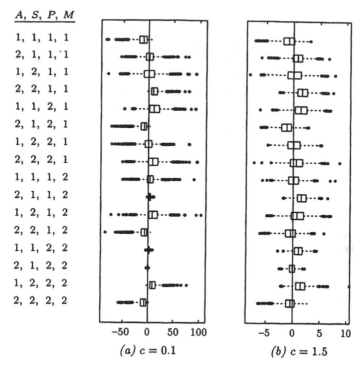

Figure 7.7. *Boxplots of simulated log-odds ratios from 1000 iterations of data augmentation under two flattening priors.*

because with $c = 1.5$ we have already added the equivalent of $1.5 \times 64 = 96$ prior observations with respect to estimation of the elements of θ. It appears that modest amounts of prior information are not sufficient to stabilize the inference; the observed data are simply too sparse to support the estimation of separate odds ratios within each cell of the $ASPM$ classification. We will deal with this problem of sparseness in Chapter 8 by fitting a simpler model that assumes a common odds ratio for all sixteen levels of $ASPM$.

7.4 Fast algorithms for near-monotone patterns

7.4.1 Factoring the likelihood and prior density

In Chapter 6 we introduced a class of algorithms called monotone data augmentation. Monotone data augmentation is similar to ordinary data augmentation except that in each I-step we impute only enough of the missing values to complete a monotone pattern. The advantage of monotone data augmentation is that it tends to converge very quickly when the observed data are nearly monotone. In this section we present monotone data augmentation for the saturated multinomial model.

Monotone data augmentation is feasible when the prior and likelihood for the complete data factor neatly into independent pieces corresponding to the marginal distribution of Y_1, the conditional distribution for Y_2 given Y_1, the conditional distribution for Y_3 given Y_1 and Y_2, and so on. Let us first consider the likelihood. Until now we have been describing the data by a single multinomial distribution for the complete-data contingency table x, but we can equivalently characterize this model as a sequence of product-multinomials. Suppose we write

$$P(Y_1, \ldots, Y_p | \theta) = P(Y_1 | \phi_1) P(Y_2 | Y_1, \phi_2) \qquad (7.44)$$
$$\cdots P(Y_p | Y_1, \ldots, Y_{p-1}, \phi_p),$$

where ϕ_j denotes the parameters governing the conditional distribution of Y_j given $(Y_1, \ldots, Y_{j-1})$. Each of the factors of the right-hand side of (7.44) corresponds to a product-multinomial distribution on a collapsed version of x.

To be more precise we need some additional notation. Suppose that $y = (y_1, y_2, \ldots, y_p)$ is a generic realization of $(Y_1, Y_2, \ldots, Y_p)$ for a single unit. Let $\mathcal{F}_j$ be a function that extracts from y the first j elements,

$$\mathcal{F}_j(y) = (y_1, \ldots, y_j),$$

and let $\mathcal{L}_j$ extract the last $p - j$ elements,

$$\mathcal{L}_j(y) = (y_{j+1}, \ldots, y_p).$$

Let F_j and L_j, respectively, be the sets over which $\mathcal{F}_j(y)$ and $\mathcal{L}_j(y)$ are allowed to vary; that is, F_j will be the Cartesian cross-product of the sets $\{1, 2, \ldots, d_k\}$ for $k = 1, \ldots, j$, and L_j the cross-product for $k = j + 1, \ldots, p$. We will write the probability of the event $Y_1 = y_1, Y_2 = y_2, \ldots, Y_j = y_j$ as

$$\xi_{\mathcal{F}_j(y)} = \sum_{\mathcal{L}_j(y) \in L_j} \theta_y,$$

and the full set of parameters governing the marginal distribution of $(Y_1, Y_2, \ldots, Y_j)$ as

$$\xi_j = \{\xi_{\mathcal{F}_j(y)} : \mathcal{F}_j(y) \in F_j\}.$$

The conditional probability of the event $Y_j = y_j$ given that $Y_1 = y_1, Y_2 = y_2, \ldots, Y_{j-1} = y_{j-1}$ will be

$$\phi_{\mathcal{F}_j(y)} = \xi_{\mathcal{F}_j(y)} / \xi_{\mathcal{F}_{j-1}(y)}, \tag{7.45}$$

and the full set of parameters governing the conditional distribution of Y_j given $(Y_1, Y_2, \ldots, Y_{j-1})$ is

$$\phi_j = \{\phi_{\mathcal{F}_j(y)} : \mathcal{F}_j(y) \in F_j\}.$$

Suppose we collapse the p-dimensional contingency table x on its last $p - j$ dimensions, producing a table that cross-classifies the units by $(Y_1, Y_2, \ldots, Y_j)$. Denote a frequency in this table by

$$z_{\mathcal{F}_j(y)} = \sum_{\mathcal{L}_j(y) \in L_j} x_y,$$

and the entire j-dimensional table by

$$z_j = \{z_{\mathcal{F}_j(y)} : \mathcal{F}_j(y) \in F_j\}.$$

By the rules for collapsing and partitioning (Section 7.2.2), z_j has a multinomial distribution with index n and parameter ξ_j. Moreover, the conditional distribution of z_j given z_{j-1} is a product-multinomial whose parameters are contained in ϕ_j. More specifically, suppose we partition z_j into a set of $d_1 \times d_2 \times \cdots d_{j-1}$ vectors, each of length d_j. Denote one of these vectors by

$$z_{j;\mathcal{F}_{j-1}(y)} = \{z_{\mathcal{F}_j(y)} : y_j = 1, 2, \ldots, d_j\},$$

which is simply the portion of z_j obtained by fixing $(y_1, \ldots, y_{j-1})$ at a specific value but letting y_j vary over $\{1, 2, \ldots, d_j\}$. The table z_j is then the collection of these vectors,

$$z_j = \{z_{j;\mathcal{F}_{j-1}(y)} : \mathcal{F}_{j-1}(y) \in F_{j-1}\}.$$

If we partition ϕ_j in the same fashion, as

$$\phi_j = \{\phi_{j;\mathcal{F}_{j-1}(y)} : \mathcal{F}_{j-1}(y) \in F_{j-1}\}$$

where

$$\phi_{j;\mathcal{F}_{j-1}(y)} = \{\phi_{\mathcal{F}_j(y)} : y_j = 1, 2, \ldots, d_j\},$$

then the conditional distribution of z_j given z_{j-1} is

$$z_{j;\mathcal{F}_{j-1}(y)} \mid z_{j-1}, \phi_j \sim M(z_{\mathcal{F}_{j-1}(y)}, \phi_{j;\mathcal{F}_{j-1}(y)}) \tag{7.46}$$

independently for all $\mathcal{F}_{j-1}(y) \in F_{j-1}$.

By these properties, it follows that the multinomial likelihood function for any ξ_j can be factored as

$$L(\xi_j \mid z_j) = L(\xi_{j-1} \mid z_{j-1}) L(\phi_j \mid z_j),$$

the product of a multinomial likelihood for ξ_{j-1} whose sufficient statistics are contained in z_{j-1} and a product-multinomial likelihood for ϕ_j whose sufficient statistics are contained in z_j. Applying this factorization recursively, first to $\xi_p = \theta$, then to ξ_{p-1}, and so on down to ξ_2, we obtain

$$L(\phi \mid Y) = \prod_{j=1}^{p} L(\phi_j \mid z_j),$$

where each factor $L(\phi_j \mid z_j)$ is a product-multinomial likelihood. The full set of parameters $\phi = (\phi_1, \phi_2, \dots, \phi_p)$ forms a one-to-one transformation of θ, and it follows from (7.45) that the back-transformation is

$$\theta_y = \phi_{\mathcal{F}_1(y)} \phi_{\mathcal{F}_2(y)} \cdots \phi_{\mathcal{F}_p(y)}. \tag{7.47}$$

Factoring the prior

Just as the likelihood function factors into independent pieces for $\phi_1, \phi_2, \dots, \phi_p$, the density function for ϕ induced by the ordinary Dirichlet prior on θ also factors into a product of independent densities. Suppose that a priori θ has a Dirichlet distribution,

$$\theta \sim D(\alpha), \tag{7.48}$$

where the hyperparameters are regarded as an array with the same dimensions as θ,

$$\alpha = \{\alpha_y : y \in \mathcal{Y}\}.$$

By the collapsing rules for the Dirichlet discussed in Section 7.2.6, the distribution for ξ_j implied by (7.48) is also Dirichlet. The parameters of this distribution, which we shall call

$$\beta_j = \{\beta_{\mathcal{F}_j(y)} : \mathcal{F}_j(y) \in F_j\},$$

are obtained by summing the elements of α in the same way the elements of θ were summed to produce ξ_j,

$$\beta_{\mathcal{F}_j(y)} = \sum_{\mathcal{L}_j(y) \in L_j} \alpha_y.$$

Moreover, by the results of Section 7.2.6, the conditional distribution of ϕ_j given ξ_{j-1} for any j is a product of independent Dirichlet distributions. That is, if we partition the j-dimensional table β_j in precisely the same manner as we partitioned ϕ_j, as

$$\beta_j = \{\beta_{j;\mathcal{F}_{j-1}(y)} : \mathcal{F}_{j-1}(y) \in F_{j-1}\}$$

where

$$\beta_{j;\mathcal{F}_{j-1}(y)} = \{\beta_{\mathcal{F}_j(y)} : y_j = 1, 2, \ldots, d_j\},$$

the conditional distribution of ϕ_j given ξ_{j-1} is

$$\phi_{j;\mathcal{F}_{j-1}(y)} \mid \xi_{j-1} \sim D(\beta_{j;\mathcal{F}_{j-1}(y)}) \qquad (7.49)$$

independently for all $\mathcal{F}_{j-1}(y) \in F_{j-1}$.

Now from (7.45) it is clear that ξ_j is a one-to-one function of $(\phi_1, \ldots, \phi_j)$ for any j. The prior density for $\phi = (\phi_1, \ldots, \phi_p)$ can thus be written

$$
\begin{aligned}
\pi(\phi) &= \pi_1(\phi_1) \prod_{j=2}^{p} \pi_j(\phi_j \mid \phi_1, \ldots, \phi_{j-1}) \\
&= \pi_1(\phi_1) \prod_{j=2}^{p} \pi_j(\phi_j \mid \xi_{j-1}).
\end{aligned}
\qquad (7.50)
$$

But notice that ξ_{j-1} does not appear on the right-hand side of (7.49); thus ϕ_j is independent of ξ_{j-1}, and (7.50) becomes

$$\pi(\phi) = \prod_{j=1}^{p} \pi_j(\phi_j), \qquad (7.51)$$

where each of the terms $\pi_j(\phi_j)$ is a product of independent Dirichlet densities whose parameters are contained in β_j.

7.4.2 Monotone data augmentation

By the factorizations described above, it immediately follows that complete-data Bayesian inferences under the saturated multinomial model and Dirichlet prior,

$$
\begin{aligned}
x \mid \theta &\sim M(n, \theta), \\
\theta &\sim D(\alpha),
\end{aligned}
$$

can be carried out as a sequence of independent Bayesian inferences for $\phi_1, \phi_2, \ldots, \phi_p$,

$$P(\phi|Y) = \prod_{j=1}^{p} P(\phi_j|z_j).$$

By combining (7.46) with (7.49), we see that the complete-data posterior distribution for any term ϕ_j is

$$\phi_{j;\mathcal{F}_{j-1}(y)} \mid z_j \sim D(\beta_{j;\mathcal{F}_{j-1}(y)} + z_{j;\mathcal{F}_{j-1}(y)}) \qquad (7.52)$$

independently for all $\mathcal{F}_{j-1}(y) \in F_{j-1}$.

This factorization of the posterior applies not only when the data are complete; more generally, it holds whenever the observed data form a monotone pattern as described in Section 6.5. Suppose that the observed data are monotone in the sense that if Y_j is missing for a unit, then $Y_{j+1}, \ldots, Y_p$ are missing as well (Figure 6.8). By essentially the same argument as was given in Section 6.5.1, the observed-data likelihood for ϕ given Y_{obs} can be factored as

$$L(\phi | Y_{obs}) = \prod_{j=1}^{p} L(\phi_j | z_j^*),$$

where z_j^* is the contingency table that cross classifies all the units for which Y_j is observed by their values of $Y_1, \ldots, Y_j$. If we denote a cell of this table by $z_{\mathcal{F}_j(y)}^*$ and let

$$z_{j;\mathcal{F}_{j-1}(y)}^* = \{ z_{\mathcal{F}_j(y)}^* : y_j = 1, 2, \ldots, d_j \}$$

be a subvector within this table, $L(\phi_j | z_j^*)$ will be the likelihood that arises from the product-multinomial distribution

$$z_{j;\mathcal{F}_{j-1}(y)}^* | z_{j-1}^*, \phi_j \sim M(z_{\mathcal{F}_{j-1}(y)}, \phi_{j;\mathcal{F}_{j-1}(y)})$$

for all $\mathcal{F}_{j-1}(y) \in F_{j-1}$. Combining this new likelihood with the prior (7.49) leads to the observed-data posterior

$$P(\phi | Y_{obs}) = \prod_{j=1}^{p} P(\phi_j | z_j^*), \tag{7.53}$$

where $P(\phi_j | z_j^*)$ is given by

$$\phi_{j;\mathcal{F}_{j-1}(y)} | z_j^* \sim D(\beta_{j;\mathcal{F}_{j-1}(y)} + z_{j;\mathcal{F}_{j-1}(y)}^*) \tag{7.54}$$

for all $\mathcal{F}_{j-1}(y) \in F_{j-1}$.

Monotone data augmentation capitalizes on (7.53) to create an efficient simulation algorithm for situations where Y_{obs} is non-monotone. Suppose that Y_{obs} is no longer monotone, but we have identified a subset Y_{mis^*} of Y_{mis} such that (Y_{obs}, Y_{mis^*}) is monotone. The monotone data augmentation algorithm alternates between the following two steps.

1. I-step: Simulate a value of Y_{mis^*} from its predictive distribution given the current value of θ,

$$Y_{mis^*}^{(t+1)} \sim P(Y_{mis^*} | Y_{obs}, \theta^{(t)}).$$

2. P-step: Draw a new value of θ from its posterior distribution given Y_{obs} and the new value of Y_{mis^*},

$$\theta^{(t+1)} \sim P(\theta|Y_{obs}, Y_{mis^*}^{(t+1)}).$$

In practice, the I-step is identical to that of ordinary data augmentation (Section 7.3.3) except that we need only draw the elements of Y_{mis^*} rather than the full Y_{mis}. The P-step is carried out by drawing $\phi_1, \ldots, \phi_p$ from the factored posterior (7.53), and then numerically transforming the resulting value of $\phi = (\phi_1, \ldots, \phi_p)$ back to the θ-scale using (7.47).

Interleaving the I- and P-steps

Notice that the simulation of ϕ_j within a P-step does not require knowledge of the most recent simulated value of the entire Y_{mis^*}; rather, it requires only the most recent value of the j-dimensional table z_j^*. This allows us to interleave portions of the I- and P-steps in the following manner. Suppose that the data are grouped by missingness pattern and sorted as shown in Figure 6.10. Let s_j denote the last pattern for which variable Y_j may need to be filled in to complete the overall monotone pattern, so that $s_p \leq s_{p-1} \leq \cdots \leq s_1$, and for convenience define $s_{p+1} = 0$. Let T_1, T_2 and T_3 be three workspace arrays, each of dimension $d_1 \times d_2 \times \cdots d_p$. Initialize T_1 and T_2 to be equal to the current parameter value $\theta^{(t)}$ and α, respectively, and initialize all the elements of T_3 to one. Then, for $j := p, p-1, \ldots, 1$, perform the following steps:

1. If $s_j > s_{j+1}$, impute the missing data for variables $Y_1, \ldots, Y_j$ within patterns $s_{j+1} + 1$ up to s_j. These data should be drawn from their predictive distribution given the observed data and the parameters stored in T_1.

2. Cross-classify the units in patterns $s_{j+1} + 1$ up to s_j by their observed or imputed values for $Y_1, \ldots, Y_j$, and add the resulting counts into the corresponding cells of the workspace T_2. Upon completion of this step, T_2 will contain β_j plus the simulated value of z_j^*.

3. Draw a value of ϕ_j from its product-multinomial posterior distribution (7.54) given the value of $\beta_j + z_j^*$ in T_2. Multiply the elements of the array T_3 by the corresponding elements of this simulated ϕ_j.

4. If $j > 1$, collapse T_1 by summing along its jth dimension, thereby reducing its size to $d_1 \times \cdots \times d_{j-1}$. Now T_1 contains

the current value of ξ_{j-1} (the parameters of the joint distribution of $Y_1, \ldots, Y_{j-1}$) which will be necessary for the next Step 1. Perform this same collapsing operation for T_2, preparing it for the next Step 2.

After all p cycles of Steps 1–4 have been completed, the workspace T_3 will contain the updated parameter $\theta^{(t+1)}$.

Running this algorithm from a starting value $\theta^{(0)}$ generates a sequence of parameter values $\{\theta^{(t)} : t = 1, 2, \ldots\}$ which converges in distribution to the correct observed-data posterior,

$$P(\theta^{(t)} | Y_{obs}, \theta^{(0)}) \to P(\theta | Y_{obs}) \text{ as } t \to \infty.$$

Convergence tends to be faster than for the ordinary data augmentation algorithm described in Section 7.3, because Y_{mis^*} contains less information about the parameter than does Y_{mis}. The most dramatic improvements are seen when Y_{obs} is nearly monotone, because then Y_{mis^*} is only a small subset of Y_{mis}. When the observed data happen to be monotone, Y_{mis^*} is empty and the algorithm converges from any starting value in a single step.

This algorithm can be used to generate proper multiple imputations of the missing data Y_{mis} as follows. First, simulate a small number of independent draws of θ from $P(\theta | Y_{obs})$, either by running multiple chains or subsampling a single chain. Then, under each of these θ values, impute the full set of missing data Y_{mis} using the ordinary data augmentation I-step (Figure 7.5).

7.4.3 Example: driver injury and seatbelt use

The data in Tables 7.4 and 7.5, previously analyzed by Hochberg (1977) and Chen (1989), concern the effectiveness of seatbelts in reducing the risk of driver injury in automobile accidents. Table 7.4 classifies 80 084 automobile accidents according to four variables obtained from police reports: driver's sex, car damage (low, high), belt use (no, yes) and injury (no, yes). At first glance, these data suggest that the use of seatbelts substantially reduces the risk of injury. The estimated odds of injury are

$$\frac{199 + 117 + 583 + 297}{3006 + 1262 + 2155 + 728} = 0.167$$

for belted drivers and

$$\frac{1687 + 1422 + 6746 + 3707}{22536 + 11199 + 17476 + 6964} = 0.233$$

Table 7.4. *Classification of accidents by police reports of driver's sex, car damage, injury and belt use*

	Male		Female	
Belt use	No	Yes	No	Yes
Low damage				
Not injured	22536	3006	11199	1262
Injured	1687	199	1422	117
High damage				
Not injured	17476	2155	6964	728
Injured	6746	583	3707	297

Source: Hochberg (1977, Table 1)

for unbelted drivers, giving an odds ratio of 0.717; an approximate 95% confidence interval for this ratio is (0.673, 0.765). This simple analysis is unconvincing, however, for a number of reasons. First, the belted and unbelted groups tend to differ with respect to a variety of characteristics (e.g. sex), and to the extent that these characteristics may be related to the risk of injury, our estimate of the effectiveness of seatbelts may be biased upward or downward.

Another difficulty with this analysis is that the data provided by the police reports are not always accurate, especially with respect to belt use and injury. Experience has shown that the police were prone to overestimate the proportion of drivers who were not injured and unbelted, and that the biases toward not injured were especially severe for low-damage accidents. Even small rates of misclassification with respect to belt use and injury can have a large impact on the estimated effect of wearing a seatbelt.

To examine the effect of misclassification errors, followup data were collected for an additional sample of 1796 accidents. Subsequent to the police reports, investigators obtained more reliable data on belt use and injury from hospital records and personal interviews. We will assume that the information obtained in this followup effort is correct. Data from the followup study are shown in Table 7.5, with the police-reported and followup values of belt use and injury indicated by (p) and (f), respectively.

The followup data in Table 7.5 may be used in a variety of ways. For example, we may ignore the police reports entirely and estimate the seatbelt effect from the followup data alone. Presumably, such estimates would be less biased than those we obtained from

Table 7.5. *Classification of accidents by driver's sex, car damage, injury and belt use obtained from police reports (p), and injury and belt use obtained from followup (f)*

| | Low damage | | | | High damage | | | |
| | Male | | Female | | Male | | Female | |
Belt (p)	No	Yes	No	Yes	No	Yes	No	Yes
Not injured (p)								
Injury/Belt (f)								
No/No	407	6	206	1	299	4	102	2
No/Yes	62	47	18	17	20	30	7	6
Yes/No	45	1	37	0	59	1	53	1
Yes/Yes	7	6	5	1	9	6	4	3
Injured (p)								
Injury/Belt (f)								
No/No	5	0	4	3	11	1	5	0
No/Yes	1	1	0	0	2	2	1	0
Yes/No	32	1	29	1	118	0	79	1
Yes/Yes	4	2	0	0	5	9	1	6

Source: Hochberg (1977, Table 2)

Table 7.4, because they would be less prone to misclassification error. On the other hand, they would have greater variability because they would be based on a much smaller sample. A more effective approach would be to combine the data from Tables 7.4 and 7.5 and analyze them as a six-variable dataset with two of the variables partially missing. Combining the two sources would allow us to make use of the police-report data for all 81 880 accidents, but would calibrate them to correct for occasional misclassification errors in keeping with the error rates seen in the followup study. In other words, a combined analysis would allow the police-report data to serve as a proxy for the followup data among the initial 80 084 cases, taking into account the fact that the correlation between the two data sources is less than perfect.

The six-variable combined dataset has a monotone pattern, with followup belt use and injury missing for 97.8% of the cases. Because of the high rate of missingness for these two variables, the EM and ordinary data augmentation algorithms described in Section 7.3 converge very slowly. To illustrate, we ran a single chain of ordinary data augmentation for 5000 steps beginning from the

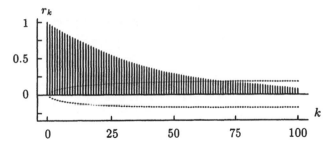

Figure 7.8. *Sample ACFs for the worst linear function of θ, estimated from 5000 iterations of ordinary data augmentation, with dashed lines indicating approximate critical values for testing $\rho_k = \rho_{k+1} = \cdots = 0$.*

ML estimate using the Jeffreys prior (all hyperparameters equal to $1/2$), and monitored the worst linear function of θ as estimated from the trajectory of EM (Section 4.4.3). The sample autocorrelation function for this parameter, plotted in Figure 7.8, reveals extreme long-range dependence. Monotone data augmentation, however, converges in a single step because the observed data are precisely monotone. A sequence of θ values generated by monotone data augmentation will be an actual independent sample from the observed-data posterior $P(\theta \mid Y_{obs})$.

Using monotone data augmentation, we simulated 1000 independent draws of θ from the observed-data posterior under the Jeffreys prior, and calculated the odds ratios relating seatbelt use to driver injury (both from the police reports and from the followup reports) within each of the four sex-by-damage cells. Boxplots of these simulated odds ratios are shown in Figure 7.9. The odds ratios based on the police reports are highly concentrated to the left of one; the beneficial effects of seatbelts thus appear to be 'statistically significant' if we ignore the problem of misclassification. The odds ratios based on followup data, however, are much more dispersed, with all of the distributions straddling one; when misclassification errors are taken into account, the evidence that seatbelts reduce the risk of injury is no longer overwhelming. Simulated posterior means, 95% interval estimates and p-values for these odds ratios are shown in Table 7.6. The p-values are simply the proportions of simulated odds ratios exceeding one; they are appropriate for testing whether a given odds ratio is one, versus the one-sided alternative that it is less than one.

Because the police-report versions of belt use and injury are

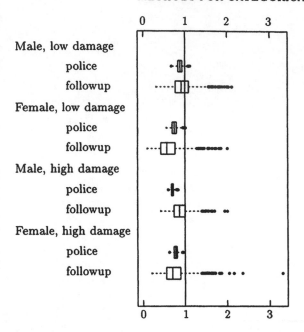

Figure 7.9. *Boxplots of 1000 simulated odds ratios showing the relationship of seatbelt use and injury within classes of damage and sex, both from police reports and from followup data.*

highly correlated with the followup versions, one might think that the rates of missing information for the followup variables should be much smaller than their actual missingness rates (98%). The fact that the followup-based intervals are so much wider than the police-based intervals, however, indicates that rates of missing information for these variables are still quite high. The main reason for this is the complexity of the saturated multinomial model. The saturated model allows for a full six-way association among the variables. The misclassification mechanism is described by the four-way table that relates the followup versions of belt-use and injury to the police versions. The saturated model estimates a full four-way association in this table; moreover, it allows the four-way association to vary freely across the four sex-by-damage cells. It is apparent that some of these high-order associations are poorly estimated, because the data in some parts of Table 7.5 are sparse. We will address this issue in Chapter 8 by applying models that are more parsimonious.

Table 7.6. *Simulated posterior means, 95% intervals and p-values for odds ratios from 1000 iterations of monotone data augmentation*

	mean	interval	p-value
Male, low damage			
police	0.89	(0.77, 1.03)	0.06
followup	0.95	(0.57, 1.59)	0.36
Female, low damage			
police	0.75	(0.62, 0.90)	0.00
followup	0.63	(0.24, 1.28)	0.09
Male, high damage			
police	0.70	(0.64, 0.77)	0.00
followup	0.89	(0.56, 1.35)	0.26
Female, high damage			
police	0.78	(0.68, 0.88)	0.00
followup	0.76	(0.37, 1.51)	0.17

CHAPTER 8

Loglinear models

8.1 Introduction

In Chapter 7 we examined methods based on the saturated multinomial model. That model was quite general, allowing the associations among the categorical variables to be arbitrarily complex. In many realistic examples, however, unless the number of variables is very small, the observed data cannot support such complexity. This chapter presents methods for a flexible class of models which allows the associations among variables to be simplified.

Loglinear models have been used extensively, particularly in the social sciences, for almost two decades. In loglinear models, the cell probabilities for the cross-classified contingency table are decomposed into multiplicative effects for each variable and for the associations among them. Eliminating certain terms from this decomposition imposes equality constraints on odds ratios in the cross-classified table. A large part of this chapter is devoted to loglinear modeling with complete data, in particular, to the classical estimation technique of iterative proportional fitting (IPF) and a new simulation algorithm known as Bayesian IPF. These methods, which will be unfamiliar to many readers, are easily extended to calculate ML estimates and simulate posterior draws of parameters and missing data. Sections 8.3 and 8.4 concentrate on IPF and Bayesian IPF, respectively, and extensions to incomplete-data problems are presented in Section 8.5.

8.2 Overview of loglinear models

8.2.1 Definition

Suppose $x = (x_1, x_2, \ldots, x_D)$ is a contingency table having a multinomial distribution,

$$x \mid \theta \sim M(n, \theta), \qquad (8.1)$$

where the cell probabilities $\theta = (\theta_1, \theta_2, \ldots, \theta_D)$ lie within the simplex

$$\Theta = \left\{ \theta : \theta_d \geq 0 \text{ for all } d \text{ and } \sum_{d=1}^{D} \theta_d = 1 \right\}.$$

A loglinear model does not alter the distributional assumption (8.1), but imposes further constraints on the elements of θ. Let

$$\eta_d = \log \theta_d, \quad d = 1, 2, \ldots, D$$

and

$$\eta = (\eta_1, \eta_2, \ldots, \eta_D)^T.$$

In the most general sense, a loglinear model is any constraint of the form

$$\eta = M\lambda, \tag{8.2}$$

where λ is an $r \times 1$ parameter vector and M is a fixed and known $D \times r$ design matrix. Thus, in addition to requiring that the elements of θ sum to one, we also require $\eta = \log \theta$ to lie in the linear subspace spanned by the columns of M. The meaning of the elements of λ will depend on the coding method used in M. In typical applications of loglinear modeling, x represents a cross-classification of sample units by categorical variables $Y_1, Y_2, \ldots, Y_p$, and M is a design matrix of the type used in the analysis of variance (ANOVA) for factorial experiments; each variable Y_j represents a 'factor,' and the elements of λ represent the 'main effects' and 'interactions' associated with the factors.

Models for three categorical variables

For expository purposes, let us temporarily assume that there are only three categorical variables ($p = 3$). This assumption is purely a matter of convenience, and all results will immediately generalize to any number of variables. Also, we will temporarily switch to a notation more consistent with that of standard texts on categorical data (e.g. Agresti, 1990); in later sections, we will return to the notation developed in Chapter 7. Suppose we have three categorical variables:

$$A \quad \text{with levels} \quad i = 1, 2, \ldots, I;$$
$$B \quad \text{with levels} \quad j = 1, 2, \ldots, J;$$
$$C \quad \text{with levels} \quad k = 1, 2, \ldots, K.$$

Let x_{ijk} denote the number of sample units for which we observe $A = i$, $B = j$, $C = k$. Let $\theta_{ijk} = P(A = i, B = j, C = k)$

and $\eta_{ijk} = \log \theta_{ijk}$. Finally, let '+' in place of a subscript denote summation over that subscript, as in

$$x_{+jk} = \sum_{i=1}^{I} x_{ijk} \quad \text{and} \quad \theta_{i++} = \sum_{j=1}^{J}\sum_{k=1}^{K} \theta_{ijk}.$$

The total sample size is $n = x_{+++}$.

As in a factorial ANOVA model, we can decompose η_{ijk} into additive terms corresponding to the 'main effects' and 'interactions' of A, B, and C,

$$\eta_{ijk} = \lambda_0 + \lambda_i^A + \lambda_j^B + \lambda_k^C + \lambda_{ij}^{AB} + \lambda_{ik}^{AC} + \lambda_{jk}^{BC} + \lambda_{ijk}^{ABC}, \quad (8.3)$$

where for identifiability the λ terms are constrained to sum to zero over any subscript,

$$\sum_{i=1}^{I} \lambda_i^A = 0, \quad \sum_{i=1}^{I} \lambda_{ij}^{AB} = \sum_{j=1}^{J} \lambda_{ij}^{AB} = 0, \quad (8.4)$$

and so on. To see how this relates to the general specification (8.2), consider the special case where $I = J = K = 2$; taking

$$\eta = \begin{bmatrix} \eta_{111} \\ \eta_{211} \\ \eta_{121} \\ \eta_{221} \\ \eta_{112} \\ \eta_{212} \\ \eta_{122} \\ \eta_{222} \end{bmatrix}, \quad M = \begin{bmatrix} 1 & 1 & 1 & 1 & 1 & 1 & 1 & 1 \\ 1 & -1 & 1 & 1 & -1 & -1 & 1 & -1 \\ 1 & 1 & -1 & 1 & -1 & 1 & -1 & -1 \\ 1 & -1 & -1 & 1 & 1 & -1 & -1 & 1 \\ 1 & 1 & 1 & -1 & 1 & -1 & -1 & -1 \\ 1 & -1 & 1 & -1 & -1 & 1 & -1 & 1 \\ 1 & 1 & -1 & -1 & -1 & -1 & 1 & 1 \\ 1 & -1 & -1 & -1 & 1 & 1 & 1 & -1 \end{bmatrix}$$

yields

$$\lambda = [\lambda_0,\ \lambda_1^A,\ \lambda_1^B,\ \lambda_1^C,\ \lambda_{11}^{AB}, \lambda_{11}^{AC},\ \lambda_{11}^{BC},\ \lambda_{111}^{ABC}]^T,$$

and the other λ terms follow from the identifiability constraints,

$$\lambda_1^A = -\lambda_2^A, \quad \lambda_{11}^{AB} = -\lambda_{12}^{AB} = -\lambda_{21}^{AB} = \lambda_{22}^{AB},$$

and so on.

In many respects the loglinear model (8.3) is like the classical linear model for a factorial experiment. There are two important differences, however, that distinguish the loglinear model from its linear counterpart. First, the term λ_0, which appears to be like the 'grand mean,' is not a free parameter but a normalizing constant chosen to make the cell probabilities sum to one,

$$\lambda_0 = -\log \left\{ \sum_{ijk} \exp \left(\lambda_i^A + \lambda_j^B + \cdots + \lambda_{ijk}^{ABC} \right) \right\}.$$

Second, the linear equation (8.3) does not represent the mean of a response variable given $A = i$, $B = j$, $C = k$; rather, it represents the log-probability of the event $A = i$, $B = j$, $C = k$ itself. The loglinear model is not a regression model describing the effects of A, B and C on an additional response variable, but a true multivariate model describing the relationships among the variables A, B and C. Thus the meaning of the λ terms is quite different from the usual interpretation of main effects and interactions in a linear model. For example, the set of terms $\lambda^{AB} = \{\lambda_{ij}^{AB}\}$ describes the *association* between A and B, not their *interaction* with respect to a third variable. The terms in λ^{AB} are essentially the log-odds ratios describing the association between A and B, and the terms $\lambda^{ABC} = \{\lambda_{ijk}^{ABC}\}$ are the differences in log-odds ratios describing how the association between any two variables varies across levels of the third. For details on the exact correspondence between the λ terms and log-odds ratios, see Bishop, Fienberg and Holland (1975) or Agresti (1990).

8.2.2 Eliminating associations

The number of free parameters in the loglinear model (8.3) can be counted in the same manner as the number of degrees of freedom in a factorial ANOVA.

Source	No. of parameters
A	$I - 1$
B	$J - 1$
C	$K - 1$
AB	$(I - 1)(J - 1)$
AC	$(I - 1)(K - 1)$
BC	$(J - 1)(K - 1)$
ABC	$(I - 1)(J - 1)(K - 1)$
Total	$IJK - 1$

Notice that the total number of free parameters in (8.3), $IJK - 1$, is the same as in the saturated multinomial; hence (8.3) is nothing more than a reparameterization of the saturated model, with the cell probabilities θ re-expressed in terms of the loglinear coefficients λ. The loglinear representation has a great advantage, however, in that it allows us to selectively eliminate associations among variables by setting groups of λ terms to zero. Suppose we set all the terms in $\lambda^{AB} = \{\lambda_{ij}^{AB}\}$, $\lambda^{AC} = \{\lambda_{ik}^{AC}\}$, $\lambda^{BC} = \{\lambda_{jk}^{BC}\}$, and $\lambda^{ABC} = \{\lambda_{ijk}^{ABC}\}$ to zero. The loglinear model can then be written as

$$\theta_{ijk} \propto \exp\left(\lambda_i^A + \lambda_j^B + \lambda_k^C\right),$$

which implies that A, B and C are mutually independent,

$$\theta_{ijk} = P(A = i)\, P(B = j)\, P(C = k).$$

Setting $\lambda^{BC} = \lambda^{AC} = \lambda^{ABC} = 0$ but allowing λ^{AB} to vary leads to

$$\theta_{ijk} = P(A = i, B = j)\, P(C = k),$$

which means that A and B may be related but requires them to be jointly independent of C. Setting $\lambda^{AB} = \lambda^{ABC} = 0$ gives

$$\theta_{ijk} = P(A = i\,|\,C = k)\, P(B = j\,|\,C = k)\, P(C = k),$$

which means that A and B are conditionally independent given C. Finally, setting $\lambda^{ABC} = 0$ results in a model of *homogeneous association*. This model does not imply any form of independence or conditional independence, but has the property that the association between any two variables (in terms of odds ratios) is constant across levels of the third.

Hierarchical models

In most applications of loglinear modeling, it would not make sense to specify a model that contains an association but omits a main effect. A model that includes λ^{AB} but omits λ^A allows A to be related to B, but requires the average log-probability across levels of B to be the same within every level of A. Under ordinary circumstances one would not expect this to happen except by chance. Similarly, it would rarely make sense to fit a model that contains the three-way association λ^{ABC} but omits one or more of the two-way associations λ^{AB}, λ^{AC} or λ^{BC}.

A loglinear model is said to be hierarchical if omitting a λ term implies that all higher-order associations containing that term are omitted as well; for example, if setting $\lambda^{AB} = 0$ requires that we also set $\lambda^{ABC} = 0$. Putting it another way, a model is hierarchical if no association is present unless all lower-order terms within that association are also present. Thus a hierarchical model containing λ^{ABC} must also contain λ^A, λ^B, λ^C, λ^{AB}, λ^{AC} and λ^{BC}. The class of hierarchical models includes models of independence and conditional independence, as well as some other models that may be of interest, e.g. the model of homogeneous association in a three-way table ($\lambda^{ABC} = 0$). Non-hierarchical models, however, rarely correspond to sensible hypotheses about the underlying categorical variables. For the remainder of this book, we will restrict our attention to hierarchical models only.

8.2.3 Sufficient statistics

The loglikelihood for the saturated model in terms of the cell probabilities θ is

$$l(\theta \,|\, x) = \sum_{ijk} x_{ijk} \log \theta_{ijk}.$$

When expressed in terms of the loglinear coefficients, the loglikelihood becomes

$$
\begin{aligned}
l(\lambda \,|\, x) &= \sum_{ijk} x_{ijk} \left(\lambda_0 + \lambda_i^A + \cdots + \lambda_{ijk}^{ABC} \right) \\
&= n\,\lambda_0 + \sum_i x_{i++} \lambda_i^A + \sum_j x_{+j+} \lambda_j^B \\
&\quad + \sum_k x_{++k} \lambda_k^C + \sum_{ij} x_{ij+} \lambda_{ij}^{AB} + \sum_{ik} x_{i+k} \lambda_{ik}^{AC} \\
&\quad + \sum_{jk} x_{+jk} \lambda_{jk}^{BC} + \sum_{ijk} x_{ijk} \lambda_{ijk}^{ABC}.
\end{aligned}
$$

We will use $x^A = \{x_{i++}\}$, $x^{AB} = \{x_{ij+}\}$, $x^{ABC} = \{x_{ijk}\}$ and so on to denote the marginal frequencies that result when units are cross-classified by subsets of variables. Following Bishop, Fienberg and Holland (1975), we will call these marginal tables *configurations*. Because the configurations x^A, x^B, x^C, x^{AB}, x^{AC}, and x^{BC} can be obtained by summing the elements of x^{ABC}, the loglikelihood for the saturated model is a linear function of the configuration x^{ABC}.

If we simplify the model by eliminating some of the λ terms, the corresponding configurations drop out of the loglikelihood. For example, if we set $\lambda^{BC} = \lambda^{ABC} = 0$, the loglikelihood becomes

$$
\begin{aligned}
l(\lambda \,|\, x) &= n\,\lambda_0 + \sum_i x_{i++} \lambda_i^A + \sum_j x_{+j+} \lambda_j^B \\
&\quad + \sum_k x_{++k} \lambda_k^C + \sum_{ij} x_{ij+} \lambda_{ij}^{AB} + \sum_{ik} x_{i+k} \lambda_{ik}^{AC}.
\end{aligned}
$$

Because x^A, x^B and x^C follow from x^{AB} and x^{AC}, the latter two configurations constitute a minimal set of sufficient statistics for this model. If a model is hierarchical, then the configuration for any set of variables present in the model can be derived from the highest-order configuration containing that set. Consequently, the configurations for these highest-order terms form a minimal set of sufficient statistics. We will call these the *sufficient configurations*. It has become standard practice to identify loglinear models by their sufficient configurations. For example, the model

Table 8.1. *Hierarchical loglinear models for three categorical variables*

Model	Omitted terms	Interpretation
(ABC)	none	saturated model
(AB, AC, BC)	λ^{ABC}	homogeneous association
(AB, AC)	$\lambda^{ABC}, \lambda^{BC}$	B, C indep. given A
(AB, BC)	$\lambda^{ABC}, \lambda^{AC}$	A, C indep. given B
(AC, BC)	$\lambda^{ABC}, \lambda^{AB}$	A, B indep. given C
(AB, C)	$\lambda^{ABC}, \lambda^{AC}, \lambda^{BC}$	(A, B) indep. of C
(AC, B)	$\lambda^{ABC}, \lambda^{AB}, \lambda^{BC}$	(A, C) indep. of B
(BC, A)	$\lambda^{ABC}, \lambda^{AB}, \lambda^{AC}$	(B, C) indep. of A
(A, B, C)	$\lambda^{ABC}, \lambda^{AB}, \lambda^{AC}, \lambda^{BC}$	mutual independence

$\lambda^{ABC} = 0$ can be denoted by (x^{AB}, x^{AC}, x^{BC}) or, more simply, (AB, AC, BC).

8.2.4 Model interpretation

The hierarchical models that can be fitted to a three-variable dataset are listed in Table 8.1, along with their sufficient configurations. This list does not include any model that omits one or more of the main effects λ^A, λ^B, λ^C. Setting a main effect to zero is equivalent to saying that the marginal distribution of the corresponding variable is uniform across its levels, a hypothesis which is rarely of interest.

Models in four or more dimensions are interpreted in a similar fashion. For example: (AB, CD) means that A and B are jointly independent of C and D; (ABC, BCD) means that A and D are conditionally independent given (B, C); (AB, AC, AD, BC, BD, CD) means that the odds ratios for any two variables are constant across levels of the other two; and (ABC, ABD, ACD, BCD) means that the associations among any three variables are constant across levels of the fourth.

Correspondence to logit models

If one of the variables is regarded as a response and the others are regarded as potential predictors, then certain loglinear models are equivalent to standard logistic regression or logit models (Goodman, 1970). Consider the saturated model for A, B and C, where

C is a binary variable considered to be a response, and let

$$\pi_{ij} = P(C = 1 \mid A = i, B = j).$$

The logit model for predicting the probability of $C = 1$ from A and B can be written as

$$\log\left(\frac{\pi_{ij}}{1 - \pi_{ij}}\right) = \log\left(\frac{\theta_{ij1}/\theta_{ij+}}{\theta_{ij2}/\theta_{ij+}}\right)$$

$$= \eta_{ij1} - \eta_{ij2},$$

where $\eta_{ijk} = \log\theta_{ijk}$. But notice that

$$\begin{aligned}
\eta_{ij1} - \eta_{ij2} &= (\lambda_1^C - \lambda_2^C) + (\lambda_{i1}^{AC} - \lambda_{i2}^{AC}) \\
&\quad + (\lambda_{j1}^{BC} - \lambda_{j2}^{BC}) + (\lambda_{ij1}^{ABC} - \lambda_{ij2}^{ABC}) \\
&= 2\lambda_1^C + 2\lambda_{i1}^{AC} + 2\lambda_{j1}^{BC} + 2\lambda_{ij1}^{ABC},
\end{aligned}$$

so this logit model is of the form

$$\log\left(\frac{\pi_{ij}}{1 - \pi_{ij}}\right) = \beta_0 + \beta_i^A + \beta_j^B + \beta_{ij}^{AB}, \qquad (8.5)$$

where the coefficients satisfy

$$\sum_i \beta_i^A = \sum_j \beta_j^B = \sum_i \beta_{ij}^{AB} = \sum_j \beta_{ij}^{AB} = 0.$$

Thus, the saturated model (ABC) implies a standard logit model for C that includes main effects for A and B as well as the AB interaction.

Notice that if we set $\lambda^{ABC} = 0$ in the loglinear model, (8.5) becomes

$$\log\left(\frac{\pi_{ij}}{1 - \pi_{ij}}\right) = \beta_0 + \beta_i^A + \beta_j^B,$$

a logit model with main effects only. Setting $\lambda^{ABC} = \lambda^{AC} = 0$ and $\lambda^{ABC} = \lambda^{BC} = 0$ removes the effects of A and B, respectively, and $\lambda^{ABC} = \lambda^{AC} = \lambda^{BC} = 0$ produces the null model

$$\log\left(\frac{\pi_{ij}}{1 - \pi_{ij}}\right) = \beta_0.$$

Omitting λ^{AB}, however, would require A and B to be conditionally independent, an assumption not found in the standard logit model. The standard logit model, like other regression models, makes no assumptions about the predictors; it allows their joint distribution to be arbitrary.

The relationships between loglinear models and logit models for three categorical variables are summarized in Table 8.2. In general,

Table 8.2. *Loglinear and corresponding logit models for three categorical variables*

Model	Implied logit model for C
(ABC)	A, B main effects and AB interaction
(AB, AC, BC)	A, B main effects only
(AB, AC)	A main effect
(AB, BC)	B main effect
(AB, C)	null model

a loglinear model is equivalent to a standard logit model provided that it includes all potential associations among the variables considered to be predictors. A two-way association between a response and a predictor in the loglinear model introduces a main effect for that predictor in the logit model; a three-way association between a response and two predictors introduces an interaction between the two predictors; and so on. The response variable need not be binary; if it has more than two categories, the loglinear model implies a generalized logit model for an unordered multinomial response (e.g. Agresti, 1990).

8.3 Likelihood-based inference with complete data

8.3.1 Maximum-likelihood estimation

To derive the ML estimates for a loglinear model, we could try to differentiate the loglikelihood with respect to some set of free parameters and set the resulting expressions to zero. However, as demonstrated by Birch (1963), we may also apply the method that leads to ML estimates for any regular exponential family model: solve the system of equations that results when the minimal sufficient statistics are set equal to their expectations (Section 3.2.1). In many cases, this system can be solved immediately to yield the ML estimates for the cell probabilities θ.

For example, consider the saturated model (ABC). Setting the elements of the sufficient configuration x^{ABC} equal to their expectations $E(x_{ijk} \mid \theta) = n\theta_{ijk}$ produces

$$\hat{\theta}_{ijk} = x_{ijk}/n$$

for all i, j and k. For the model (AB, C), the moment equations are

$$x_{ij+} = n\hat{\theta}_{ij+},$$
$$x_{++k} = n\hat{\theta}_{++k}.$$

But because this model implies $\theta_{ijk} = \theta_{ij+}\theta_{++k}$, we obtain

$$\hat{\theta}_{ijk} = (x_{ij+}x_{++k})/n^2.$$

The model (AB, BC) gives

$$x_{ij+} = n\hat{\theta}_{ij+},$$
$$x_{+jk} = n\hat{\theta}_{+jk},$$

and because this model implies

$$\theta_{ijk} = \theta_{+j+}\left(\frac{\theta_{ij+}}{\theta_{+j+}}\right)\left(\frac{\theta_{+jk}}{\theta_{+j+}}\right),$$

the ML estimates are

$$\hat{\theta}_{ijk} = (x_{ij+}x_{+jk})/(n\,x_{+j+}).$$

The model (AB, AC, AC), however, produces

$$x_{ij+} = n\hat{\theta}_{ij+},$$
$$x_{i+k} = n\hat{\theta}_{i+k},$$
$$x_{+jk} = n\hat{\theta}_{+jk},$$

a system for which there is no closed-form solution.

It turns out that (AB, AC, BC) is the only hierarchical model in three dimensions for which the ML estimates cannot be written in closed form. In four or more dimensions, however, there are many more models for which this is so. When the moment equations do not yield explicit ML estimates for θ, they may be solved numerically by the method of iterative proportional fitting.

8.3.2 Iterative proportional fitting

Iterative proportional fitting (IPF) is a simple and intuitive method for solving the moment equations. First, start with an arbitrary value of θ that satisfies the loglinear constraints, typically a uniform table (all cell probabilities equal). Then proportionately adjust the elements of θ to satisfy the moment equations for a single configuration. Do this for each sufficient configuration in turn, and repeat the entire process until the elements of θ stabilize.

For example, consider the model (AB, AC, BC). Given the current estimate $\theta^{(t)}$, IPF updates it as follows:

$$\theta_{ijk}^{(t+1/3)} = \theta_{ijk}^{(t+0/3)} \left(\frac{x_{ij+}/n}{\theta_{ij+}^{(t+0/3)}} \right) \quad \text{for all } i, j, k; \qquad (8.6)$$

$$\theta_{ijk}^{(t+2/3)} = \theta_{ijk}^{(t+1/3)} \left(\frac{x_{i+k}/n}{\theta_{i+k}^{(t+1/3)}} \right) \quad \text{for all } i, j, k; \qquad (8.7)$$

$$\theta_{ijk}^{(t+3/3)} = \theta_{ijk}^{(t+2/3)} \left(\frac{x_{+jk}/n}{\theta_{+jk}^{(t+2/3)}} \right) \quad \text{for all } i, j, k. \qquad (8.8)$$

Notice that $\theta^{(t+1/3)}$ satisfies the required conditions for x^{AB} but not necessarily those for x^{AC} or x^{BC}. Similarly, $\theta^{(t+2/3)}$ satisfies those for x^{AC} but not necessarily for x^{AB} or x^{BC}, and $\theta^{(t+3/3)}$ satisfies those for x^{BC} but not necessarily x^{AB} or x^{BC}. Repeating the cycle (8.6)–(8.8) produces a sequence $\theta^{(1)}, \theta^{(2)}, \ldots$ which converges to a value $\theta^{(\infty)} = \hat{\theta}$ satisfying all three sets of moment equations simultaneously; this is the unique ML estimate of θ.

This IPF algorithm immediately generalizes to loglinear models of any dimension. When the moment equations can be solved in closed form, IPF may still be used, and it typically converges to the correct ML estimates in a single cycle. In other cases, IPF exhibits linear convergence near the mode. Proofs of the convergence of IPF are given by Bishop, Fienberg and Holland (1975) and their references. Because IPF operates on the cell probabilities θ, it does not automatically yield explicit estimates of the loglinear coefficients λ. Estimates of λ may be obtained in a variety of ways. One simple way is to define a full-rank design matrix M such that $\log \theta = M\lambda$, and calculate the ordinary least-squares estimates

$$\hat{\lambda} = (M^T M)^{-1} M^T \log \hat{\theta}$$

using standard regression software. Except for rounding errors, the regression model will have perfect fit because $\log \hat{\theta}$ is required to lie in the space spanned by the columns of M. Another way to obtain the elements of λ is to express them as linear contrasts of the elements of $\log \theta$; see Bishop, Fienberg and Holland (1975) for details.

Comparison with other methods

IPF has been in existence for more than half a century. Deming and Stephan (1940) discussed *raking*, a method of proportionately adjusting survey data to make the observed distributions of certain variables agree with census totals; their algorithm is essentially equivalent to IPF. Early work on loglinear modeling (e.g. Bishop, Fienberg and Holland, 1975) relied almost exclusively on IPF, but more recent books emphasize other methods. Software packages capable of fitting loglinear models typically use Newton-Raphson or Fisher scoring (e.g. Agresti, 1990). These methods tend to be quicker than IPF because their convergence behavior is quadratic; moreover, they provide asymptotic standard errors as an automatic byproduct, because they make use of the loglikelihood function's second derivatives. Standard errors can be obtained with IPF, but computing them requires additional formulas that are not an integral part of the fitting algorithm. Yet IPF maintains some advantages because of its simplicity and computational stability. In this text, we focus on IPF because of its intimate relationships to ECM and the simulation algorithms described later in this chapter.

Random and structural zeroes

If the contingency table contains random zeroes, $\hat{\theta}$ may lie on the boundary of its parameter space with estimated probabilities of zero in one or more cells. When this occurs, some of the IPF equations may be undefined at $\hat{\theta}$ because they may involve division by zero. This difficulty is easily overcome by the following modification: if any probability falls below a small positive constant ϵ, set it to zero and omit that cell from further iterations.

Structural zeroes, whose cell probabilities are taken to be zero a priori, can also be handled quite easily. The usual way of handling them is to omit them from the model and assume that the loglinear specification (8.2) holds for the remaining cells. With IPF, we simply choose a starting value of θ that has zeroes in the structural-zero cells and uniform values elsewhere. Because $0 < \epsilon$, the estimated probabilities for these cells will remain at zero for all iterations.

An implementation in pseudocode

Returning now to the general notation of Chapter 7, suppose that $Y_1, Y_2, \ldots, Y_p$ are categorical variables recorded for a sample of n units, where Y_j takes values $1, 2, \ldots, d_j$. Let $y = (y_1, \ldots, y_p)$ denote a generic realization of $(Y_1, \ldots, Y_p)$; let $\mathcal{Y}$ be the set of all possible values of y; and let x_y and θ_y be the frequency and cell probability, respectively, associated with cell y of the p-dimensional

```
for each sufficient configuration C do
    for all C(y) do
        sum1 := 0
        sum2 := 0
        for all C'(y) do
            sum1 := sum1 + θy
            sum2 := sum2 + xy
        end do
        sum2 := sum2/n
        for all C'(y) do
            if θy > ε then
                θy := θy sum2/sum1
            else
                θy := 0
            end if
        end do
    end do
end do•
```

Figure 8.1. *Single cycle of iterative proportional fitting.*

cross-classified table. Let C be a subset of $\{1, 2, \ldots, p\}$ identifying a generic configuration; for example, $C = \{1, 3\}$ indicates the configuration $Y_1 Y_3$. For brevity, we will also use C to denote the function that extracts from $y = (y_1, \ldots, y_p)$ the elements corresponding to the configuration C; for example, if $C = \{2, 4\}$ then $C(y) = (y_2, y_4)$. Finally, a generic marginal count within C and its corresponding marginal probability will be denoted by

$$x_{C(y)} = \sum_{C'(y)} x_y \quad \text{and} \quad \theta_{C(y)} = \sum_{C'(y)} \theta_y,$$

respectively, where C' is the complement of C.

Pseudocode for a general implementation of IPF is shown in Figure 8.1. Given the observed counts in the workspace x and the current parameter $\theta^{(t)}$ in θ, this code performs one cycle of IPF, overwriting $\theta^{(t)}$ with the updated cell means $n\theta^{(t+1)}$. Prior to execution, the values stored in θ need not sum to one; we will obtain the same result if this workspace contains $c\theta^{(t)}$ for any constant c. Therefore, the updated cell means $n\theta^{(t+1)}$ from one cycle may be used directly as input to the next cycle; there is no need to rescale them to sum to one at each cycle.

8.3.3 Hypothesis testing and goodness of fit

A loglinear model's quality of fit may be assessed by its deviance. The deviance, typically denoted by G^2, is the likelihood-ratio statistic for testing the current model against the alternative of a saturated model,

$$G^2 = 2 \sum_{y \in \mathcal{Y}^*} x_y \log \frac{x_y}{n\hat{\theta}_y}, \tag{8.9}$$

where $\hat{\theta} = \{\hat{\theta}_y : y \in \mathcal{Y}^*\}$ is the maximizer of the likelihood under the current model, and $\mathcal{Y}^*$ is the set of all cells excluding structural zeroes. The deviance is asymptotically equivalent to the well-known goodness-of-fit statistic due to Pearson,

$$X^2 = \sum_{y \in \mathcal{Y}^*} \frac{(x_y - n\hat{\theta}_y)^2}{n\hat{\theta}_y}. \tag{8.10}$$

If the sample size is sufficiently large, G^2 and X^2 are distributed approximately as χ^2_{df} under the null hypothesis that the current model is true, where df is equal to the difference in the number of free parameters in the saturated and current models. An approximate p-value for testing the current model against a general alternative is thus $P(\chi^2_{df} \geq G^2)$ or $P(\chi^2_{df} \geq X^2)$. The chisquare approximation for these goodness-of-fit tests is traditionally regarded as accurate if $n\hat{\theta}_y \geq 5$ for all $y \in \mathcal{Y}^*$; in addition, some empirical studies have shown that it may be reasonably accurate if a small proportion of the cells have $n\hat{\theta}_y$ as small as 2 or even 1; see Agresti (1990, pp. 246–247) for further details.

The G^2 and X^2 statistics also provide a basis for general comparisons between models that are nested. Suppose we want to test the null hypothesis that Model A is true against the alternative that Model B is true, where Model A is a special case of Model B. Then

$$\Delta G^2 = G^2 \text{ for Model A} - G^2 \text{ for Model B}$$

and

$$\Delta X^2 = X^2 \text{ for Model A} - X^2 \text{ for Model B}$$

are distributed approximately as chisquare with degrees of freedom equal to

$$\Delta df = df \text{ for Model A} - df \text{ for Model B}.$$

Large values of ΔG^2 or ΔX^2 indicate that Model B fits the data substantially better than Model A. Asymptotic arguments suggest that the chisquare approximations for ΔG^2 and ΔX^2 may be quite accurate even when the approximations for the individual goodness-of-fit statistics for Model A and Model B are poor. Consequently, ΔG^2 and ΔX^2 can be useful even with sparse tables, provided that (a) the number of observations is large relative to Δdf, and (b) the observed frequencies are of approximately the same order of magnitude (Haberman, 1977).

Effects of random zeroes and boundary estimates

Notice that the presence of a random zero ($x_y = 0$) will cause G^2 to be undefined. This problem can be overcome by taking $0 \log 0$ to be 0. When a pattern of random zeroes causes the ML estimate to lie on the boundary ($\theta_y = 0$ for some y), however, neither G^2 nor X^2 can be calculated directly. In these situations, it is customary to omit the cells with zero estimates from consideration and adjust the degrees of freedom to reflect the fact that some parameters may not be estimable. Rules for adjusting the degrees of freedom (e.g. Bishop, Fienberg and Holland, 1975) are quite complicated and are difficult to implement in general-purpose computer code. Users of general-purpose software for loglinear modeling should be wary of these adjustments, because situations exist for which nearly every popular software package gives misleading results (Clogg *et al.*, 1991). When sparseness in the data table x leads to boundary estimates, a simpler and more reliable procedure is to introduce a small amount of prior information to smooth the data and move $\hat{\theta}$ away from the boundary; see Clogg *et al.* (1991) and Section 8.4.2 below.

8.3.4 Example: misclassification of seatbelt use and injury

Recall the data of Table 7.5 from a followup study on misclassification error in seatbelt use and injury in automobile accidents. Hochberg (1977) and Chen (1989) investigated loglinear models for the six dichotomous variables:

Code	Variable
D	car damage (1=low, 2=high)
S	driver's sex (1=male, 2=female)
B_1	belt use, police report (1=no, 2=yes)
I_1	injury, police report (1=no, 2=yes)
B_2	belt use, followup study (1=no, 2=yes)
I_2	injury, followup study (1=no, 2=yes)

Table 8.3. *Goodness-of-fit statistics for nine loglinear models fitted to the automobile accident followup data*

Model	G^2	X^2	df
1. (DSB_2I_2, E_BE_I)	1056.46	1726.43	45
2. $(DSB_2I_2, B_2I_2E_BE_I)$	64.59	62.14	36
3. $(DSB_2I_2, B_2I_2E_BE_I, DE_B)$	60.40	57.09	35
4. $(DSB_2I_2, B_2I_2E_BE_I, DE_I)$	57.51	57.67	35
5. $(DSB_2I_2, B_2I_2E_BE_I, DE_B, DE_I)$	53.99	53.47	34
6. $(DSB_2I_2, B_2I_2E_BE_I, DE_BE_I)$	53.05	51.99	33
7. $(DSB_2I_2, B_2I_2E_BE_I, DE_B, DE_I, SE_B)$	53.90	53.03	33
8. $(DSB_2I_2, B_2I_2E_BE_I, DE_B, DE_I, SE_I)$	52.48	51.29	33
9. $(DSB_2I_2, B_2I_2E_BE_I, DSE_I)$	52.37	51.07	32

Instead of working with these six variables directly, let us consider models for D, S, B_2, I_2 and the two error indicators

$$E_B = 1 \text{ if } B_1 = B_2, \text{ 0 otherwise};$$
$$E_I = 1 \text{ if } I_1 = I_2, \text{ 0 otherwise.}$$

Working with D, S, B_2, I_2, E_B and E_I rather than the six original variables may result in a model for the misclassification mechanism that is easier to interpret, because the associations between the underlying 'true' state of an accident DSB_2I_2 and the error indicators E_BE_I may be somewhat simpler than the associations between DSB_2I_2 and the police report B_1I_1. Regarding E_B and E_I as response variables and D, S, B_2, and I_2 as potential predictors, perhaps the simplest loglinear model worth considering is (DSB_2I_2, E_BE_I), which states that the bivariate response is unrelated to the predictors. Goodness-of-fit statistics for this model and eight other loglinear models are shown in Table 8.3.

None of the nine models shown in Table 8.3 produced ML estimates on the boundary of the parameter space, but all of them had estimated expected counts falling below 1.0 for some cells; p-values based on the chisquare approximations for G^2 and X^2 are not shown because they are not trustworthy. Chisquare approximations for comparisons among these models are probably more accurate, however, and results from hypothesis tests for various pairs of nested models are shown in Table 8.4. Model 1, the null model of no relationships between the response and predictors, appears to fit the data very poorly. The fit improves dramatically when the actual belt use/injury status B_2I_2 is allowed to influ-

Table 8.4. *Hypothesis tests for various pairs of nested models*

Comparison	Δdf	ΔG^2	p	ΔX^2	p
2 versus 1	9	991.87	0.00	1664.28	0.00
3 versus 2	1	4.19	0.04	5.06	0.02
4 versus 2	1	7.07	0.01	4.47	0.03
5 versus 3	1	6.41	0.01	3.61	0.06
5 versus 4	1	3.52	0.06	4.20	0.04
6 versus 5	1	0.94	0.33	1.48	0.22
7 versus 5	1	0.09	0.76	0.44	0.51
8 versus 5	1	1.52	0.22	2.18	0.14
9 versus 8	1	0.11	0.74	0.22	0.64

ence the response (Model 2). In addition, the data provide fairly strong evidence for the associations DE_B, DE_I, and perhaps SE_I. Among these nine, the simplest models that capture the essential relationships between the response and the predictors appear to be Models 5 and 8.

8.4 Bayesian inference with complete data

8.4.1 Prior distributions for loglinear models

In our work with the saturated multinomial model in the last chapter, we adopted the simple Dirichlet prior distribution $\theta \sim D(\alpha)$, with the elements of α typically chosen to be equal. This prior is 'naive' in the sense that it treats the cell probabilities in an unordered fashion, i.e. it does not describe the special structure that exists in a cross-classified contingency table. This was not regarded as a serious drawback, because the saturated multinomial model does not make use of this cross-classified structure either. The fundamental quality of loglinear models, however, is that they take this structure into account.

Many alternative types of prior distributions have been proposed to sensibly incorporate prior information about the structure of a loglinear model. Bishop, Fienberg and Holland (1975) decomposed the Dirichlet hyperparameters α into 'main effects' and 'associations' in a loglinear fashion. Good (1967) proposed a second-stage prior distribution on α, resulting in a mixture of Dirichlet priors that can potentially reflect a cross-classified structure. Several authors have applied normal prior distributions to the loglinear coefficients λ; variations of this approach are discussed by Good (1956), Leonard (1975), Laird (1978), and Knuiman and Speed (1988). The normal priors, although conceptually attractive, lead to nonnormal posteriors that are computationally more difficult to handle than the Dirichlet.

The constrained Dirichlet prior

For our purposes, it will be convenient to adopt a prior distribution that has the same functional form as the Dirichlet, but which requires the parameters to satisfy the constraints imposed by a loglinear model. Let M denote the design matrix for a loglinear model

$$\log \theta = M\lambda, \tag{8.11}$$

and let Θ_M denote the set of all parameters $\theta = \{\theta_y : y \in \mathcal{Y}\}$ that lie in the simplex and satisfy (8.11) for some λ. Let us take the prior density for θ to be

$$\pi(\theta) \propto \prod_{y \in \mathcal{Y}} \theta_y^{\alpha_y - 1}$$

for $\theta \in \Theta_M$ and zero elsewhere. We will call this the *constrained Dirichlet prior* with hyperparameter $\alpha = \{\alpha_y : y \in \mathcal{Y}\}$. This is not a Dirichlet distribution per se, but the conditional distribution of $\theta \sim D(\alpha)$ given that the event $\theta \in \Theta_M$ has occurred. The normalizing constant

$$\int_{\Theta_M} \prod_{y \in \mathcal{Y}} \theta_y^{\alpha_y - 1} \, d\theta$$

is not generally tractable, but this will not be a problem because in the algorithms to follow this integral will not be explicitly evaluated.

The advantage of the constrained Dirichlet prior is that it retains the same functional form as the multinomial likelihood and thus forms a conjugate class; the posterior distribution of θ given the contingency table x is another constrained Dirichlet with updated hyperparameters $\alpha' = \alpha + x$. A potential disadvantage is that this prior makes the strong assumption that the given loglinear model is true; it assigns zero probability to values of θ not satisfying (8.11). Just as in likelihood-based inference, however, it will be possible to examine the adequacy of a model by performing goodness-of-fit tests against alternative models that are more general.

8.4.2 Inference using posterior modes

Under the constrained Dirichlet prior, the complete-data posterior density for θ is

$$P(\theta \mid x) \propto \prod_{y \in \mathcal{Y}} \theta_y^{x_y + \alpha_y - 1} \tag{8.12}$$

for $\theta \in \Theta_M$ and zero elsewhere. Notice that this is equivalent to the likelihood function for θ given a modified contingency table with cell counts $x'_y = x_y + \alpha_y - 1$. Any algorithm that computes ML estimates for loglinear models can thus be trivially modified to find posterior modes for θ as well; all we need to do is to augment each cell count x_y by the amount $\alpha_y - 1$. In particular, the IPF algorithm of Section 8.3.2 will find posterior modes if we simply replace each x_y by $x'_y = x_y + \alpha_y - 1$.

It might seem natural to call this modified IPF algorithm 'Bayesian IPF.' However, we will reserve that name for another algorithm, to be discussed shortly, for simulating random draws from a constrained Dirichlet distribution.

Notice that the posterior mode for θ is identical to the ML estimate under the uniform prior $\alpha = (1, 1, \ldots, 1)$. A prior $\alpha = (c, c, \ldots, c)$ for some $c > 1$ has a 'flattening' effect; the posterior mode under this prior will represent a compromise between the ML estimate and a uniform table in which all cell probabilities are equal (Section 7.2.5). Flattening priors can be especially useful for ensuring that the mode lies within the interior of the parameter space Θ_M, avoiding complications that arise with sparse data when ML estimates lie on the boundary.

Posterior modes and goodness of fit

The goodness-of-fit statistics G^2 and X^2 defined in Section 8.3.3 can be used with posterior modes. One possibility is to use the same expressions (8.9)–(8.10) and simply replace the ML estimate $\hat{\theta}$ with a posterior mode. In many situations, however, it will be more natural to work with statistics that are based on the augmented cell counts $x'_y = x_y + \alpha_y - 1$. For a given loglinear model, let $\tilde{\theta} = \{\tilde{\theta}_y : y \in \mathcal{Y}^*\}$ represent the posterior mode under the constrained Dirichlet prior with hyperparameter α, where $\mathcal{Y}^*$ is the set of all cells excluding structural zeroes. The posterior mode under the saturated model and the unrestricted $D(\alpha)$ prior occurs at

$$\theta_y = \frac{x'_y}{n'}, \quad n' = \sum_{y \in \mathcal{Y}^{\bullet}} x'_y. \tag{8.13}$$

The statistic

$$G^2 = 2 \sum_{y \in \mathcal{Y}^{\bullet}} x'_y \log \frac{x'_y}{n' \tilde{\theta}_y} \tag{8.14}$$

represents twice the increase in the log-posterior density as we move from the mode under the current model to the mode under the saturated model. Like its likelihood-based counterpart, the modified statistic (8.14) is approximately distributed as χ^2_{df} over repeated samples, where df is the difference in the number of free parameters under the two models. This result holds because as the sample size grows, the cell counts x_y become appreciably larger than the hyperparameters α_y, and the influence of the prior becomes negligible. The analogue of (8.14) corresponding to Pearson's goodness-of-fit statistic is

$$X^2 = \sum_{y \in \mathcal{Y}^{\bullet}} \frac{(x'_y - n'\tilde{\theta}_y)^2}{n'\tilde{\theta}_y}. \tag{8.15}$$

One attractive feature of (8.14) and (8.15) is that these two statistics are easy to calculate; they will be generated automatically by standard software for loglinear modeling if the cell counts x_y are replaced by x'_y. Moreover, if all the hyperparameters α_y are greater than one, both $\tilde{\theta}$ and the unrestricted mode (8.13) are guaranteed to lie in the interior of the parameter space, and there is no need to worry about adjusting df for estimates on the boundary (Clogg et al., 1991).

8.4.3 Inference by Bayesian IPF

Here we present a clever but still relatively unknown technique for simulating random draws from a constrained Dirichlet posterior (8.12). This iterative method, first presented by Gelman et al. (1995), bears a striking resemblance to iterative proportional fitting and has thus been named Bayesian IPF. For simplicity, we describe Bayesian IPF for three categorical variables A, B and C under the model of homogeneous association (AB, AC, BC). Following the notation of Section 8.2, let x_{ijk}, θ_{ijk} and α_{ijk} denote the observed frequency, probability and prior hyperparameter, respectively, corresponding to the event $(A = i, B = j, C = k)$. Let $\theta^{(t)}$

denote the simulated value of the parameter $\theta = \{\theta_{ijk}\}$ at cycle t. Bayesian IPF updates the parameter in three steps: first,

$$\theta_{ijk}^{(t+1/3)} = \theta_{ijk}^{(t+0/3)} \left(\frac{g_{ij+}/g_{+++}}{\theta_{ij+}^{(t+0/3)}} \right) \quad \text{for all } i, j, k, \qquad (8.16)$$

where the g_{ij+} are independent random variates drawn from standard gamma distributions with shape parameters

$$\alpha'_{ij+} = \sum_k (\alpha_{ijk} + x_{ijk})$$

(Section 7.2.3), and $g_{+++} = \sum_{ij} g_{ij+}$ is their sum; second,

$$\theta_{ijk}^{(t+2/3)} = \theta_{ijk}^{(t+1/3)} \left(\frac{g_{i+k}/g_{+++}}{\theta_{i+k}^{(t+1/3)}} \right) \quad \text{for all } i, j, k, \qquad (8.17)$$

where the g_{i+k} are standard gamma variates with shape parameters

$$\alpha'_{i+k} = \sum_j (\alpha_{ijk} + x_{ijk})$$

drawn independently of those in (8.16), and $g_{+++} = \sum_{ik} g_{i+k}$ is the new sum; and third,

$$\theta_{ijk}^{(t+3/3)} = \theta_{ijk}^{(t+2/3)} \left(\frac{g_{+jk}/g_{+++}}{\theta_{+jk}^{(t+2/3)}} \right) \quad \text{for all } i, j, k, \qquad (8.18)$$

where the g_{+jk} are standard gamma variates with shape parameters

$$\alpha'_{+jk} = \sum_i (\alpha_{ijk} + x_{ijk})$$

drawn independently of those in the first two steps, and $g_{+++} = \sum_{jk} g_{+jk}$ is the new sum. Given any starting value $\theta^{(0)}$ that satisfies the constraints of the loglinear model (AB, AC, BC), these three steps (8.16)–(8.18) define a Markov chain $\{\theta^{(t)} : t = 1, 2, \ldots\}$ which converges in distribution to the constrained Dirichlet posterior with hyperparameters $\alpha'_{ijk} = \alpha_{ijk} + x_{ijk}$; a heuristic argument for this result will be given below. Thus, for a suitably large value of t, we can regard $\theta^{(t)}$ as a random draw from the correct posterior $P(\theta \mid x)$. The subsequent output stream $\theta^{(t+1)}, \theta^{(t+2)}, \ldots$ represents a dependent sample from $P(\theta \mid x)$ which can be summarized by any of the methods described in Chapter 4.

Relationship to conventional IPF

It is easy to see the relationship between this algorithm and conventional IPF. Consider the first step of conventional IPF under the constrained Dirichlet prior,

$$\theta_{ijk}^{(t+1/3)} = \left(\frac{\theta_{ijk}^{(t+0/3)}}{\theta_{ij+}^{(t+0/3)}} \right) \left(\frac{x'_{ij+}}{n'} \right) \quad \text{for all } i, j, k, \qquad (8.19)$$

where $x'_{ijk} = x_{ijk} + \alpha_{ijk} - 1$ and $n' = \sum_{ijk} x'_{ijk}$. The first term in parentheses on the right-hand side of (8.19) is the estimate of the conditional probability of $C = k$ given $(A = i, B = j)$ from the previous step. The second term in parentheses is the posterior mode of the marginal probability of $(A = i, B = j)$. Thus (8.19) represents the marriage between an old estimate of $P(C = k \mid A = i, B = j)$ and a new estimate of $P(A = i, B = j)$. Now consider the first step of Bayesian IPF,

$$\theta_{ijk}^{(t+1/3)} = \left(\frac{\theta_{ijk}^{(t+0/3)}}{\theta_{ij+}^{(t+0/3)}} \right) \left(\frac{g_{ij+}}{g_{+++}} \right) \quad \text{for all } i, j, k. \qquad (8.20)$$

The first term in (8.20) is the old simulated value of $P(C = k \mid A = i, B = j)$. The second term, g_{ij+}/g_{+++}, simulates new values of the marginal probabilities $\theta_{ij+} = \sum_k \theta_{ijk}$ from the Dirichlet distribution with parameters $\{\alpha'_{ij+}\}$, the marginal posterior distribution of θ_{ij+} given the data. Thus (8.19) represents the marriage between an old draw of $P(C = k \mid A = i, B = j)$ and a new draw of $P(A = i, B = j)$. The second and third steps of Bayesian IPF continue in a similar vein, updating the parameters by taking new random draws of the marginal probabilities $P(A = i, C = k)$ and $P(B = j, C = k)$, respectively.

An implementation in pseudocode

Like its conventional counterpart, Bayesian IPF generalizes immediately to hierarchical loglinear models for any number of variables. Pseudocode for a general implementation of Bayesian IPF is shown in Figure 8.2. This code, which uses the same notation as that of Figure 8.1, performs one cycle of Bayesian IPF and overwrites θ with its updated value. The starting value of θ must lie in the interior of the parameter space; in particular, it must satisfy the following requirements. (a) If any structural zeroes are present, the starting value must have zeroes in those positions. (b) All other elements of the starting value must be nonzero. (c) The starting

```
for each sufficient configuration C do
    sum3:= 0
    for all C(y) do
        sum1:= 0
        sum2:= 0
        zflag:= 0
        for all C'(y) do
            sum1:= sum1 + θ_y
            if y ∈ 𝒴* then
                sum2:= sum2 + x_y + α_y
                zflag:= 1
            end if
        end do
        if zflag = 1 then
            draw g ~ G(sum2)
            sum3:= sum3 + g
        end if
        for all C'(y) do θ_y := θ_y g/sum1
    end do
    for y ∈ 𝒴* do θ_y := θ_y/sum3
end do
```

Figure 8.2. *Single cycle of Bayesian iterative proportional fitting.*

value must satisfy the constraints of the loglinear model. One way to create a starting value with these properties is to fill θ with zeroes corresponding to the structural zeroes and uniform values elsewhere. Another good choice is a posterior mode under a constrained Dirichlet prior with all hyperparameters $\alpha_y > 1$, which can be obtained from conventional IPF.

One unusual feature of Bayesian IPF is that if a cell probability θ_y ever becomes zero, it remains at zero for all subsequent iterations. In theory, this should never happen for a non-structural-zero cell, because true gamma random variates are always positive. In practice, however, if the prior hyperparameters α_y are close to zero and the observed contingency table contains random zeroes, the pseudorandom number generator used in

$$\text{draw } g \sim G(\text{sum2}) \tag{8.21}$$

may ocasionally produce a value with a floating-point representation of zero. The resulting value of θ will then fall on the boundary and remain trapped there for all future iterations, and the Markov chain will fail to converge to the correct posterior distribution. The problem is that boundary values are absorbing states, whose presence violates the regularity conditions necessary for an iterative simulation algorithm to converge (Section 3.5.2). In principle the probability of ever reaching the boundary should be zero, but due to the limitations of computer arithmetic, the chance of falling within machine precision of the boundary might be non-negligible. This difficulty is easily overcome by adding a very small positive constant (say 10^{-20}) to the value of g in (8.21), the effect of which will be imperceptible in the statistical inference.

8.4.4 Why Bayesian IPF works

Here we present heuristic arguments to establish that Bayesian IPF does indeed converge to the constrained Dirichlet posterior for the given loglinear model. For simplicity, let us consider the homogeneous-association model for three variables, (AB, AC, BC), where each of the variables A, B and C is binary; extensions to other loglinear models will be immediate. The relationships among the log-cell probabilities $\eta = \log \theta$ can be expressed as $\eta = M\lambda$, where

$$
\eta = \begin{bmatrix} \eta_{111} \\ \eta_{211} \\ \eta_{121} \\ \eta_{221} \\ \eta_{112} \\ \eta_{212} \\ \eta_{122} \\ \eta_{222} \end{bmatrix}, \quad
M = \begin{bmatrix}
1 & 1 & 1 & 1 & 1 & 1 & 1 \\
1 & -1 & 1 & 1 & -1 & -1 & 1 \\
1 & 1 & -1 & 1 & -1 & 1 & -1 \\
1 & -1 & -1 & 1 & 1 & -1 & -1 \\
1 & 1 & 1 & -1 & 1 & -1 & -1 \\
1 & -1 & 1 & -1 & -1 & 1 & -1 \\
1 & 1 & -1 & -1 & -1 & -1 & 1 \\
1 & -1 & -1 & -1 & 1 & 1 & -1
\end{bmatrix},
$$

and

$$
\lambda = \left[\, \lambda_0,\ \lambda_1^A,\ \lambda_1^B,\ \lambda_1^C,\ \lambda_{11}^{AB}, \lambda_{11}^{AC},\ \lambda_{11}^{BC} \,\right]^T.
$$

The remaining loglinear coefficients follow from the identifiability constraints

$$
\lambda_1^A = -\lambda_2^A, \quad \lambda_{11}^{AB} = -\lambda_{12}^{AB} = -\lambda_{21}^{AB} = \lambda_{22}^{AB},
$$

and so on.

Until now we have been assuming that the cell frequencies x follow a multinomial distribution,

$$
x \mid \theta \sim M(n, \theta),
$$

where the sample size $n = x_{+++}$ is considered fixed, and the cell probabilities $\theta = \{\theta_{ijk}\}$ follow a Dirichlet distribution with hyperparameters $\alpha = \{\alpha_{ijk}\}$. With the restrictions imposed by the loglinear model, $\eta = \log \theta$ must lie in $\mathcal{R}(M)$, the seven-dimensional linear space spanned by the columns of M; in addition, θ must satisfy $\theta_{+++} = 1$. This combination of linear and loglinear constraints on the elements of θ makes the parameter space somewhat difficult to visualize and understand. The geometric features can be simplified, however, if we expand the model by allowing the total sample size n to vary.

The Poisson/gamma representation

Consider an expanded model in which the cell counts are Poisson,

$$x_{ijk} \mid \mu \sim \text{Poisson}(\mu_{ijk}) \tag{8.22}$$

independently for all i, j, k, and the cell means $\mu = \{\mu_{ijk}\}$ are a priori distributed as independent gamma variates

$$\mu_{ijk} \sim c\,G(\alpha_{ijk}) \tag{8.23}$$

with a common scaling factor c. By well-known properties of the Poisson model, (8.22) implies that

$$n \mid \mu \sim \text{Poisson}(\mu_{+++})$$

and

$$x \mid n, \mu \sim M(n, \theta),$$

where $\mu_{+++} = \sum_{ijk} \mu_{ijk}$ and $\theta_{ijk} = \mu_{ijk}/\mu_{+++}$ (e.g. Agresti, 1990). Moreover, it can be shown that the product-gamma prior (8.23) implies that μ_{+++} and θ are independently distributed as

$$\mu_{+++} \sim c\,G(\alpha_{+++})$$

and

$$\theta \sim D(\alpha),$$

respectively; the proof is a standard exercise in transformation and will be left to the reader.

Thus the expanded model (8.22)–(8.23) for x and μ implies our usual multinomial-Dirichlet model for x and θ; the only difference is that the expanded model allows estimation of an overall intensity parameter μ_{+++} which is independent of θ in both the prior and the posterior distributions. By standard Bayesian arguments, the posterior distributions of the cell means μ are

$$\mu_{ijk} \mid x \sim c'G(\alpha'_{ijk}) \tag{8.24}$$

where $\alpha'_{ijk} = \alpha_{ijk} + x_{ijk}$ and $c' = c/(c+1)$, and the posterior distribution of the intensity parameter is

$$\mu_{+++} \mid x \sim c'G(\alpha'_{+++})$$

where $\alpha'_{+++} = \sum_{ijk} \alpha_{ijk} + n$. As before, the posterior distribution of θ is $D(\alpha')$, $\alpha' = \alpha + x$.

The Poisson/gamma representation is geometrically convenient because, unlike θ, the cell means μ are not required to sum to any particular value. The loglinear model for the cell probabilities, $\log \theta = M\lambda$, implies a similar model for the cell means,

$$\log \mu = M\lambda^*, \tag{8.25}$$

where

$$\lambda^* = \begin{bmatrix} \lambda_0^*, \ \lambda_1^A, \ \lambda_1^B, \ \lambda_1^C, \ \lambda_{11}^{AB}, \lambda_{11}^{AC}, \ \lambda_{11}^{BC} \end{bmatrix}^T$$

and $\lambda_0^* = \lambda_0 + \log \mu_{+++}$. Unlike λ_0, the new intercept λ_0^* is a free parameter that can take any value on the real line. Thus the parameter space for μ is simpler than the space for θ, because $\log \mu$ is allowed to lie anywhere in $\mathcal{R}(M)$.

The cell-means version of Bayesian IPF

Under the expanded model, we can define a version of Bayesian IPF that operates on the cell means μ. It is similar to the version for θ except that we do not rescale the parameters to sum to one at every step. The cell-means version is

$$\mu_{ijk}^{(t+1/3)} = \mu_{ijk}^{(t+0/3)} \left(\frac{c'g_{ij+}}{\mu_{ij+}^{(t+0/3)}} \right) \quad \text{for all } i,j,k, \quad (8.26)$$

$$\mu_{ijk}^{(t+2/3)} = \mu_{ijk}^{(t+1/3)} \left(\frac{c'g_{i+k}}{\mu_{i+k}^{(t+1/3)}} \right) \quad \text{for all } i,j,k, \quad (8.27)$$

$$\mu_{ijk}^{(t+3/3)} = \mu_{ijk}^{(t+2/3)} \left(\frac{c'g_{+jk}}{\mu_{+jk}^{(t+2/3)}} \right) \quad \text{for all } i,j,k, \quad (8.28)$$

where the g_{ij+}, g_{i+k} and g_{+jk} are independent gamma variates as before. To see the relationship to the previous version, notice that we can rewrite the first step as

$$\mu_{ijk}^{(t+1/3)} = \left(\frac{\theta_{ijk}^{(t+0/3)}}{\theta_{ij+}^{(t+0/3)}} \right) \left(\frac{g_{ij+}}{g_{+++}} \right) c'g_{+++}$$

$$= \theta_{ijk}^{(t+1/3)} \, c'g_{+++},$$

and similarly for the second and third steps. The value of θ at every step is the same under the new version; the only difference is that the intensity parameter

$$\mu_{+++} = \sum_{i,j,k} \theta_{ijk} \, c'g_{+++} = c'g_{+++}$$

is updated at every step to be a random draw from $c'G(\alpha'_{+++})$.

Without constraints, the product-gamma posterior (8.24) for μ implies that the posterior distribution of θ is $D(\alpha')$. Constraining μ and θ to lie in $\mathcal{R}(M)$ does not change the functional form of the densities for μ or θ, but only their normalizing constants; so if we are able to show that the cell-means version of Bayesian IPF converges to the constrained product-gamma posterior over $\mathcal{R}(M)$, then we have successfully shown that the original version converges to the constrained Dirichlet posterior over $\mathcal{R}(M)$.

Heuristic argument for convergence

The three steps (8.26)–(8.28) define the transition rule of a Markov chain for μ. To show that a particular distribution F is the stationary distribution for this chain, one must establish two facts. First, one must show that the chain 'maps F onto itself,' in other words, that $\mu^{(t)} \sim F$ implies $\mu^{(t+1)} \sim F$. Second, one must show that the chain is *ergodic*, containing no periodicities or absorbing states: it must be possible for $\mu^{(t)}$ to reach any value in the support of F for a sufficiently large t, and for every step thereafter, from any starting value $\mu^{(0)}$ within the support.

To establish the first condition, notice that the first step (8.26) combines conditional probabilities $P(C = k \mid A = i, B = j)$ from the previous cycle with updated values for the $(A = i, B = j)$ marginal rates,

$$\mu_{ijk}^{(t+1/3)} = \theta_{(ij)k}^{(t+0/3)} \, \mu_{ij+}^{(t+1/3)},$$

where

$$\theta_{(ij)k}^{(t+0/3)} = \frac{\theta_{ijk}^{(t+0/3)}}{\theta_{ij+}^{(t+0/3)}} = \frac{\mu_{ijk}^{(t+0/3)}}{\mu_{ij+}^{(t+0/3)}}$$

and

$$\mu_{ij+}^{(t+1/3)} \sim c'G(\alpha'_{ij+}) \qquad (8.29)$$

independently for all i, j. Because (8.29) is the marginal distribution of $\{\mu_{ij+}\}$ implied by (8.24), this first step represents a draw from the conditional posterior of μ with $\{\theta_{(ij)k}\}$ fixed at its previous value,

$$\mu^{(t+1/3)} \sim P(\mu \mid x, \{\theta_{(ij)k}\} = \{\theta_{(ij)k}^{(t+0/3)}\}).$$

Now if the old value of μ is drawn from the actual posterior distribution,

$$\mu^{(t+0/3)} \sim P(\mu \mid x),$$

then the old values of $\theta_{(ij)k}$ are drawn from their actual posterior as well,

$$\{\theta_{(ij)k}^{(t+0/3)}\} \sim P(\{\theta_{(ij)k}\} \mid x),$$

which implies

$$\mu^{(t+1/3)} \sim P(\mu \mid x).$$

Thus we have established that the first step (8.26) maps $P(\mu \mid x)$ onto itself. By similar arguments this result holds for the second and third steps (8.27)–(8.28) as well.

To establish ergodicity, we must examine the structure of the design matrix M in the loglinear model (8.25) for μ. Let

$$
M_1 = \begin{bmatrix}
1 & 1 & 1 & 1 \\
1 & -1 & 1 & -1 \\
1 & 1 & -1 & -1 \\
1 & -1 & -1 & 1 \\
1 & 1 & 1 & 1 \\
1 & -1 & 1 & -1 \\
1 & 1 & -1 & -1 \\
1 & -1 & -1 & 1
\end{bmatrix}, \quad
M_2 = \begin{bmatrix}
1 & 1 & 1 & 1 \\
1 & -1 & 1 & -1 \\
1 & 1 & 1 & 1 \\
1 & -1 & 1 & -1 \\
1 & 1 & -1 & -1 \\
1 & -1 & -1 & 1 \\
1 & 1 & -1 & -1 \\
1 & -1 & -1 & 1
\end{bmatrix},
$$

and

$$
M_3 = \begin{bmatrix}
1 & 1 & 1 & 1 \\
1 & 1 & 1 & 1 \\
1 & -1 & 1 & -1 \\
1 & -1 & 1 & -1 \\
1 & 1 & -1 & -1 \\
1 & 1 & -1 & -1 \\
1 & -1 & -1 & 1 \\
1 & -1 & -1 & 1
\end{bmatrix}
$$

denote the portions of M corresponding to the AB, AC and BC effects, respectively. The space spanned by the columns of M_1 is the same as that of

$$M_1^* = \begin{bmatrix} 1 & 0 & 0 & 0 \\ 0 & 1 & 0 & 0 \\ 0 & 0 & 1 & 0 \\ 0 & 0 & 0 & 1 \\ 1 & 0 & 0 & 0 \\ 0 & 1 & 0 & 0 \\ 0 & 0 & 1 & 0 \\ 0 & 0 & 0 & 1 \end{bmatrix}.$$

Similarly, the range spaces of M_2 and M_3 are the same as those of

$$M_2^* = \begin{bmatrix} 1 & 0 & 0 & 0 \\ 0 & 1 & 0 & 0 \\ 1 & 0 & 0 & 0 \\ 0 & 1 & 0 & 0 \\ 0 & 0 & 1 & 0 \\ 0 & 0 & 0 & 1 \\ 0 & 0 & 1 & 0 \\ 0 & 0 & 0 & 1 \end{bmatrix} \quad \text{and } M_3^* = \begin{bmatrix} 1 & 0 & 0 & 0 \\ 1 & 0 & 0 & 0 \\ 0 & 1 & 0 & 0 \\ 0 & 1 & 0 & 0 \\ 0 & 0 & 1 & 0 \\ 0 & 0 & 1 & 0 \\ 0 & 0 & 0 & 1 \\ 0 & 0 & 0 & 1 \end{bmatrix},$$

respectively. Notice that the first step of Bayesian IPF represents a proportionate adjustment for each group of cells that contributes to a mean μ_{ij+} for the AB marginal table. This first step can thus be written in terms of the log-cell means as

$$\log \mu^{(t+1/3)} = \log \mu^{(t+0/3)} + M_1^* \log \gamma_1,$$

where γ_1 is a vector of four gamma variates. Similarly, the second and third steps can be written

$$\log \mu^{(t+2/3)} = \log \mu^{(t+1/3)} + M_2^* \log \gamma_2,$$
$$\log \mu^{(t+3/3)} = \log \mu^{(t+2/3)} + M_3^* \log \gamma_3.$$

The complete cycle consisting of all three steps is thus

$$\log \mu^{(t+1)} = \log \mu^{(t)} + M^* \log \gamma \qquad (8.30)$$

where $M^* = (M_1^*, M_2^*, M_3^*)$ and $\gamma = (\gamma_1^T, \gamma_2^T, \gamma_3^T)^T$. Because the columns of M^* span the same space as those of M, and the elements of γ are random gamma variates whose logarithms can lie anywhere on the real line, (8.30) ensures that $\mu^{(t+1)}$ has a nonzero chance of falling anywhere in $\mathcal{R}(M)$ provided that $\mu^{(t)} \in \mathcal{R}(M)$. Thus it follows that this Markov chain can reach any state in a single cycle from any state in the parameter space of μ, and ergodicity is established.

Further notes

Bayesian IPF was first presented by Gelman *et al.* (1995) who gave brief arguments for convergence under a Poisson/gamma loglinear model. Our version (8.26)–(8.28) differs from theirs in that we have included a factor c' arising from the scaling parameter in the prior distribution (8.23). Without this factor, the resulting posterior could give misleading inferences about the overall intensity μ_{+++}. Inferences about the cell probabilities $\theta_{ijk} = \mu_{ijk}/\mu_{+++}$, however, will be the same under both versions.

Bayesian IPF bears an interesting relationship to Gibbs sampling (Section 3.4.1). In Gibbs sampling, we partition a random vector Z into non-overlapping subvectors $(Z_1, Z_2, \ldots, Z_J)$ and draw from the full conditionals $P(Z_j \mid \{Z_k : k \neq j\})$ for $j = 1, \ldots, J$ in turn. In Bayesian IPF, however, the vector is partitioned differently at each step of the cycle; in our example we partition μ as

$$(\{\mu_{ij+}\}, \{\mu_{ijk}/\mu_{ij+}\}) \quad \text{at Step 1,}$$
$$(\{\mu_{i+k}\}, \{\mu_{ijk}/\mu_{i+k}\}) \quad \text{at Step 2,}$$
$$(\{\mu_{+jk}\}, \{\mu_{ijk}/\mu_{+jk}\}) \quad \text{at Step 3.}$$

As noted by several authors (e.g. Gelfand and Smith, 1990), any partitioning scheme will work provided that the complete cycle is ergodic, allowing the random vector to eventually reach any state from any other state.

8.4.5 Example: misclassification of seatbelt use and injury

In Section 8.3.4 we examined loglinear models pertaining to errors in police reporting of seatbelt use and injury in automobile accidents. Regarding the error indicators E_B and E_I as response variables and D, S, B_2 and I_2 as predictors, we found convincing evidence for the associations $B_2 I_2 E_B E_I$, DE_B, DE_I and mild evidence for SE_I. This evidence was based on p-values from chisquare approximations for the test statistics ΔG^2 and ΔX^2. Using Bayesian IPF, we can make Bayesian inferences about these associations directly without large-sample approximations. To illustrate, we ran Bayesian IPF under Model 8,

$$(DSB_2 I_2, B_2 I_2 E_B E_I, DE_B, DE_I, SE_I). \tag{8.31}$$

Recall that the ML estimate for this model lies in the interior of the parameter space. Taking the ML estimate from IPF as a starting value, we ran 5100 cycles of Bayesian IPF under the Jeffreys

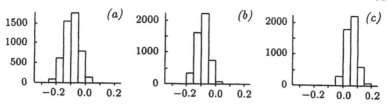

Figure 8.3. *Histograms of 5000 simulated values of (a)* $\lambda_{11}^{DE_B}$, *(b)* $\lambda_{11}^{DE_I}$ *and (c)* $\lambda_{11}^{SE_I}$, *respectively, from Bayesian IPF.*

prior with hyperparameters 0.5; ignoring the first 100 cycles, we stored the results of the remaining 5000. Bayesian IPF appears to converge very quickly in this example; autocorrelation plots of a variety of parameters revealed no significant correlations beyond lag 5. This behavior is consistent with that of ordinary IPF, which converged in only 11 cycles.

Let us consider how to draw inferences about the coefficients λ of the loglinear model. The output of each cycle of Bayesian IPF is a table of simulated cell probabilities θ, and each coefficient in λ is a linear contrast among the elements of $\log \theta$. Consider the terms in λ^{DE_B}, which pertain to the effect of damage on errors in the police report of belt use. If we average the elements of the 2^6 array $\log \theta$ over the dimensions corresponding to S, B_2, I_2 and E_I, all the coefficients pertaining to these variables drop out due to the linear constraints imposed on them. The result of this averaging is a 2×2 table with elements

$$\gamma_{ij}^{DE_B} = \lambda_0 + \lambda_i^D + \lambda_j^{E_B} + \lambda_{ij}^{DE_B}$$

for $i, j = 1, 2$. The loglinear coefficients can then be obtained as

$$\lambda_0 = \tfrac{1}{4} \sum_{ij} \gamma_{ij}^{DE_B},$$
$$\lambda_i^D = \tfrac{1}{2} \sum_j \gamma_{ij}^{DE_B} - \lambda_0,$$
$$\lambda_j^{E_B} = \tfrac{1}{2} \sum_i \gamma_{ij}^{DE_B} - \lambda_0,$$
$$\lambda_{ij}^{DE_B} = \gamma_{ij}^{DE_B} - \lambda_i^D - \lambda_j^{E_B} - \lambda_0.$$

By similar manipulations of the elements of $\log \theta$ we can derive any coefficient in the loglinear model. Histograms of the 5000 simulated values of $\lambda_{11}^{DE_B}$, $\lambda_{11}^{DE_I}$, and $\lambda_{11}^{SE_I}$ are shown in Figure 8.3 (a), (b) and (c), respectively.

Notice that the distribution in Figure 8.3 (a) is located primarily to the left of zero, providing evidence that errors in reporting of belt use ($E_B = 2$) tend to occur more frequently for accidents with low damage ($D = 1$) than those with high damage ($D = 2$). Among the 5000 simulated values of $\lambda_{11}^{DE_B}$, 182 fell above zero, so a two-tailed Bayesian p-value for testing the current model (8.31) against the reduced model that sets $\lambda^{DE_B} = 0$ is $2 \times 182/5000 = 0.07$. Similarly, Figures 8.3 (b) and (c) show that low damage ($D = 1$) and female drivers ($S = 2$) are associated with higher rates of reporting errors for injury ($E_I = 2$); two-tailed Bayesian p-values for testing $\lambda^{DE_I} = 0$ and $\lambda^{SE_I} = 0$ are 0.03 and 0.13, respectively.

8.5 Loglinear modeling with incomplete data

8.5.1 ML estimates and posterior modes

The two algorithms we have discussed thus far, IPF and Bayesian IPF, can be extended quite easily to handle missing values in the original data matrix. With conventional IPF, the extension is an example of the ECM algorithm, a generalization of EM discussed briefly in Chapter 3.

EM for loglinear models

Let us now return to our general notation, with $Y_1, Y_2, \ldots, Y_p$ representing categorical variables, and $x = \{x_y : y \in \mathcal{Y}\}$ and $\theta = \{\theta_y : y \in \mathcal{Y}\}$ the cell counts and probabilities, respectively, in the p-dimensional cross-classified contingency table. As described in Section 7.3, the actual cell counts x are not observed when the data are incomplete; rather, we observe a table $z^{(s)}$ of potentially smaller dimension for each missingness pattern $s = 1, 2, \ldots, S$, where $z^{(s)}$ contains marginal frequencies for the variables observed in pattern s. The basic EM algorithm (Section 7.3.2) updates the estimate of θ in two steps: the E-step, in which we calculate the predicted mean of x given $z^{(1)}, \ldots, z^{(S)}$ under the current estimate of θ; and the M-step, in which we re-estimate θ from the predicted mean of x. Under the saturated multinomial model, the M-step has a particularly simple form because the complete-data ML estimates are $\hat{\theta} = x_y/n$ for all $y \in \mathcal{Y}$.

Now consider what happens to EM when we move from the saturated model to a loglinear model, which requires the parameter θ to lie in a restricted space Θ_M. The E-step, which is performed under an assumed value of θ, does not change at all, because the conditional expectation of x given $z^{(1)}, \ldots, z^{(S)}$ and θ has the same form whether $\theta \in \Theta_M$ or $\theta \notin \Theta_M$. The M-step, however, becomes a constrained maximization of the (expected) complete-data loglikelihood or log-posterior over Θ_M. For loglinear models, this maximization cannot in general be carried out in closed form, but requires an iterative technique such as IPF. A general EM algorithm for loglinear models would thus be doubly iterative, requiring iteration to convergence within each M-step.

The ECM algorithm

In many situations, EM for loglinear models is not unduly cumbersome, especially in modern computing environments. Several authors speculated, however, that it might not be necessary to iterate until full convergence at each M-step; rather, running only a single cycle of IPF might be enough (e.g. Fuchs, 1982). As shown by Meng and Rubin (1993), this modification produces an example of an algorithm called Expectation-Conditional Maximization or ECM. ECM possesses the same reliable convergence properties as EM, increasing the observed-data loglikelihood at each step. The key idea of ECM is that the full M-step is replaced by a quicker CM-step, a single cycle of constrained maximizations which, if repeated over and over, would eventually result in a maximization over the full parameter space Θ_M.

Each step in a cycle of IPF is a constrained maximization. Consider the three steps of IPF for the model (AB, AC, BC). The first step (8.6) is based on a factorization of the complete-data likelihood for the cell probabilities $\theta_{ijk} = P(A = i, B = j, C = k)$ into independent factors corresponding to the conditional probabilities for C given A and B,

$$P(C = k \mid A = i, B = j) = \theta_{ijk}/\theta_{ij+},$$

and the marginal probabilities for A and B,

$$P(A = i, B = j) = \theta_{ij+}.$$

The first step fixes $\{\theta_{ijk}/\theta_{ij+}\}$ at its previous value but replaces $\{\theta_{ij+}\}$ by an ML estimate or posterior mode; thus it represents a constrained maximization of the likelihood or posterior density for θ. Similarly, the second and third steps (8.7)–(8.8) represent maximizations subject to fixed values of $\{\theta_{ijk}/\theta_{i+k}\}$ and $\{\theta_{ijk}/\theta_{+jk}\}$, respectively.

For a cycle of constrained maximizations to form a valid CM-step, it must satisfy a set of technical requirements known as the *space-filling conditions* (Meng and Rubin, 1993). These conditions, which have been demonstrated to hold for a single cycle of IPF

(Meng and Rubin, 1991b), are similar to those needed to establish ergodicity in a Markov chain (Section 8.4.4). The fact that IPF can reach any point in Θ_M from any other point in a single cycle ensures that the ECM algorithm will eventually converge to an unconstrained maximum rather than a constrained one.

To obtain a general ECM algorithm for loglinear models, we only need to replace the M-step of the basic EM (the last line of pseudocode in Figure 7.2) by a single call to the IPF algorithm presented in Figure 8.1. As in ordinary IPF, the starting value for θ should lie in the interior of the parameter space; one choice that always works is to assign zeroes to the structural-zero cells and uniform values elsewhere.

8.5.2 Goodness-of-fit statistics

The goodness-of-fit statistics G^2 and X^2 can be readily extended to handle incomplete data. Using the notation of Section 7.3, let $y = (y_1, y_2, \ldots, y_p)$ denote a generic realization of the variables $(Y_1, Y_2, \ldots, Y_p)$, and let $\mathcal{O}_s(y)$ and $\mathcal{M}_s(y)$, respectively, denote the subvectors of y corresponding to the variables that are observed and missing in pattern s. Let O_s and M_s denote the sets over which $\mathcal{O}_s(y)$ and $\mathcal{M}_s(y)$ can vary, excluding structural zeroes. The marginal table $z^{(s)}$ that we observe for pattern s has counts

$$z^{(s)}_{\mathcal{O}_s(y)} = \sum_{\mathcal{M}_s(y) \in M_s} x^{(s)}_y \quad \text{for all } \mathcal{O}_s(y) \in O_s, \qquad (8.32)$$

and the marginal probabilities corresponding to these counts are

$$\beta_{\mathcal{O}_s(y)} = \sum_{\mathcal{M}_s(y) \in M_s} \theta_y. \qquad (8.33)$$

The most obvious way to extend G^2 is to take

$$G^2_{raw} = 2 \sum_{s=1}^{S} \sum_{\mathcal{O}_s(y) \in O_s} z^{(s)}_{\mathcal{O}_s(y)} \log \frac{z^{(s)}_{\mathcal{O}_s(y)}}{n_s \beta_{\mathcal{O}_s(y)}}, \qquad (8.34)$$

where n_s represents the total sample size in pattern s. This statistic, when evaluated at an ML estimate $\hat{\theta}$, increases as the observed frequencies deviate from their estimated expected values. The corresponding extension of Pearson's X^2 is

$$X^2_{raw} = \sum_{s=1}^{S} \sum_{\mathcal{O}_s(y) \in O_s} \frac{(z^{(s)}_{\mathcal{O}_s(y)} - n_s \beta_{\mathcal{O}_s(y)})^2}{n_s \beta_{\mathcal{O}_s(y)}}. \qquad (8.35)$$

As noted by Fuchs (1982) and Little and Rubin (1987), these statistics differ from their complete-data counterparts in that they are typically nonzero even when evaluated at the ML estimate for the saturated model. The reason, which is somewhat technical, is buried in the definition of the observed-data likelihood in Chapter 2. The marginal probabilities (8.33) are not really the expected proportions for the observed counts (8.32) within each missingness pattern, unless the missingness happens to be MCAR. Under the less restrictive assumption of MAR, the true expected proportions may differ from (8.33), because MAR does not require the distribution of observed data to be identical across patterns. Using the same cell probabilities θ in the calculation of (8.33) for all patterns is merely a matter of convenience, because, as argued in Section 2.3, likelihood-based inferences for parameters of the complete-data model are identical under any ignorable mechanism.

The practical effect of using a common θ for all patterns is that G^2_{raw} and X^2_{raw} as defined above may be drastically different from zero even when evaluated at the ML estimate for the saturated model. In fact, if the sample is large enough, these statistics can be used to test the null hypothesis that the missingness data are MCAR against the alternative of MAR. In most situations, such a test will not be of great interest, because we are concerned primarily with the parameters of the complete-data model; the parameters of the missingness mechanism are a nuisance. Moreover, in all but the most trivial real data examples, the expected cell counts within missingness patterns are rarely large enough for the chisquare approximation to work well. For these reasons, we will not attempt to interpret a value of G^2_{raw} or X^2_{raw} from the saturated model, except as a baseline for assessing the fit of a smaller model.

Adjusted goodness-of-fit statistics

Let G^2_0 denote the value of (8.34) evaluated at the ML estimate for the saturated model. Consider the adjusted goodness-of-fit measure

$$G^2 = 2 \sum_{s=1}^{S} \sum_{O_s(y) \in O_s} z^{(s)}_{O_s(y)} \log \frac{z^{(s)}_{O_s(y)}}{n_s \beta_{O_s(y)}} - G^2_0 \qquad (8.36)$$

regarded as a function of θ. This represents twice the difference in the observed-data loglikelihood evaluated at the current value of θ and at the global maximum over the entire simplex Θ. When evaluated at the ML estimate for the saturated model, (8.36) is zero. When evaluated at the ML estimate for a non-saturated loglinear model, it becomes the likelihood-ratio statistic for testing the fit of the model against the saturated alternative. Because this statistic behaves in much the same manner as the deviance (8.9) for complete data, we will adopt (8.36) as our definition for the deviance with incomplete data. The Pearson counterpart to (8.36) is

$$X^2 = \sum_{s=1}^{S} \sum_{O_s(y) \in O_s} \frac{(z_{O_s(y)}^{(s)} - n_s \beta_{O_s(y)})^2}{n_s \beta_{O_s(y)}} - X_0^2, \qquad (8.37)$$

where X_0^2 represents the raw version (8.35) evaluated at the MLE for the saturated model.

Just as in the complete-data case, the chisquare approximation for the distributions of G^2 and X^2 may be poor when the data are sparse. Even with sparse data, however, chisquare approximations for the differences ΔG^2 and ΔX^2 can be quite reliable for nested model comparisons, particularly when Δdf is small. Finally, just as with complete data, G^2 and X^2 become problematic when ML estimates lie on the boundary. The easiest way to handle such situations is to add a small amount of prior information, e.g. in the form of a Dirichlet prior with all hyperparameters greater than one, to smooth the posterior mode away from the boundary.

8.5.3 Data augmentation and Bayesian IPF

We have seen that IPF can be extended in a straightforward way to handle missing data, resulting in an ECM algorithm. In a similar fashion, we can extend Bayesian IPF to create an algorithm for parameter simulation and multiple imputation.

Recall the basic data augmentation procedure for the saturated multinomial model (Section 7.3.3). In this algorithm, the observed marginal counts $z^{(s)}$ for missingness patterns $s = 1, 2, \dots, S$ are randomly allocated to the cells of the full p-dimensional table x under an assumed value for θ (the I-step). Then a new value of θ is drawn from its complete-data Dirichlet posterior given the simulated version of x (the P-step). Repeating the I- and P-steps a large number of times eventually produces a draw of θ from its observed-data posterior $P(\theta \mid Y_{obs})$.

As we move from the saturated model to a loglinear model, the I-step remains unchanged, because the random allocation procedure has the same form regardless of the value of θ. The P-step, however, must in general be carried out iteratively, because creating posterior draws of θ under a loglinear model requires multiple cycles of Bayesian IPF. True data augmentation, like a true EM algorithm, would thus require undesirable nested iterations.

Suppose, however, that instead of iterating to full convergence within each P-step, we perform only a single cycle of Bayesian IPF. The resulting algorithm, which we call *data augmentation-Bayesian IPF* (DABIPF), still converges to the observed-data posterior under the constrained Dirichlet prior. Although we are not drawing from the correct conditional distribution $P(\theta \mid x)$ in this modified P-step, we are simulating one step from the transition rule of a Markov chain whose stationary distribution is $P(\theta \mid x)$. DABIPF is neither a true data augmentation algorithm nor a Gibbs sampler, but a hybrid algorithm of the type described in Section 3.4.5 with the same basic convergence properties. Combining the data augmentation I-step (Section 7.3.3) with the implementation of Bayesian IPF in Figure 8.2 produces a single iteration of DABIPF. The algorithm may be used for parameter simulation or (when combined with the imputation code in Figure 7.5) for multiple imputation of the unit-level missing data.

Factorizations for near-monotone patterns

In the last chapter, we derived a monotone data augmentation procedure for the saturated model that tends to converge faster than ordinary data augmentation for near-monotone missingness patterns (Section 7.4). The algorithm was based on a factorization of the multinomial likelihood into a sequence of multinomial likelihoods pertaining to the distribution of each variable given the previous ones. For loglinear models, we can again exploit factorizations of the likelihood to improve the performance of DABIPF, but only in certain special cases. For many loglinear models, the parameters corresponding to the sequence of conditional distributions are not distinct, due to the loglinear restrictions; we cannot always separate the complete-data inference into a sequence of independent inferences corresponding to the near-monotone pattern in the dataset. For this reason, we will not consider further the possible monotone versions of DABIPF.

8.6 Examples

8.6.1 Protective Services Project for Older Persons

Recall the data introduced in the last chapter (Section 7.3.5) regarding the impact of social services on elderly clients. In this six-

Table 8.5. *Parameters in the model*
$(ASPMG, ASPMD, GD)$

Source	No. of parameters
$ASPM$	$2^4 - 1 = 15$
GD	$2^2 - 1 = 3$
$ASPM \times G$	$15 \times (2 - 1) = 15$
$ASPM \times D$	$15 \times (2 - 1) = 15$
Total	$15 + 15 + 15 + 3 = 48$

variable dataset, the main question of interest pertained to the effect of the treatment-group indicator G on survival D, controlling for the possible confounding effects of the covariates age A, sex S, physical status P and mental status M. With only $n = 164$ clients in the study, some of whom had missing values for P and M, the data were too sparse to allow for estimation of individual GD associations within each of the sixteen covariate patterns. Now we will fit a loglinear model that constrains these associations to be the same.

Consider the model $(ASPMG, ASPMD, GD)$. The presence of the association $ASPMG$ allows the distribution of G to vary freely across the sixteen $ASPM$ covariate patterns; similarly, $ASPMD$ allows the distribution of D to vary freely across the covariate patterns. The GD association allows G to have a direct influence on D beyond that provided by their mutual associations with A, S, P and M. The absence of any association between GD and $ASPM$, however, requires the conditional GD odds ratios within the sixteen covariate patterns to be equal. The number of free parameters in this model, 48, can be counted as shown in Table 8.5. Notice that the saturated model has $2^6 - 1 = 63$ free parameters; the difference is $63 - 48 = 15$ because the saturated model fits 16 conditional GD odds ratios rather than just one. By pooling information across covariate patterns, the reduced model can provide a stable estimate of a common GD effect even though the information within any single pattern may be weak. With complete data, inferences about the conditional GD association under this model would be similar to those given by the well known Mantel-Haenszel test (Mantel and Haenszel, 1959; Agresti, 1990).

Using the tools of Section 8.5, we can draw inferences about the effect of interest in two ways. First, we can perform a sin-

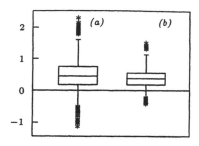

Figure 8.4. *Posterior draws of GD log-odds ratios under prior hyperparameters of (a) 0.1 and (b) 1.5, simulated from 5000 cycles of DABIPF.*

gle degree-of-freedom test of the null model $(ASPMG, ASPMD)$ against the $(ASPMG, ASPMD, GD)$ alternative using a large-sample approximation to ΔX^2 or ΔG^2. Under both of these models, the ECM algorithm converges to ML estimates on the boundary. To move the estimates away from the boundary, we re-ran ECM for each model using prior hyperparameters of 1.1. Comparing the observed-data loglikelihood at the two posterior modes, we find $\Delta G^2 = 0.826$. The corresponding p-value is 0.36, so there is essentially no evidence of any conditional GD association given A, S, P and M.

A second method, which does not rely on large-sample approximations, is to simulate posterior draws of the parameters under the larger model $(ASPMG, ASPMD, GD)$ and examine the marginal distribution of the conditional GD association. Starting from the posterior mode that we obtained from ECM, we ran 5000 cycles of DABIPF after a burn-in period of 100 cycles. We did this under two alternative priors, setting the prior hyperparameters to 0.1 and 1.5, respectively; the first results in very little smoothing, whereas the second pulls the estimates rather strongly toward a uniform table. Boxplots of the simulated log-odds ratios under these two priors are shown in Figure 8.4. Simulated posterior means and interval estimates for the odds ratio in (a) are 1.74 and $(0.68, 3.75)$, respectively; the corresponding estimates for (b) are 1.50 and $(0.82, 2.51)$. Thus there is no evidence to suggest that enriched social services are beneficial to clients. On the contrary, we find weak evidence that membership in the experimental group $(G = 1)$ is associated with an increased rate of mortality $(D = 1)$. The effects are not 'statistically significant,' however; simulated two-tailed Bayesian p-values are 0.26 for (a) and 0.20 for (b).

Recall that when we tried to draw inferences about the conditional GD associations under the saturated model (Section 7.3.5), we encountered difficulty because the parameters were so poorly estimated. Comparing the new boxplots in Figure 8.4 to the old ones in Figure 7.7, we see that the new inferences are much more plausible, and also much less sensitive to the choice of prior hyperparameters; pooling across covariate patterns to estimate a common odds ratio was indeed helpful.

8.6.2 Driver injury and seatbelt use

In the last chapter (Section 7.4.3) we examined data from a large sample of 80 084 automobile accidents and found apparently convincing evidence that seatbelt use reduces the risk of injury. Those data, however, were marred by errors in the police reports of injury and belt use. A followup study of an additional 1796 accidents provided information on error rates in the police reports. We attempted to use the followup data to calibrate the larger dataset, correcting the inference for potential biases due to misclassification. Those efforts were hindered by the complexity of the saturated model, the only model available to us at the time. Let us re-examine these data by applying a more parsimonious loglinear model to the combined sample of 81 880 accidents.

Our loglinear modeling of the 1796 followup cases (Section 8.3.4) provides some insight into the misclassification mechanism. Among various models relating damage D, driver sex S, true belt use B_2 and true injury I_2 to the error indicators for belt use E_B and injury E_I, we found that

$$(DSB_2I_2, B_2I_2E_BE_I, DE_B, DE_I, SE_I)$$

seemed to provide a good fit. For modeling the combined dataset of 81 880 cases, however, it is more convenient to work with D, S, B_2, I_2 and the original police-report variables B_1 and I_1, because E_B and E_I are not determined for the accidents not included in the followup study. Because E_B is a function of B_1 and B_2, and E_I is a function of I_1 and I_2, all the associations in the above model are present in

$$(DSB_2I_2, B_1I_1B_2I_2, DB_1B_2, DI_1I_2, SI_1I_2).$$

Furthermore, we expect the full four-way association DSB_1I_1 to be well estimated because these four variables are recorded for all cases in the combined dataset. Therefore, we will fit the model

$$(DSB_1I_1, DSB_2I_2, B_1I_1B_2I_2, DB_1B_2, DI_1I_2, SI_1I_2),$$

which has a total of 39 free parameters.

Under this model, both ECM and DABIPF converge rather slowly. This is not surprising, because B_2 and I_2 are missing for about 98% of the cases in the combined dataset. Because of the slow convergence, it would be difficult to draw inferences by parameter simulation; consecutive draws from DABIPF are so highly correlated that a very large number of cycles would be needed to obtain good posterior summaries. Instead of storing draws of parameters, we created ten multiple imputations of the followup belt use B_2 and injury status I_2. These imputations were created by running ten parallel chains of DABIPF for 2500 cycles each, using the ML estimate as a starting value and setting the prior hyperparameters equal to 0.5. The ten imputations are shown in Figure 8.6. The imputed variables, denoted by B and I, represent true belt use and injury, and the variation among the ten imputations reflects the uncertainty due to misclassification in the original data. After imputation the followup cases were removed, so that only the original 80 084 accidents are represented in the imputed data.

Using these ten imputations, we calculated point and interval estimates for the odds ratios relating seatbelt use to injury. The estimation was carried out on the logarithmic scale, as described in Section 6.4.2. Results for the overall odds ratio, and for the conditional odds ratios within each of the four $D \times S$ cells, are summarized in Table 8.7. Over the entire population, seatbelt use appears to reduce the odds of injury by about $1 - 0.73 = 27\%$, and the effect is statistically significant (p-value $= 0.04$). This marginal analysis, however, ignores the possible confounding effects due to the covariates D and S. Within the four $D \times S$ cells, the estimated odds ratios are all less than one, but the interval estimates are very wide; none of the effects is statistically significant. After controlling for damage and sex of driver, the evidence for any beneficial effect of seatbelt use is very weak.

The fact that all four of the conditional odds ratios are less than one suggests that we may be able to strengthen our conclusions by assuming a common odds ratio across the four $D \times S$ cells; that is, by fitting the loglinear model (DSB, DSI, BI), we may be able to find a significant BI association. The loglinear model (DSB, DSI, BI) implies a logit model for I that includes main effects for D and S, a $D \times S$ interaction and a main effect

Table 8.6. *Multiple imputations of accident frequencies by damage D (1=low, 2=high), sex of driver S (1=male, 2=female), actual belt use B (1=no, 2=yes), and actual injury I (1=not injured, 2=injured), reflecting errors of classification*

D	S	B	I	Imputations 1–5				
				1	2	3	4	5
1	1	1	1	18275	17698	18344	18570	18132
2	1	1	1	14667	15195	13739	14817	14218
1	2	1	1	9254	8735	8618	9341	8525
2	2	1	1	4311	4631	4565	4271	4516
1	1	2	1	5212	4954	4719	4865	4986
2	1	2	1	2558	2446	2860	2664	2670
1	2	2	1	2018	1471	1923	1607	1653
2	2	2	1	762	633	456	1117	703
1	1	1	2	3142	3847	3414	3173	3356
2	1	1	2	7912	7824	9113	8133	8499
1	2	1	2	2428	3544	3048	2740	3366
2	2	1	2	6165	5968	5897	5865	5741
1	1	2	2	799	929	951	820	954
2	1	2	2	1823	1495	1248	1346	1573
1	2	2	2	300	250	411	312	456
2	2	2	2	458	464	778	443	736

D	S	B	I	Imputations 6–10				
				1	2	3	4	5
1	1	1	1	18562	18433	18019	17766	18302
2	1	1	1	13612	14601	13405	13911	14021
1	2	1	1	8832	8671	9748	9157	8991
2	2	1	1	4149	4191	4395	4097	4535
1	1	2	1	4840	4742	5365	4966	5022
2	1	2	1	2979	2823	2907	3055	2862
1	2	2	1	2005	1724	1325	1585	1597
2	2	2	1	592	566	945	956	660
1	1	1	2	3346	3275	3142	3591	3422
2	1	1	2	9096	8413	9303	8454	8174
1	2	1	2	2966	3013	2506	2770	2821
2	2	1	2	6285	6088	5818	6042	5744
1	1	2	2	680	978	902	1105	682
2	1	2	2	1273	1123	1345	1540	1903
1	2	2	2	197	592	421	488	591
2	2	2	2	670	851	538	601	757

Table 8.7. *Multiple-imputation inferences for odds ratios relating to belt use to injury, overall and within cells of damage by sex of driver: estimates, intervals, p-values and percent missing information*

	est.	interval	p-value	% missing
Overall	0.73	(0.54, 0.98)	0.04	98
low damage, male	0.95	(0.66, 1.37)	0.76	95
high damage, male	0.87	(0.46, 1.67)	0.65	99
low damage, female	0.70	(0.23, 2.12)	0.49	99
high damage, female	0.63	(0.20, 1.99)	0.39	99

Table 8.8. *Multiple-imputation inferences for logistic-regression coefficients for predicting injury, assuming a common effect of belt use across classes of damage and sex*

	est.	interval	p-value	% missing
intercept	−1.66	(−1.85, −1.47)	0.00	96
damage	1.15	(0.87, 1.44)	0.00	98
sex	0.51	(0.24, 0.79)	0.00	96
damage × sex	0.27	(−0.05, 0.59)	0.09	95
belt use	−0.19	(−0.51, 0.13)	0.22	98

for B. We fit this logit model to each of the imputed datasets, coding dummy variables for the main effects of D (1 if high damage, 0 otherwise), S (1 if female, 0 otherwise), B (1 if belt used, 0 otherwise) and the $D \times S$ interaction (1 if high damage and female, 0 otherwise). The results of the multiply-imputed logit analysis are shown in Table 8.8. The estimate of the common odds ratio is $\exp(-0.19) = 0.83$ and the 95% interval ranges from $\exp(-0.51) = 0.60$ to $\exp(0.13) = 1.14$, so the evidence is still weak. Accounting for occasional errors in the police reports greatly increases our uncertainty about the relationship between belt use and injury. These results are consistent with those of Chen (1989), who reached similar conclusions using likelihood-based methods.

CHAPTER 9

Methods for mixed data

9.1 Introduction

Chapters 5–8 pertained to datasets in which the variables were either all continuous or all categorical. In practice, however, statistical analyses involving variables of both types are extremely common: analysis of variance, analysis of covariance, logistic regression with continuous predictors, and so on. Sample surveys often contain variables of both types. This chapter develops general tools for incomplete multivariate data matrices containing both continuous and categorical variables. Such a dataset is shown in Figure 9.1, with missing values denoted by question marks.

The statistical literature on multivariate methods tends to emphasize models for variables that are all of the same type; relatively

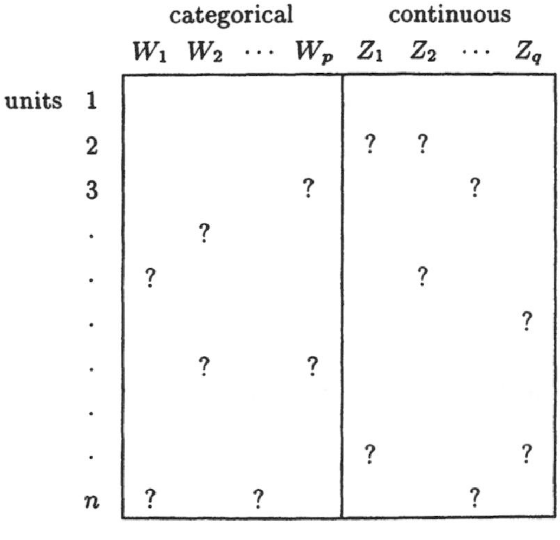

Figure 9.1. *Mixed dataset with missing values.*

little attention has been paid to models for mixed data. One notable exception is the model that underlies classical discriminant analysis, which contains a single categorical response and one or more continuous predictors. We begin with a version of this model called the general location model (Section 9.2) and discuss methods for keeping the number of parameters manageable (Section 9.3). Algorithms for incomplete mixed data are presented in Section 9.4, and Section 9.5 concludes with several data examples.

9.2 The general location model

9.2.1 Definition

As in Figure 9.1, let $W_1, W_2, \ldots, W_p$ denote a set of categorical variables and $Z_1, Z_2, \ldots, Z_q$ a set of continuous ones. If these variables are recorded for a sample of n units, the result is an $n \times (p+q)$ data matrix $Y = (W, Z)$, where W and Z represent the categorical and continuous parts, respectively.

The categorical data W may be summarized by a contingency table. Let us suppose that W_j takes possible values $1, 2, \ldots, d_j$, so that each unit can be classified into a cell of a p-dimensional table with total number of cells equal to $D = \prod_{j=1}^{p} d_j$. A generic response pattern for the categorical variables will be denoted by $w = (w_1, w_2, \ldots, w_p)$, and the frequencies in the complete-data contingency table will be

$$x = \{x_w : w \in \mathcal{W}\}, \qquad (9.1)$$

where x_w is the number of units for which $(W_1, W_2, \ldots, W_p) = w$, and $\mathcal{W}$ is the set of all possible w. We may also arrange the cells of the contingency table in a linear order indexed by $d = 1, 2, \ldots, D$, for example, the anti-lexicographical storage order in which w_1 varies the fastest, w_2 varies the next fastest, and so on (Appendix B). Then we can replace the vector subscript in x_w by a single subscript d,

$$x = \{x_d : d = 1, 2, \ldots, D\}. \qquad (9.2)$$

Depending on the context, we will regard x either as a multidimensional array (9.1) or a vector (9.2).

Finally, it will be helpful to introduce one additional characterization of W. Let U be an $n \times D$ matrix with rows u_i^T, $i = 1, 2, \ldots, n$, where u_i is a D-vector containing a 1 in position d if unit i falls into cell d, and 0s in all other positions. Hence each row of U contains a single 1, and $U^T U$ is

$$U^T U = \text{diag}(x) = \begin{bmatrix} x_1 & 0 & \cdots & 0 \\ 0 & x_2 & \cdots & 0 \\ \vdots & \vdots & \ddots & \vdots \\ 0 & 0 & \cdots & x_D \end{bmatrix}. \tag{9.3}$$

Because the sample units are assumed to be independent and identically distributed, all relevant statistical information in W is contained in x, U or $U^T U$. The continuous data are characterized simply by Z.

The general location model, so named by Olkin and Tate (1961), is most easily defined in terms of the marginal distribution of W and the conditional distribution of Z given W. The former is described by a multinomial distribution on the cell counts x,

$$x \mid \pi \sim M(n, \pi), \tag{9.4}$$

where $\pi = \{\pi_w : w \in \mathcal{W}\} = \{\pi_d : d = 1, 2, \ldots, D\}$ is an array of cell probabilities corresponding to x. Given W, the rows $z_1^T, z_2^T, \ldots, z_n^T$ of Z are then modeled as conditionally multivariate normal. Let E_d denote a D-vector containing a 1 in position d and 0s elsewhere. We assume

$$z_i \mid u_i = E_d, \mu_d, \Sigma \sim N(\mu_d, \Sigma) \tag{9.5}$$

independently for $i = 1, 2, \ldots, n$, where μ_d is a q-vector of means corresponding to cell d, and Σ is a $q \times q$ covariance matrix. The means of $Z_1, Z_2, \ldots, Z_q$ are allowed to vary freely from cell to cell, but a common covariance structure Σ is assumed for all cells. When $D = 2$, this reduces to the model that underlies classical discriminant analysis (e.g. Anderson, 1984).

The parameters of the general location model will be written

$$\theta = (\pi, \mu, \Sigma),$$

where $\mu = (\mu_1, \mu_2, \ldots, \mu_D)^T$ is a $D \times q$ matrix of means. For the moment, we will impose no prior restrictions on θ other than the necessary positive definiteness for Σ and $\sum_{w \in \mathcal{W}} \pi_w = 1$. The number of free parameters in the unrestricted model is thus

$$(D - 1) + Dq + q(q + 1)/2.$$

Notice that the model for Z given W may also be regarded as a classical multivariate regression,

$$Z = U\mu + \epsilon, \tag{9.6}$$

where ϵ is an $n \times q$ matrix of errors whose rows are independently distributed as $N(0, \Sigma)$. The columns of U contain dummy variables for each of the cells $d = 1, 2, \ldots, D$. Because U has the same rank as $U^T U = \mathrm{diag}(x)$, this will be a full-rank regression provided that there are no random zeroes in x. Structural zeroes may be handled simply by omitting them from the columns of U. A model of the form (9.6) is sometimes called a *standard multivariate regression*; in this model the same matrix of regressors U is used to predict each column of the response Z.

9.2.2 Complete-data likelihood

Combining (9.4) with (9.5), we can write the complete-data likelihood as the product of multinomial and normal likelihoods,

$$L(\theta \mid Y) \propto L(\pi \mid W)\, L(\mu, \Sigma \mid W, Z). \tag{9.7}$$

The likelihood factors are $L(\pi \mid W) \propto \prod_{d=1}^{D} \pi_d^{x_d}$ and

$$L(\mu, \Sigma \mid W, Z) \propto |\Sigma|^{-\frac{n}{2}} \exp\left\{ -\tfrac{1}{2} \sum_{d=1}^{D} \sum_{i \in B_d} (z_i - \mu_d)^T \Sigma^{-1} (z_i - \mu_d) \right\},$$

where $B_d = \{i : u_i = E_d\}$ is the set of all units belonging to cell d. After some algebraic manipulation, the second factor may be written as

$$L(\mu, \Sigma \mid W, Z) \propto |\Sigma|^{-\frac{n}{2}} \exp\left\{ -\tfrac{1}{2} \operatorname{tr} \Sigma^{-1} Z^T Z \right. \tag{9.8}$$
$$\left. + \operatorname{tr} \Sigma^{-1} \mu^T U^T Z - \tfrac{1}{2} \operatorname{tr} \Sigma^{-1} \mu^T U^T U \mu \right\},$$

revealing that the complete-data loglikelihood is linear in the elements of the sufficient statistics

$$T_1 = Z^T Z, \quad T_2 = U^T Z, \quad \text{and} \quad T_3 = U^T U = \mathrm{diag}(x). \tag{9.9}$$

Maximum-likelihood estimates

Because the parameters associated with the two factors in (9.7) are distinct, complete-data ML estimates may be found by maximizing each factor separately. The result for π is the usual ML estimate for an unrestricted multinomial model,

$$\hat{\pi}_d = \frac{x_d}{n}, \quad d = 1, 2, \ldots, D.$$

The estimate for μ follows from the least-squares regression of Z on U,

$$\hat{\mu} = (U^T U)^{-1} U^T Z = T_3^{-1} T_2, \qquad (9.10)$$

and the estimate for Σ is

$$\hat{\Sigma} = \frac{1}{n} \hat{\epsilon}^T \hat{\epsilon} = \frac{1}{n} \left(T_1 - T_2^T T_3^{-1} T_2 \right), \qquad (9.11)$$

where $\hat{\epsilon} = Z - U\hat{\mu}$ is the matrix of estimated residuals. Notice that (9.11) differs from the classical unbiased estimate in that it uses a denominator of n rather than $n - D$.

These estimates can be further understood by noting that

$$(U^T U)^{-1} = \begin{bmatrix} x_1^{-1} & 0 & \cdots & 0 \\ 0 & x_2^{-1} & \cdots & 0 \\ \vdots & \vdots & \ddots & \vdots \\ 0 & 0 & \cdots & x_D^{-1} \end{bmatrix}$$

and that $U^T Z$ is a $D \times q$ matrix with $\sum_{i \in B_d} z_i^T$ in the dth row. The rows of $\hat{\mu}$ are thus

$$\hat{\mu}_d^T = x_d^{-1} \sum_{i \in B_d} z_i^T, \quad d = 1, 2, \ldots, D,$$

the within-cell averages of the rows of Z. The rows of the residual matrix $\hat{\epsilon}$ are the deviations of the rows of Z from their cell-specific means, so the estimated covariance matrix can be written as

$$\hat{\Sigma} = \frac{1}{n} \sum_{d=1}^{D} \sum_{i \in B_d} (z_i - \hat{\mu}_d)(z_i - \hat{\mu}_d)^T.$$

Random zeroes and sparse data

If any cell in x is randomly zero, the matrix of regressors U has deficient rank and the least-squares estimate (9.10) is no longer defined. When this happens, the mean vector μ_d corresponding to the empty cell drops out of the likelihood function and becomes inestimable; the likelihood takes the same value regardless of μ_d, and the ML estimate is no longer unique.

Clearly, the unrestricted general location model will tend to be useful only when n is large relative to D, when enough observations are present in each cell to estimate all the components of μ. When the data are sparse, restricted versions of the model that contain fewer free parameters (to be discussed below) will be more appropriate.

Table 9.1. *Classification of subjects by foreign language studied and sex*

LAN	SEX		
	male	female	total
French	35	31	66
Spanish	45	32	77
German	62	52	114
Russian	9	11	20
total	151	126	277

9.2.3 Example

In Section 6.3 we examined data pertaining to the validity of the Foreign Language Attitude Scale (FLAS), a test instrument for predicting achievement in foreign language study; the raw data are reproduced in Appendix A. We will now apply the unrestricted general location model to a portion of this dataset. As shown in Table 6.5, the variables LAN and FLAS had no missing values, and SEX and HGPA were missing for only one subject each. For the moment, let us discard those two subjects to obtain an apparently complete dataset with four variables and 277 observations. The variables FLAS and HGPA are continuous, whereas LAN and SEX are categorical with four and two levels, respectively. The frequencies for the LAN by SEX classification are shown in Table 9.1. Adopting a columnwise storage order, the cell counts are

$$U^T U = \text{diag}(35, 45, 62, 9, 31, 32, 52, 11),$$

and dividing these counts by $n = 277$ yields the ML estimate

$$\hat{\pi} = (0.126, 0.162, 0.224, 0.032, 0.112, 0.116, 0.188, 0.040).$$

The sufficient statistics pertaining to HGPA and FLAS are

$$U^T Z = \begin{bmatrix} 94.45 & 2841 \\ 121.08 & 3397 \\ 170.78 & 4987 \\ 26.35 & 694 \\ 82.63 & 2759 \\ 83.12 & 2719 \\ 153.41 & 4517 \\ 29.86 & 907 \end{bmatrix}, \quad Z^T Z = \begin{bmatrix} 2199.69 & 62894.18 \\ 62894.18 & 1934421 \end{bmatrix}.$$

Dividing the rows of $U^T Z$ by the cell counts yields the estimated matrix of means,

$$\hat{\mu} = \begin{bmatrix} 2.70 & 81.2 \\ 2.69 & 75.5 \\ 2.75 & 80.4 \\ 2.93 & 77.1 \\ 2.67 & 89.0 \\ 2.60 & 85.0 \\ 2.95 & 86.9 \\ 2.71 & 82.4 \end{bmatrix},$$

and the ML estimate of the covariance matrix is

$$\hat{\Sigma} = n^{-1} \left(Z^T Z - Z^T U (U^T U)^{-1} U^T Z \right)$$

$$= \begin{bmatrix} 0.367 & 0.411 \\ 0.411 & 176.9 \end{bmatrix}.$$

9.2.4 Complete-data Bayesian inference

The factorization (9.7) which simplified the problem of ML estimation is also convenient from a Bayesian point of view: if we apply independent prior distributions to π and (μ, Σ), these parameter sets will be independent in the posterior distribution as well. For simplicity, we will apply a Dirichlet prior to the cell probabilities,

$$\pi \sim D(\alpha),$$

where $\alpha = \{\alpha_w : w \in \mathcal{W}\} = \{\alpha_d : d = 1, 2, \ldots, D\}$ is an array of user-specified hyperparameters; the complete-data posterior distribution of π is then

$$\pi \sim D(\alpha'),$$

where $\alpha' = \alpha + x$. For discussion on choosing values for the hyperparameters, see Section 7.2.5.

Inferences for μ and Σ under a noninformative prior

With regard to μ and Σ, let us first consider what happens when we apply an improper uniform prior to the elements of μ and the standard noninformative prior to the covariance matrix Σ,

$$P(\mu, \Sigma) \propto |\Sigma|^{-\left(\frac{q+1}{2}\right)}. \tag{9.12}$$

With a little algebra, the likelihood factor (9.8) for μ and Σ can be written in terms of the least-squares estimates,

$$L(\mu, \Sigma \mid W, Z) \propto |\Sigma|^{-\frac{n}{2}} \exp\left\{ -\tfrac{1}{2} \operatorname{tr} \Sigma^{-1} \hat{\epsilon}^T \hat{\epsilon} \right. \tag{9.13}$$

$$\left. -\tfrac{1}{2} \operatorname{tr} \Sigma^{-1} (\mu - \hat{\mu})^T U^T U (\mu - \hat{\mu}) \right\}.$$

The diagonal form of $U^T U$ then allows us to rewrite (9.13) as

$$L(\mu, \Sigma \mid Z, W) \propto |\Sigma|^{-\frac{n}{2}} \exp\left\{ -\tfrac{1}{2} \operatorname{tr} \Sigma^{-1} \hat{\epsilon}^T \hat{\epsilon} \right.$$

$$\left. -\tfrac{1}{2} \sum_{d=1}^{D} x_d (\mu_d - \hat{\mu}_d)^T \Sigma^{-1} (\mu_d - \hat{\mu}_d) \right\},$$

which is equivalent to

$$L(\mu, \Sigma \mid Z, W) \propto |\Sigma|^{-\left(\frac{n-D}{2}\right)} \exp\left\{ -\tfrac{1}{2} \operatorname{tr} \Sigma^{-1} \hat{\epsilon}^T \hat{\epsilon} \right\} \tag{9.14}$$

$$\times \prod_{d=1}^{D} |x_d^{-1} \Sigma|^{-\frac{1}{2}} \exp\left\{ -\tfrac{1}{2} (\mu_d - \hat{\mu}_d)^T (x_d^{-1} \Sigma)^{-1} (\mu_d - \hat{\mu}_d) \right\}.$$

Combining (9.14) with the prior (9.12) leads to

$$P(\mu, \Sigma \mid Z, W) \propto |\Sigma|^{-\left(\frac{n-D+q+1}{2}\right)} \exp\left\{ -\tfrac{1}{2} \operatorname{tr} \Sigma^{-1} \hat{\epsilon}^T \hat{\epsilon} \right\}$$

$$\times \prod_{d=1}^{D} |x_d^{-1} \Sigma|^{-\frac{1}{2}} \exp\left\{ -\tfrac{1}{2} (\mu_d - \hat{\mu}_d)^T (x_d^{-1} \Sigma)^{-1} (\mu_d - \hat{\mu}_d) \right\},$$

which, by inspection, is the product of independent multivariate normal densities for $\mu_1, \mu_2, \ldots, \mu_D$ given Σ and an inverted-Wishart density for Σ,

$$\mu_d \mid \Sigma, Y \sim N(\hat{\mu}_d, x_d^{-1} \Sigma), \tag{9.15}$$

$$\Sigma \mid Y \sim W^{-1}(n - D, (\hat{\epsilon}^T \hat{\epsilon})^{-1}). \tag{9.16}$$

For this posterior to be proper, we need $n \geq D + q$ and $x_d > 0$ for all d, structural zeroes excluded; also, the matrix $\hat{\epsilon}^T \hat{\epsilon}$ of residual sums of squares and cross-products should have full rank.

Informative priors

The preceding arguments can easily be extended to incorporate prior knowledge about μ and Σ. The most convenient way to specify prior information for μ would be in the form of independent multivariate normal distributions for $\mu_1, \mu_2, \ldots, \mu_D$ with covariance matrices proportional to Σ; prior information for Σ could then be expressed through an inverted-Wishart distribution. The resulting complete-data posterior would again be the product of independent normal distributions for $\mu_1, \mu_2, \ldots, \mu_D$ given Σ and an inverted-Wishart distribution for Σ, and the updated hyperparameters would be obtained by calculations similar to those given in Section 5.2.2.

For typical applications of the general location model, strong prior information about μ or Σ will not be available; in all our examples, we will use the noninformative prior (9.12). The use of an improper prior can lead to difficulties, especially in sparse-data situations. For many datasets, particularly if the number of cells D in the contingency table is large, we may find that portions of μ or Σ are poorly estimated or inestimable, and the posterior may be improper. When this happens, we will not attempt to stabilize the inference through informative priors for μ or Σ; rather, we will specify a more parsimonious regression model for Z given W, reducing the number of free parameters and enforcing simpler relationships between $Z_1, Z_2, \ldots, Z_q$ and $W_1, W_2, \ldots, W_p$.

9.3 Restricted models

9.3.1 Reducing the number of parameters

The unrestricted general location model tends to work well when the sample size n is appreciably larger than the total number of cells D. When this is not the case, the data may contain little or no information about certain aspects of π, μ or Σ, and it would be wise to reduce the number of free parameters. As shown by Krzanowski (1980, 1982) and Little and Schluchter (1985), the general location model is amenable to certain types of restrictions on the parameter space. Because we defined the complete-data distribution and likelihood as the product of two distinct factors, the marginal distribution of W and the conditional distribution of Z given W, we will impose restrictions on the parameter sets π and (μ, Σ) separately to keep them distinct.

Loglinear models for the cell probabilities

For the cell probabilities π, we may require them to satisfy a loglinear model

$$\log \pi = M\lambda \tag{9.17}$$

where M is a user-specified matrix. Because the contingency table is a cross-classification by $W_1, W_2, \ldots, W_p$, M will typically reflect this structure, containing 'main effects' for $W_1, W_2, \ldots, W_p$ and 'interactions' among them. If the first column of M is constant, the first element of λ (the intercept) is not a free parameter but a normalizing constant that scales π to sum to one. The total number of free parameters in this loglinear model is rank $(M) - 1$. Our fitting procedures will operate directly on the elements of π; there will be no need to explicitly create M or estimate λ unless the loglinear coefficients are of intrinsic interest.

Linear models for the within-cell means

In the unrestricted general location model, the conditional distribution of Z given W is specified by the multivariate regression

$$Z = U\mu + \epsilon, \qquad (9.18)$$

where U is an $n \times D$ matrix of dummy indicators recording the cell location $1, 2, \ldots, D$ of each sample unit. The means of Z_1, Z_2, $\ldots$, Z_q are allowed to vary freely among cells. As a result, (9.18) is equivalent to a multivariate analysis of variance (MANOVA) model for $(Z_1, Z_2, \ldots, Z_q)$ with main effects for $W_1, W_2, \ldots, W_p$ and all interactions among them. In practice, many of these interactions may be poorly estimated, and it is advantageous to eliminate them from the model.

To simplify the model, we could directly replace U by another matrix with fewer columns. For notational purposes, however, it is helpful to retain the present definition of U because of its role in the complete-data sufficient statistics. Instead, let us restrict μ to be of the form

$$\mu = A\beta \qquad (9.19)$$

for some β, where A is a constant matrix of dimension $D \times r$. Each of the q columns of μ, corresponding to the variables $Z_1, Z_2, \ldots, Z_q$, is thus required to lie in the linear subspace of $\mathcal{R}^D$ spanned by the columns of A. The regression model becomes

$$Z = UA\beta + \epsilon,$$

with a reduced set of regression coefficients in β. By taking $A = I$ (the identity matrix) we obtain the unrestricted model (9.18) as a special case.

If A has full rank, then each of the $r \times q$ elements of β represents a free parameter. More generally, the number of free parameters in β is $q \times \text{rank}(A)$. If the contingency table contains no random zeroes, then all of the regression coefficients will be estimable. If the table does contain zeroes, the coefficients may still all be estimable, because estimability now depends on the rank of UA rather than U itself. To keep matters simple, let us proceed under the assumption that there are no deficiencies in the rank of A or UA,

$$\text{rank}(A) = \text{rank}(UA) = r.$$

In practice we can ensure that this is satisfied by defining A to have full rank, and then checking the rank of UA by seeing whether $A^T U^T UA$ is invertible.

Choosing the design matrix

The design matrix A defines the regression that relates the cells of the contingency table to the means of the continuous variables. This matrix is created in the same way that one creates a design matrix for a factorial ANOVA. Thinking of the categorical variables $W_1, W_2, \ldots, W_p$ as 'factors' of the experiment, we first list all the possible combinations of levels of these factors, using the linear storage order that we adopted for our contingency table; these identify the rows of A. Then we create columns for the main effects of $W_1, W_2, \ldots, W_p$, and perhaps interactions among them, using any coding scheme that is convenient. In most applications, the first column of A will contain 1s for an intercept and the remaining columns will contain dummy codes or contrasts for the desired effects of $W_1, W_2, \ldots, W_p$ and their interactions.

For example, consider a model with $p = 2$ categorical variables, W_1 and W_2, taking $d_1 = 2$ and $d_2 = 3$ levels, respectively, so that the contingency table has $D = 6$ cells. Let us adopt the anti-lexicographical storage order

$$(W_1, W_2) = (1,1), (2,1), (1,2), (2,2), (1,3), (2,3).$$

One possible design matrix is

$$A = \begin{bmatrix} 1 & 1 & 1 & 0 \\ 1 & -1 & 1 & 0 \\ 1 & 1 & 0 & 1 \\ 1 & -1 & 0 & 1 \\ 1 & 1 & -1 & -1 \\ 1 & -1 & -1 & -1 \end{bmatrix},$$

whose columns correspond to the intercept, a main-effect contrast for W_1 and two main-effect contrasts for W_2. We may also add contrasts for the W_1W_2 interaction by including the products of the second column with the third and fourth. If the interaction were included, the resulting model would have the same number of parameters and give the same fit as the unrestricted version (9.18).

9.3.2 Likelihood inference for restricted models

The two sets of restrictions that we have imposed, the loglinear restrictions on π and the linear restrictions on μ, do not interfere with each other; the joint parameter space for $\theta = (\pi, \mu, \Sigma)$ is still the product of the individual spaces for π and (μ, Σ). Therefore, the problem of maximizing the joint likelihood for θ still separates into two unrelated maximizations. The ML estimate for π may be found by conventional IPF (Section 8.3). For μ and Σ, the estimates come from the least-squares fit of the reduced regression model $Z = UA\beta + \epsilon$, which gives

$$
\begin{aligned}
\hat{\beta} &= (A^T U^T U A)^{-1} A^T U^T Z \\
&= (A^T T_3 A)^{-1} A^T T_2,
\end{aligned}
\tag{9.20}
$$

$$
\begin{aligned}
n\hat{\Sigma} &= (Z - UA\hat{\beta})^T (Z - UA\hat{\beta}) \\
&= T_1 - T_2^T A (A^T T_3 A)^{-1} A^T T_2.
\end{aligned}
\tag{9.21}
$$

The corresponding ML estimate of μ is $\hat{\mu} = A\hat{\beta}$. For the covariance matrix, most statisticians would tend to use the unbiased estimate $n(n-r)^{-1}\hat{\Sigma}$ rather than $\hat{\Sigma}$. Notice that AT_3A is not diagonal, so in general the estimation of μ and Σ now requires the inversion of an $r \times r$ matrix.

Example: Foreign Language Attitude Scale

Returning to the example of Section 9.2.3, let us fit a reduced model to this four-variable dataset in which (a) SEX and LAN are marginally independent, and (b) the linear model for HGPA and FLAS has only main effects for SEX and LAN. Let x_{ij} denote a count in the LAN $\times$ SEX contingency table (Table 9.1) and π_{ij} the corresponding cell probability. The ML estimates of the cell probabilities for the independence model are available in closed form as $\hat{\pi}_{ij} = x_{i+}x_{+j}/n^2$, which gives

$$
\hat{\pi} = (0.130, 0.152, 0.224, 0.039, 0.108, 0.126, 0.187, 0.033).
$$

Using the dummy-coded design matrix

$$A = \begin{bmatrix} 1 & 1 & 0 & 0 & 1 \\ 1 & 0 & 1 & 0 & 1 \\ 1 & 0 & 0 & 1 & 1 \\ 1 & 0 & 0 & 0 & 1 \\ 1 & 1 & 0 & 0 & 0 \\ 1 & 0 & 1 & 0 & 0 \\ 1 & 0 & 0 & 1 & 0 \\ 1 & 0 & 0 & 0 & 0 \end{bmatrix},$$

the least-squares regression of Z on UA yields

$$\hat{\beta} = \begin{bmatrix} 2.825 & 83.435 \\ -0.125 & 5.403 \\ -0.154 & 0.390 \\ 0.036 & 4.024 \\ -0.032 & -7.522 \end{bmatrix}, \quad \hat{\Sigma} = \begin{bmatrix} 0.372 & 0.385 \\ 0.385 & 177.3 \end{bmatrix}.$$

The corresponding ML estimate of the cell-means matrix is

$$\hat{\mu} = A\hat{\beta} = \begin{bmatrix} 2.67 & 81.3 \\ 2.64 & 76.3 \\ 2.83 & 79.9 \\ 2.79 & 75.9 \\ 2.70 & 88.8 \\ 2.67 & 83.8 \\ 2.86 & 87.5 \\ 2.82 & 83.4 \end{bmatrix}$$

We can check the plausibility of this restricted model against the unrestricted alternative by means of a likelihood-ratio test. Plugging $\hat{\pi}$, $\hat{\mu}$ and $\hat{\Sigma}$ into the formula for the complete-data log-likelihood,

$$l(\pi, \mu, \Sigma \mid Y) = \sum_{d=1}^{D} x_d \log \pi_d - \tfrac{n}{2} \log |\Sigma| - \tfrac{1}{2} \operatorname{tr} \Sigma^{-1} T_1$$
$$+ \operatorname{tr} \Sigma^{-1} \mu^T T_2 - \tfrac{1}{2} \operatorname{tr} \Sigma^{-1} \mu^T T_3 \mu, \qquad (9.22)$$

yields a value of -1394.83. The parameter estimates from the unrestricted model (Section 9.2.3) give a slightly higher loglikelihood of -1391.86. The two models are separated by $(4-1) \times (2-1) = 3$ parameters for the marginal association between SEX and LAN, plus $3 \times 2 = 6$ coefficients for the LAN×SEX interaction in the linear model for HGPA and FLAS. The deviance statistic is $2 \times (-1391.86 + 1394.83) = 5.94$, and the corresponding p-value is $P(\chi_9^2 \geq 5.94) = 0.75$. The reduced model thus appears to fit the data quite adequately. Because the complete-data likelihood factors into distinct pieces for π and (μ, Σ), we can also separate this goodness-of-fit test into two tests, one for the marginal model for LAN and SEX (3 degrees of freedom), another for the conditional model for HGPA and FLAS (6 degrees of freedom), and the two deviance statistics will add up to the overall deviance.

9.3.3 Bayesian inference

Bayesian inference for the restricted model proceeds most easily if we apply independent prior distributions to the parameter sets π and (μ, Σ), so that they remain independent in the complete-data posterior distribution. In keeping with the methods developed in the last chapter, let us apply a constrained Dirichlet prior to the elements of π, with prior density

$$P(\pi) \propto \prod_{d=1}^{D} \pi_d^{\alpha_d - 1}$$

for values of π that satisfy the loglinear constraints and $P(\pi) = 0$ elsewhere. The complete-data posterior density will then be constrained Dirichlet with updated hyperparameters $\alpha_d' = \alpha_d + x_d$. Posterior modes can be calculated using conventional IPF (Section 8.3), and simulated posterior draws of π can be obtained with Bayesian IPF (Section 8.4).

Bayesian inference for β and Σ under a noninformative prior

Bayesian inference for the standard multivariate regression model is covered in many texts on multivariate analysis; a good source is Press (1982). The likelihood function for Σ and the free coefficients β is

$$L(\beta, \Sigma \mid Y) \propto |\Sigma|^{-\frac{n}{2}} \exp\left\{ -\tfrac{1}{2} \operatorname{tr} \Sigma^{-1} (Z - UA\beta)^T (Z - UA\beta) \right\}.$$

Following some algebraic manipulation, this likelihood function can be rewritten in terms of the least-squares estimates as

$$|\Sigma|^{-\frac{n}{2}} \exp\left\{ -\tfrac{1}{2} \operatorname{tr} \Sigma^{-1} \hat{\epsilon}^T \hat{\epsilon} - \tfrac{1}{2} (\beta - \hat{\beta})^T [\Sigma \otimes V]^{-1} (\beta - \hat{\beta}) \right\}, \quad (9.23)$$

where $\hat{\beta}$ is the matrix of estimated coefficients, $\hat{\epsilon} = Z - UA\hat{\beta}$ is the matrix of estimated residuals and $V = (A^T U^T UA)^{-1}$. The symbol

$\otimes$ denotes the Kronecker product,

$$\Sigma \otimes V = \begin{bmatrix} \sigma_{11}V & \sigma_{12}V & \cdots & \sigma_{1q}V \\ \sigma_{12}V & \sigma_{22}V & \cdots & \sigma_{2q}V \\ \vdots & \vdots & \ddots & \vdots \\ \sigma_{q1}V & \sigma_{q2}V & \cdots & \sigma_{qq}V \end{bmatrix}.$$

In (9.23), the columns of β and $\hat{\beta}$ have been implicitly stacked to form vectors of length rq, so that $(\beta - \hat{\beta})^T [\Sigma \otimes V]^{-1} (\beta - \hat{\beta})$ is meaningful. For some elementary properties of Kronecker products, see Mardia, Kent and Bibby (1979).

Let us first consider what happens when we apply an improper uniform prior to β and the standard Jeffreys prior to Σ,

$$P(\beta, \Sigma) \propto |\Sigma|^{-\left(\frac{q+1}{2}\right)}. \tag{9.24}$$

When $A = I$, we have $\beta = \mu$, and this reduces to the noninformative prior (9.12) that we used in the unrestricted model. Combining (9.24) with the likelihood function (9.23), and using the fact that

$$|\Sigma \otimes V| = |\Sigma|^r \, |V|^q,$$

we obtain the posterior density

$$P(\beta, \Sigma | Y) \quad \propto \quad |\Sigma|^{-\left(\frac{n-r+q+1}{2}\right)} \exp\left\{ -\tfrac{1}{2} \operatorname{tr} \Sigma^{-1} \hat{\epsilon}^T \hat{\epsilon} \right\} \tag{9.25}$$

$$\times \; |\Sigma \otimes V|^{-\frac{1}{2}} \exp\left\{ -\tfrac{1}{2} (\beta - \hat{\beta})^T [\Sigma \otimes V]^{-1} (\beta - \hat{\beta}) \right\}.$$

By inspection, this is the product of a multivariate normal density for β given Σ and an inverted-Wishart density for Σ,

$$\beta \,|\, \Sigma, Y \quad \sim \quad N(\hat{\beta}, \, \Sigma \otimes V), \tag{9.26}$$

$$\Sigma \,|\, Y \quad \sim \quad W^{-1}(n-r, \, (\hat{\epsilon}^T \hat{\epsilon})^{-1}). \tag{9.27}$$

Given Σ, the posterior distribution of each column of β is multivariate normal, centered at the corresponding column of $\hat{\beta}$ and with covariance matrix proportional to V. Marginally, the columns of β have multivariate t-distributions with $n - r$ degrees of freedom. Notice that for (9.25) to be a proper posterior density, we need $n \geq q + r$, and $\hat{\epsilon}^T \hat{\epsilon}$ must have full rank.

Informative priors for β and Σ

One may extend the above arguments to incorporate more substantial prior information about β and Σ. To obtain a convenient posterior distribution for (β, Σ) within the normal inverted-Wishart family, however, the prior distribution must have a particular form: Σ must be inverted-Wishart, and β given Σ must be multivariate normal with a patterned covariance matrix similar to that of (9.26). The limitations of this family of priors are discussed by Press (1982). In most practical applications of the general location model, it will be difficult to quantify prior knowledge about β and Σ; all our examples will use the noninformative prior (9.24). If the posterior distribution under this prior is not proper, then we may interpret it as a sign that the model is too complex to be supported by the data, and the model should be simplified by choosing a design matrix A with fewer columns.

9.4 Algorithms for incomplete mixed data

Thus far we have reviewed the basic methods of likelihood and Bayesian inference for the parameters of the unrestricted (Section 9.2) and restricted (Section 9.3) general location models. Now we extend these methods to handle mixed datasets with arbitrary patterns of missing values. These algorithms are built from portions of the code for normal and categorical data given in Chapters 5–8. The reader who is less interested in computational details than in applications may wish to lightly skim this section to see what algorithms are available, and then proceed directly to the data examples in Section 9.5.

9.4.1 Predictive distributions

A row of the data matrix may have missing values for any or all of the variables $W_1, \ldots, W_p, Z_1, \ldots, Z_q$. Before we can derive estimation and simulation algorithms for the general location model, we must be able to characterize the joint distribution of any subset of these variables given the rest, so that we can obtain the predictive distribution of the missing data in any row of the data matrix given the observed data.

Categorical variables completely missing

Let us first consider the conditional distribution of the categorical variables given the continuous ones, which is needed when $Z_1, \ldots, Z_q$ are observed but $W_1, \ldots, W_p$ are missing. We can represent the complete data for row i by (u_i, z_i), where z_i^T is the realized value of $(Z_1, \ldots, Z_q)$, and u_i is a vector of length D containing a single 1 in the cell position corresponding to the realized values of $W_1, \ldots, W_p$ and 0s elsewhere. Let E_d be the D-vector with 1 in position d and 0s elsewhere. By definition, the joint density of (u_i, z_i) under the general location model is

$$P(u_i = E_d, z_i \mid \theta) \propto \pi_d \, |\Sigma|^{-\frac{1}{2}} \exp\left\{-\tfrac{1}{2}(z_i - \mu_d)^T \Sigma^{-1}(z_i - \mu_d)\right\}.$$

The conditional distribution of u_i given z_i is thus

$$P(u_i = E_d \mid z_i, \theta) = \frac{\pi_d \, \exp\left\{-\tfrac{1}{2}(z_i - \mu_d)^T \Sigma^{-1}(z_i - \mu_d)\right\}}{\displaystyle\sum_{d'=1}^{D} \pi_{d'} \, \exp\left\{-\tfrac{1}{2}(z_i - \mu_{d'})^T \Sigma^{-1}(z_i - \mu_{d'})\right\}}.$$

The portions of the numerator and denominator involving the quadratic term $z_i^T \Sigma^{-1} z_i$ cancel out, leading to a well-known result from classical multivariate analysis: the conditional probability that unit i belongs to cell d is

$$P(u_i = E_d \mid z_i, \theta) \propto \exp(\delta_{d,i}),$$

where $\delta_{d,i}$ denotes the value of the *linear discriminant function* of z_i with respect to μ_d,

$$\delta_{d,i} = \mu_d^T \Sigma^{-1} z_i - \tfrac{1}{2} \mu_d^T \Sigma^{-1} \mu_d + \log \pi_d. \tag{9.28}$$

When $Z_1, \ldots, Z_q$ are observed but $W_1, \ldots, W_p$ are missing, the predictive distribution of $W_1, \ldots, W_p$ is obtained by calculating the terms $\pi_d \exp(\delta_{d,i})$ for cells $d = 1, 2, \ldots, D$ and normalizing them to sum to one.

Continuous variables partially missing

Now consider what happens if $W_1, \ldots, W_p$ and an arbitrary subset of $Z_1, \ldots, Z_q$ are missing. Denote the observed components of z_i by $z_{i(obs)}$ and the missing components by $z_{i(mis)}$. The conditional distribution of u_i given $z_{i(obs)}$ and θ is obtained by integrating both the numerator and denominator of

$$P(u_i = E_d \mid z_i, \theta) = \frac{P(u_i = E_d, z_i \mid \theta)}{P(z_i \mid \theta)}$$

over all possible values of $z_{i(mis)}$. The result is

$$P(u_i = E_d \mid z_{i(obs)}, \theta) \propto \exp(\delta_{d,i}^*), \tag{9.29}$$

where $\delta_{d,i}^*$ is a linear discriminant based on the reduced information in $z_{i(obs)}$ rather than z_i. This new discriminant is

$$\delta_{d,i}^* = \mu_{d,i}^{*\,T}\Sigma_i^{*-1}z_{i(obs)} - \tfrac{1}{2}\mu_{d,i}^{*\,T}\Sigma_i^{*-1}\mu_{d,i}^* + \log\pi_d, \qquad (9.30)$$

where $\mu_{d,i}^*$ and Σ_i^* denote the subvector and square submatrix of μ_d and Σ, respectively, corresponding to the observed elements of z_i. (When all continuous variables are missing, define $\delta_{d,i}^* = \log\pi_d$ so that (9.29) reduces to π_d.) Moreover, because

$$z_i \mid u_i = E_d, \theta \sim N(\mu_d, \Sigma),$$

the conditional distribution of the missing elements of z_i given $u_i = E_d$ and the observed elements of z_i is also multivariate normal; the parameters of this distribution can be obtained by applying the sweep operator to μ_d and Σ (Section 5.2). This conditional normal distribution, along with the probabilities (9.29), characterize the joint predictive distribution of $W_1, \ldots, W_p$ and the missing elements of $Z_1, \ldots, Z_q$.

Continuous and categorical variables partially missing

Finally, let us now consider the general case in which arbitrary subsets of $W_1, \ldots, W_p$ and $Z_1, \ldots, Z_q$ are missing. This differs from the case we have just examined in that the predictive distribution must now take into account any additional information in the observed members of $W_1, \ldots, W_p$. When some of these categorical variables are observed, the unit is known to lie within a particular subset of the cells of the contingency table; the cell probabilities are still of the form (9.29), but must be normalized to sum to one over this reduced set.

More specifically, let $w_{i(obs)}$ and $w_{i(mis)}$ denote the observed and missing parts, respectively, of the categorical data for unit i. Rather than indexing the cells of the contingency table by their linear positions $d = 1, 2, \ldots, D$, let us now identify them by their corresponding response patterns $w = (w_1, w_2, \ldots, w_p)$, $w_j = 1, 2, \ldots, d_j$. Let $\mathcal{O}_i(w)$ and $\mathcal{M}_i(w)$ denote the subvectors of w corresponding to the observed and missing parts, respectively, of the categorical data for unit i. The predictive probability of falling into cell w given the observed data is now

$$P(u_i = E_w \mid w_{i(obs)}, z_{i(obs)}, \theta) = \frac{\exp(\delta_{w,i}^*)}{\displaystyle\sum_{\mathcal{M}_i(w)} \exp(\delta_{w,i}^*)} \qquad (9.31)$$

over the cells w for which $\mathcal{O}_i(w)$ agrees with $w_{i(obs)}$, and zero for all other cells. Once again, the conditional predictive distribution of $z_{i(mis)}$ given $u_i = E_w$ is a multivariate normal whose parameters can be obtained by sweeping μ_w and Σ on the positions corresponding to $z_{i(obs)}$.

Predictive distributions and sweep

As shown by Little and Schluchter (1985), the discriminants $\delta^*_{w,i}$ and the parameters of the conditional normal distribution of $z_{i(mis)}$ can be neatly obtained by a single application of the sweep operator. Suppose we arrange the parameters of the general location model into a matrix,

$$\theta = \begin{bmatrix} \Sigma & \mu^T \\ \mu & P \end{bmatrix}, \tag{9.32}$$

where P is a $D \times D$ matrix with elements

$$p_w = 2 \log \pi_w$$

on the diagonal and zeroes elsewhere. If we sweep this θ-matrix on the positions in Σ corresponding to $z_{i(obs)}$, we obtain a transformed version of the parameter,

$$\theta^* = \begin{bmatrix} \Sigma^* & \mu^{*T} \\ \mu^* & P^* \end{bmatrix}. \tag{9.33}$$

The diagonal element of P^* corresponding to cell w is

$$p_w^* = -\mu^{*T}_{w,i} \Sigma^{*-1}_i \mu^*_{w,i} + 2 \log \pi_w,$$

which is twice the sum of the final two terms in the linear discriminant function (9.30). The coefficients of $z_{i(obs)}$ in this discriminant, $\mu^{*T}_{w,i} \Sigma^{*-1}_i$, are found in row w of μ^*, in the columns corresponding to the variables in $z_{i(obs)}$. The remaining elements of μ^* and Σ^* contain the parameters of the multivariate regression of $z_{i(mis)}$ on $z_{i(obs)}$ for all cells w. The intercepts, which vary from cell to cell, are found in μ^*; the slopes and residual covariances, which are assumed to be equal for all cells, are found in Σ^*.

Although we have depicted θ as a $(q + D) \times (q + D)$ matrix, in practice we do not actually need $(q+D)^2$ memory locations to store it. The off-diagonal elements of P^* are not really of interest, nor are they needed to reverse-sweep θ^* back to its original form. Thus we can minimize computation and memory requirements by retaining only μ, the diagonal elements of P and the upper-triangular portion of Σ in packed storage.

9.4.2 EM for the unrestricted model

We are now ready to describe an EM algorithm for obtaining ML estimates for the unrestricted general location model (Little and Schluchter, 1985). In Section 9.2.2, we saw that the complete-data loglikelihood is a linear function of the sufficient statistics

$$T_1 = Z^T Z, \quad T_2 = U^T Z, \quad \text{and} \quad T_3 = U^T U = \text{diag}(x).$$

The ML estimates for the unrestricted model were shown to be

$$\hat{\pi} = n^{-1} x, \tag{9.34}$$

$$\hat{\mu} = T_3^{-1} T_2, \tag{9.35}$$

$$\hat{\Sigma} = n^{-1} \left(T_1 - T_2^T T_3^{-1} T_2 \right). \tag{9.36}$$

The M-step is a simple matter of calculating (9.34)–(9.36) using the expected versions of T_1, T_2 and T_3, rather than the sufficient statistics themselves. The complicated part is the E-step, where we must find the conditional expectations of T_1, T_2 and T_3 given the observed parts of the data matrix and an assumed value of θ.

The E-step

First, consider the expectation of the diagonal elements of T_3. Notice that the complete-data contingency table can be written as $x = \sum_{i=1}^{n} u_i$. The elements of u_i are Bernoulli indicators of $u_i = E_w$ for all cells w, so their expectations are just the predictive probabilities given by (9.31). Thus, the expectation of u_i can be found by the following steps. (a) Sweep the θ-matrix on positions corresponding to $z_{i(obs)}$ to obtain θ^*. (b) From $z_{i(obs)}$ and θ^*, calculate the discriminants for all cells w for which $\mathcal{O}_i(w)$ agrees with $w_{i(obs)}$. The discriminant for cell w is

$$\delta^*_{w,i} = \tfrac{1}{2} p^*_w + \sum_{j \in \mathcal{O}_i} \mu^*_{w,j} z_{ij},$$

where $\mu^*_{w,j}$ is the (w,j)th element of μ^*, and $\mathcal{O}_i$ is the subset of $\{1, 2, \ldots, q\}$ corresponding to the variables in $z_{i(obs)}$. (We have already been using $\mathcal{O}_i$ and $\mathcal{M}_i$ as operators that extract the observed and missing components of $w = (w_1, \ldots, w_p)$, and for convenience we will continue to do so; the dual usage should not create any confusion.) (c) Normalize the terms $\exp(\delta^*_{w,i})$ for these cells to obtain the predictive probabilities

$$\pi_{w,i}^* = \frac{\exp(\delta_{w,i}^*)}{\sum_{\mathcal{M}_i(w)} \exp(\delta_{w,i}^*)}. \tag{9.37}$$

These predictive probabilities also play an important role in the expectation of T_2. Row w of T_2 is $\sum_{i=1}^{n} u_{w,i} z_i^T$, where $u_{w,i} = 1$ if unit i falls into cell w and $u_{w,i} = 0$ otherwise. If the observed data in $w_{i(obs)}$ indicate that unit i cannot possibly belong to cell w, then

$$E(u_{w,i} z_i \mid Y_{obs}, \theta) = 0.$$

On the other hand, if $w_{i(obs)}$ agrees with $\mathcal{O}_i(w)$, then

$$E(u_{w,i} z_i \mid Y_{obs}, \theta) = \pi_{w,i}^* z_{w,i}^*, \tag{9.38}$$

where $z_{w,i}^*$ is the predicted mean of z_i given the observed values in $z_{i(obs)}$, and given that unit i falls into cell w. The parts of $z_{w,i}^*$ corresponding to $z_{i(obs)}$ are identical to $z_{i(obs)}$, whereas the parts corresponding to $z_{i(mis)}$ are the predicted values from the multivariate regression of $z_{i(mis)}$ on $z_{i(obs)}$ within cell w,

$$z_{w,ij}^* = \begin{cases} z_{ij} & \text{if } j \in \mathcal{O}_i, \\ \mu_{w,j}^* + \sum_{k \in \mathcal{O}_i} \sigma_{jk}^* z_{ik} & \text{if } j \in \mathcal{M}_i, \end{cases}$$

where σ_{jk}^* is the (j,k)th element of Σ^*.

Finally, consider the expectation of the sums of squares and cross-products matrix,

$$T_1 = Z^T Z = \sum_{i=1}^{n} z_i z_i^T.$$

The (j,k)th element of this matrix is $\sum_{i=1}^{n} z_{ij} z_{ik}$. But notice that a single element of this sum can be written as

$$z_{ij} z_{ik} = \sum_{w} u_{w,i} z_{ij} z_{ik},$$

so the expectation of this element is

$$E(z_{ij} z_{ik} \mid Y_{obs}, \theta) = \sum_{\mathcal{M}_i(w)} \pi_{w,i}^* E(z_{ij} z_{ik} \mid Y_{obs}, \theta, u_{w,i} = 1),$$

$$\tag{9.39}$$

where the sum is taken over all cells w for which $\mathcal{O}_i(w)$ agrees with $w_{i(obs)}$. The form of $E(z_{ij} z_{ik} \mid Y_{obs}, \theta, u_{w,i} = 1)$ depends on whether z_{ij} and z_{ik} are observed. If both are observed, this expectation is simply $z_{ij} z_{ik}$. If z_{ij} is observed but z_{ik} is missing, the expectation is $z_{ij} z_{w,ik}^*$. Finally, if both are missing, the expectation becomes $z_{w,ij}^* z_{w,ik}^* + \sigma_{jk}^*$.

Organizing the computations

To carry out the E-step, we must cycle through the units $i = 1, 2, \ldots, n$ in the dataset, sweeping θ on the positions corresponding to $z_{i(obs)}$ and summing the contributions (9.37), (9.38) and (9.39) of unit i to the expectations of the sufficient statistics. The number of forward and reverse-sweeps can be reduced by grouping together rows of the data matrix having the same pattern of missingness for $Z_1, \ldots, Z_q$, because the same version of θ^* can then be used for all units in the pattern. The expected sufficient statistics can be accumulated into a workspace of the same size and shape as θ,

$$
T = \begin{bmatrix} T_1 & T_2^T \\ T_2 & T_3 \end{bmatrix}.
$$

Once the E-step is complete, the M-step proceeds by applying (9.34)–(9.36) to T, which gives the updated estimate of θ.

Evaluating the observed-data loglikelihood

One can show that the contribution of observation i to the observed-data loglikelihood is

$$
- \tfrac{1}{2} \log |\Sigma_i^*| + \log \left\{ \sum_w \exp \left(\delta_{w,i}^* - \tfrac{1}{2} z_{i(obs)}^T \Sigma_i^{*-1} z_{i(obs)} \right) \right\},
$$

where the sum is taken over all cells w for which $\mathcal{O}_i(w)$ agrees with $w_{i(obs)}$. The procedure for evaluating the observed-data loglikelihood at any particular value of θ is very similar to the E-step. In addition to the linear discriminant $\delta_{w,i}^*$, we need to evaluate the quadratic term

$$
z_{i(obs)}^T \Sigma_i^{*-1} z_{i(obs)}
$$

and the determinant of Σ_i^{*-1}. The latter can be obtained along with θ^* as an immediate byproduct of sweep (Section 5.2.4). To calculate the former, note that $-\Sigma_i^{*-1}$ is contained in the rows and columns of Σ^* corresponding to the variables in $z_{i(obs)}$.

9.4.3 Data augmentation

With fairly minor modifications, the EM algorithm described above can be converted to data augmentation, enabling us to simulate posterior draws of θ or multiple imputations of Y_{mis}. For the I-step, we must create a random draw of (T_1, T_2, T_3) from its predictive distribution given the observed data and an assumed value for θ. Just as in the E-step, we cycle through the units $i = 1, 2, \ldots, n$, sweeping θ to obtain the parameters of the predictive distribution of the missing variables given the observed variables; we then draw the missing data for unit i from their predictive distribution, and accumulate the resulting complete-data sufficient statistics into T_1, T_2 and T_3. Once the I-step is complete, the P-step proceeds by drawing a new value of θ from its posterior given T_1, T_2 and T_3. Details of these steps are given below.

The I-step

It is convenient to draw the missing data for unit i in two stages: first by drawing u_i, which indicates the cell to which unit i belongs, and then by drawing $z_{i(mis)}$ given u_i. The predictive distribution of u_i is that of a single multinomial trial over the cells w for which $\mathcal{O}_i(w)$ agrees with $w_{i(obs)}$; the cell probabilities are given by (9.37). A simple way to simulate this multinomial trial is by table sampling: cycle through the cells, summing up their probabilities, and assign the unit to the first cell for which the cumulative probability exceeds the value of a $U(0, 1)$ random variate. Pseudocode for a similar table-sampling algorithm appears in Figure 7.4. When a unit is assigned to cell w, its contribution to T_3 is reflected by adding 1 to the wth diagonal element.

After assigning unit i to cell w, we may then draw the missing continuous variables in $z_{i(mis)}$ according to their multivariate regression on $z_{i(obs)}$. The regression prediction for an element of $z_{i(mis)}$ is

$$z^*_{w,ij} = \mu^*_{w,j} + \sum_{k \in \mathcal{O}_i} \sigma^*_{jk} z_{ik}.$$

To these predictions, we must add simulated residuals drawn from a multivariate normal distribution. The residual covariances are found in Σ^*, in the rows and columns corresponding to $z_{i(mis)}$. To draw the residuals, we will need to extract the appropriate submatrix from Σ^* and calculate its Cholesky factor (Section 5.4.1). Adding the simulated residuals to the $z^*_{w,ij}$ produces a simulated draw of $z_{i(mis)}$. The contribution of the completed version of z_i to the sufficient statistics is then reflected by adding z_i into the wth row of T_2, and adding $z_i z_i^T$ into the matrix T_1.

The P-step

In Section 9.2.4, we showed that under the improper prior distribution

$$P(\pi, \mu, \Sigma) \propto \left(\prod_w \pi_w^{\alpha_w - 1} \right) |\Sigma|^{-\left(\frac{q+1}{2} \right)},$$

the complete-data posterior is

$$\pi \mid Y \ \sim \ D(\alpha + x), \tag{9.40}$$

$$\Sigma \mid \pi, Y \ \sim \ W^{-1}(n - D, (\hat{\epsilon}^T \hat{\epsilon})^{-1}), \tag{9.41}$$

$$\mu_w \mid \pi, \Sigma, Y \ \sim \ N(\hat{\mu}_w, x_w^{-1}\Sigma), \tag{9.42}$$

where $\alpha = \{\alpha_w\}$ is an array of user-specified hyperparameters. The P-step is simply a matter of drawing from these distributions in turn, given the simulated values of T_1, T_2 and T_3 from the I-step. This can be done as follows.

1. For each cell w, draw the probability π_w from a standard gamma distribution with shape parameter $x_w + \alpha_w$, where x_w is the wth diagonal element of T_3, and normalize the π_w to sum to one.

2. Draw an upper-triangular matrix B whose elements are independently distributed as

$$b_{jj} \ \sim \ \sqrt{\chi^2_{n - D - j + 1}}, \ \ j = 1, \dots, q,$$

$$b_{jk} \ \sim \ N(0, 1), \ \ j < k,$$

and take $\Sigma = M^T M$, where $M = (B^T)^{-1} C$ and C is the upper-triangular Cholesky factor of

$$\hat{\epsilon}^T \hat{\epsilon} = T_1 - T_2^T T_3^{-1} T_2.$$

3. Calculate $\hat{\mu} = T_3^{-1} T_2$ and take $\mu = \hat{\mu} + T_3^{-1/2} HM$, where H is a $D \times q$ matrix of independent $N(0, 1)$ random variates, and $T_3^{-1/2}$ is the matrix with elements $x_w^{-1/2}$ on the diagonal and zeroes elsewhere.

9.4.4 Algorithms for restricted models

An ECM algorithm

Little and Schluchter (1985) discussed an EM algorithm for ML estimation under restricted versions of the general location model. The E-step is identical to that described above for the unrestricted model, because the expectations of T_1, T_2 and T_3 have the same form regardless of where $\theta = (\pi, \mu, \Sigma)$ lies in the parameter space. The only difference is found in the M-step, which is now a constrained maximization subject to loglinear restrictions on π and linear restrictions on μ. As discussed in Section 9.3, the constrained maxima for π and μ may be found by conventional IPF and least squares, respectively.

In the same article, Little and Schluchter also conjectured that the full maximization of the likelihood for π in each M-step, which may require many IPF cycles, could be replaced by a single IPF cycle, thus avoiding undesirable nested iterations. The resulting algorithm would no longer be EM, but it would have the same essential property that the observed-data loglikelihood would be non-decreasing. Their conjecture turned out to be correct. This algorithm is a special case of ECM, exhibiting the same reliable convergence properties as EM; see Sections 3.2.5 and 8.5.1 for further details and references. A single cycle of ECM for the restricted general location model proceeds as follows.

1. *E-step:* Given the current estimate $\theta^{(t)} = (\pi^{(t)}, \mu^{(t)}, \Sigma^{(t)})$, calculate the expectations of T_1, T_2 and T_3 as described in Section 9.4.2.

2. *CM-step:* Using the expected value of x (the diagonal elements of T_3), perform a single cycle of conventional IPF from the starting value $\pi^{(t)}$ to obtain $\pi^{(t+1)}$. Then calculate $\beta^{(t+1)}$ and $\Sigma^{(t+1)}$ as in (9.20)–(9.21) using the expected values of T_1, T_2 and T_3, and take $\mu^{(t+1)} = A\beta^{(t+1)}$.

Data augmentation-Bayesian IPF

In a similar fashion, the data augmentation algorithm for the unrestricted model can be adapted to restricted models. The I-step remains the same; only the P-step must be changed to accommodate the restrictions on the parameter space.

Under the family of prior distributions discussed in Section 9.3.3, the complete-data posterior distribution for π is constrained Dirichlet, and the complete-data posterior for (β, Σ) is

$$\Sigma \mid Y \quad \sim \quad W^{-1}(n-r, (\hat{\epsilon}^T \hat{\epsilon})^{-1}), \qquad (9.43)$$

$$\beta \mid \Sigma, Y \quad \sim \quad N(\hat{\beta}, \Sigma \otimes V), \qquad (9.44)$$

where $V = (A^T U^T U A)^{-1}$. Random draws from the constrained Dirichlet can be simulated by Bayesian IPF (Section 8.4), and drawing from (9.43) is straightforward. In many applications the dimension of β can be quite large, but simulating draws from (9.44) is not difficult if we exploit the patterned covariance structure. Let G and H denote the upper-triangular Cholesky factors of Σ and V, respectively, so that $\Sigma = G^T G$ and $V = H^T H$. Using elementary properties of Kronecker products,

$$\begin{aligned}
\Sigma \otimes V &= (G^T G) \otimes (H^T H) \\
&= (G^T \otimes H^T)(G \otimes H) \\
&= (G \otimes H)^T (G \otimes H),
\end{aligned}$$

and thus $G \otimes H$ is an upper-triangular square root for $\Sigma \otimes V$. Therefore, to simulate a multivariate normal random vector with covariance matrix $\Sigma \otimes V$, we may simply premultiply a vector of standard normal variates by $(G \otimes H)^T$.

A data augmentation-Bayesian IPF (DABIPF) algorithm for the restricted general location model proceeds as follows.

1. *I-step:* Given the current values of the parameters $\pi^{(t)}$, $\mu^{(t)} = A\beta^{(t)}$ and $\Sigma^{(t)}$, draw the missing data from their predictive distribution as described in Section 9.4.3, and accumulate the simulated values of the sufficient statistics T_1, T_2 and T_3.

2. *Bayesian IPF:* Using the simulated value of x (the diagonal elements of T_3), perform a single cycle of Bayesian IPF from the starting value $\pi^{(t)}$ to obtain $\pi^{(t+1)}$.

3. *P-step for Σ:* Draw an upper-triangular matrix B whose elements are independently distributed as

$$b_{jj} \quad \sim \quad \sqrt{\chi^2_{n-r-j+1}}, \quad j = 1, \ldots, q,$$

$$b_{jk} \quad \sim \quad N(0,1), \quad j < k,$$

and take $\Sigma^{(t+1)} = M^T M$, where $M = (B^T)^{-1} C$ and C is the upper-triangular Cholesky factor of

$$\hat{\epsilon}^T \hat{\epsilon} = T_1 - T_2^T A (A^T T_3 A)^{-1} A^T T_2.$$

4. *P-step for β:* Draw $\beta^{(t+1)}$ from a multivariate normal distribution with mean $\hat{\beta} = (A^T T_3 A)^{-1} A^T T_2$ and covariance ma-

trix $\Sigma^{(t+1)} \otimes V$, where $V = (A^T T_3 A)^{-1}$. This can be done in the following manner. Let β_j and $\hat{\beta}_j$ denote the jth columns of $\beta^{(t+1)}$ and $\hat{\beta}$, respectively. Calculate $G = \text{Chol}(\Sigma^{(t+1)})$ and $H = \text{Chol}(V)$, and take

$$\beta_1 = \hat{\beta}_1 + g_{11} H^T \kappa_1,$$

$$\beta_2 = \hat{\beta}_2 + g_{21} H^T \kappa_1 + g_{22} H^T \kappa_2,$$

$$\vdots$$

$$\beta_q = \hat{\beta}_q + g_{q1} H^T \kappa_1 + g_{q2} H^T \kappa_2 + \cdots + g_{qq} H^T \kappa_q,$$

where g_{ij} is the (i,j)th element of G, and where $\kappa_1, \kappa_2, \ldots, \kappa_q$ are vectors of independent $N(0,1)$ random variates of length r.

This DABIPF algorithm is not true data augmentation, but a hybrid that substitutes a single cycle of Bayesian IPF for the full simulation of π in the P-step.

9.5 Data examples

9.5.1 St. Louis Risk Research Project

Little and Schluchter (1985) presented data from the St. Louis Risk Research Project, an observational study to assess the effects of parental psychological disorders on various aspects of child development. In a preliminary cross-sectional study, data were collected on 69 families having two children each. The families were classified into three risk groups for parental psychological disorders. The children were classified into two groups according to the number of adverse psychiatric symptoms they exhibited. Standardized reading and verbal comprehension scores were also collected for the children. Each family is thus described by three continuous and four categorical variables:

Variable	Levels	Code
Parental risk group	1=low, 2=moderate, 3=high	G
Symptoms, child 1	1=low, 2=high	D_1
Symptoms, child 2	1=low, 2=high	D_2
Reading score, child 1	continuous	R_1
Verbal score, child 1	continuous	V_1
Reading score, child 2	continuous	R_2
Verbal score, child 2	continuous	V_2

Data from this preliminary study are displayed in Table 9.2. Missing values occur on all variables except G. Only twelve families have values recorded for all seven variables.

The unrestricted model

The unrestricted general location model for this dataset has 69 free parameters: 11 for the $3 \times 2 \times 2$ contingency table that cross-classifies families by G, D_1 and D_2, 48 for the within-cell means of R_1, V_1, R_2 and V_2, and 10 for the within-cell covariance matrix. As pointed out by Little and Schluchter (1985), all of the parameters of this model are technically estimable. There are no zero counts in the table for the 29 families that can be fully classified on G, D_1 and D_2. The only family known to belong to the $G = 2$, $D_1 = 2$, $D_2 = 1$ cell has missing values for V_1, R_2 and V_2; there are three other partially classified families that can possibly belong to this cell, however, and two of these families have all their continuous variables recorded. Similarly, the only family known to have $G = 1$, $D_1 = 2$, $D_2 = 2$ has a missing value for R_1, but there are two other partially classified families for whom R_1 is known who may belong to this cell. These partially classified families contribute 'fractional observations' of the continuous variables to certain cells. With respect to the means of these cells, the observed-data likelihood is not flat, but some of the means may be estimated with precision equivalent to sample sizes of less than one.

Using the EM algorithm described in Section 9.4.2, Little and Schluchter (1985) discovered that the observed-data likelihood for this example is multimodal. They found that EM converges to different parameter estimates from different starting values, and the loglikelihood values at these estimates are not identical. The data augmentation algorithm of Section 9.4.3, when used in conjunction with EM, provides an additional tool to help us explore the observed-data likelihood. Starting at a mode, we ran several hundred iterations of data augmentation, and used the final simulated value of the parameter as a new starting value for EM. By repeating this process, we were quickly able to identify ten distinct modes, and would have undoubtedly found more had we continued further. The unusual shape of the observed-data loglikelihood suggests that some of the parameters of the unrestricted model are very poorly estimated. This is not surprising, given that we are trying to estimate 69 parameters from only 69 incomplete observations. Time-series plots of some parameters across the iterations of

Table 9.2. Data from the St. Louis Risk Research Project

Low risk (G = 1)						Moderate risk (G = 2)						High risk (G = 3)					
R_1	V_1	D_1	R_2	V_2	D_2	R_1	V_1	D_1	R_2	V_2	D_2	R_1	V_1	D_1	R_2	V_2	D_2
110	165	1	—	150	1	88	85	2	76	78	—	98	110	—	112	103	2
118	145	2	—	130	2	—	98	—	114	133	2	127	138	1	92	118	1
116	—	—	114	125	—	108	103	2	90	100	2	113	—	—	—	—	—
—	—	—	126	—	—	113	—	2	95	115	2	107	93	—	92	75	2
118	140	1	118	123	—	—	65	—	97	68	2	—	—	1	101	—	2
—	120	—	105	138	—	118	—	2	—	—	—	114	—	—	87	98	2
—	—	—	96	113	—	92	—	2	110	—	—	56	58	2	88	105	1
138	163	1	130	140	—	90	—	1	96	88	2	96	95	1	87	100	2
115	153	1	—	—	—	98	123	—	112	115	—	126	135	2	118	133	—
—	145	2	139	185	2	113	110	—	114	120	—	—	—	—	130	195	—
126	138	1	105	133	1	102	130	2	130	135	—	—	—	—	116	—	2
120	160	—	109	150	—	89	113	2	91	75	2	64	45	2	82	53	2
—	133	—	98	108	—	90	80	—	109	88	2	128	—	2	121	—	2
—	—	—	115	140	2	—	—	—	88	73	1	—	120	1	108	118	—
115	158	2	—	135	1	75	63	1	—	—	—	—	—	—	100	140	2
112	115	2	93	140	—	93	—	1	115	138	2	105	138	1	74	75	1
133	168	1	126	158	2	—	—	—	115	123	2	88	118	—	84	103	—
118	180	1	116	148	—	123	170	1	104	123	2						
123	—	1	110	155	1	114	130	2	113	—	2						
100	—	1	101	120	1	—	—	2	—	103	—						
118	138	1	—	110	1	113	—	—	82	—	—						
103	108	—	—	—	—	117	—	1	114	—	2						
121	155	1	—	100	—	122	—	1	—	—	1						
—	—	—	—	—	2	105	—	2									
—	—	—	104	118	2												
—	—	—	87	85	1												
—	—	—	—	63	—												

Source: Little and Schluchter (1985)

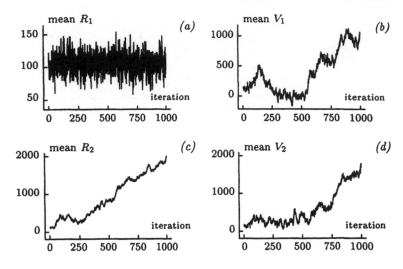

Figure 9.2. *Time-series plots of the conditional means of* R_1, V_1, R_2 *and* V_2 *given* $(G = 2, D_1 = 2, D_2 = 1)$ *for 1000 iterations of data augmentation under the unrestricted general location model.*

data augmentation show erratic behavior. Plots of the simulated means of the four continuous variables within the $G = 2$, $D_1 = 2$, $D_2 = 1$ cell are shown in Figure 9.2. The means for V_1, R_2 and V_2 are highly unstable, wandering well outside the plausible range of reading and verbal scores. The use of the unrestricted model is not recommended for this dataset, as it is clearly overparameterized.

Restricted models

Because the ultimate purpose of the St. Louis Risk study was to examine the relationship of parental psychological disorders on child development, we now examine two restricted models that focus attention on the effects of greatest interest, namely, the associations between parental risk G and the child development variables D_1, R_1, V_1, D_2, R_2 and V_2.

The first model, which will be called the 'null model', allows the six development variables to be interrelated, but assumes that they are collectively independent of G. The loglinear model for the categorical variables is $(G, D_1 D_2)$. The design matrix specifying the regression of the four continuous variables on the categorical ones is shown in Table 9.3 (a); it includes an intercept, main effects for D_1 and D_2 and the $D_1 D_2$ interaction. This model fits 5 free

Table 9.3. *Design matrix for the null model, and the linear contrast for G included in the alternative model*

Cell			(a) Design matrix				(b) G effect
G	D_1	D_2	int.	D_1	D_2	$D_1 D_2$	linear
1	1	1	1	−1	−1	1	−1
2	1	1	1	−1	−1	1	0
3	1	1	1	−1	−1	1	1
1	2	1	1	1	−1	−1	−1
2	2	1	1	1	−1	−1	0
3	2	1	1	1	−1	−1	1
1	1	2	1	−1	1	−1	−1
2	1	2	1	−1	1	−1	0
3	1	2	1	−1	1	−1	1
1	2	2	1	1	1	1	−1
2	2	2	1	1	1	1	0
3	2	2	1	1	1	1	1

parameters to the contingency table, 16 regression coefficients and 10 covariances for a total of 31 free parameters.

The second model, which we call the 'alternative model', adds simple associations between G and each of the six development variables. The loglinear model is now $(GD_1, GD_2, D_1 D_2)$, and the association between G and the continuous variables is specified by adding columns to the design matrix for G. To conserve parameters, we add only a single column for a linear contrast, as shown in Table 9.3 (b). The alternative model has 9 parameters for the contingency table, 20 regression coefficients and 10 covariances for a total of 39 parameters.

ML estimates under these two models were computed using the ECM algorithm of Section 9.4.4. As with the unrestricted model, the observed-data loglikelihood functions are not unimodal; we found two modes under the null model and two modes under the alternative. The likelihood-ratio test statistic based on the two major modes is 21.9 with 8 degrees of freedom. It appears that the alternative model may fit the data substantially better than the null model, but we cannot assign an accurate p-value to this difference due to the unusual shape of the likelihood function.

Adopting a Bayesian approach, however, we can demonstrate rather conclusively that G is indeed related to each of the six development variables. Using the DABIPF algorithm, we simulated

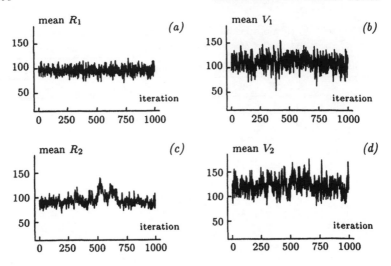

Figure 9.3. *Time-series plots of the conditional means of R_1, V_1, R_2 and V_2 given $(G = 2, D_1 = 2, D_2 = 1)$ for 1000 iterations of DABIPF under the alternative model.*

5000 correlated draws from the observed-data posterior under the alternative model and stored the values of parameters of interest. Time-series plots of the parameters, shown in Figure 9.3, did not exhibit the same instability found in plots for the unrestricted model, so the algorithm appears to be converging reliably. By examining the simulated values of the parameters pertaining to the associations between G and the other variables, we may proceed to make Bayesian inferences about these parameters directly without appealing to large-sample approximations.

Risk and adverse psychological symptoms

Let π_{ijk} denote the marginal probability of the event $G = i$, $D_1 = j$, $D_2 = k$. The association between G and D_1 can be described by two odds ratios, say

$$\omega_1 = \frac{\pi_{11k}\pi_{22k}}{\pi_{21k}\pi_{12k}}, \quad \omega_2 = \frac{\pi_{21k}\pi_{32k}}{\pi_{31k}\pi_{22k}}.$$

These express the increase in odds of adverse symptoms in the first child as we move from low to moderate risk, and from moderate to high risk, respectively. Notice that these odds ratios do not depend on k; they are identical for $k = 1$ and $k = 2$ because the loglinear model omits the three-way association GD_1D_2. Similarly,

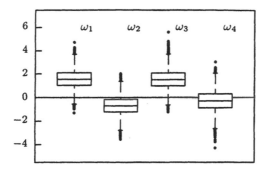

Figure 9.4. *Boxplots of simulated log-odds ratios from 5000 iterations of DABIPF under the alternative model.*

Table 9.4. *Simulated posterior percentiles and p-values for odds ratios*

	percentile					
	2.5	25	50	75	97.5	p
ω_1	1.09	2.79	4.68	8.11	22.97	0.04
ω_2	0.11	0.29	0.49	0.84	2.27	0.37
ω_3	0.97	2.66	4.50	7.90	23.67	0.05
ω_4	0.12	0.41	0.74	1.35	4.31	0.75

the association between G and D_2 can be described by

$$\omega_3 = \frac{\pi_{1j1}\pi_{2j2}}{\pi_{2j1}\pi_{1j2}}, \quad \omega_4 = \frac{\pi_{2j1}\pi_{3j2}}{\pi_{3j1}\pi_{2j2}},$$

which express the increase in odds of adverse symptoms in the second child as we move from low to moderate and from moderate to high risk.

Boxplots of the logarithms of the four odds ratios from 5000 cycles of DABIPF are shown in Figure 9.4. The logs of ω_1 and ω_3 are nearly all positive, providing strong evidence that children in moderate-risk families ($G = 2$) have higher rates of adverse symptoms that children in low-risk families ($G = 1$). The logs of ω_2 and ω_4, however, lie on both sides of zero; there is no evidence that the adverse-symptom rates differ for children in moderate- ($G = 2$) and high-risk ($G = 3$) families. Simulated percentiles of

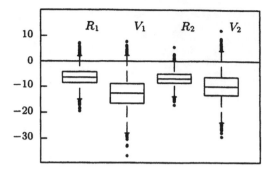

Figure 9.5. *Boxplots of simulated regression coefficients from 5000 iterations of DABIPF under the alternative model.*

Table 9.5. *Simulated posterior percentiles and p-values for regression coefficients*

	percentile					
	2.5	25	50	75	97.5	p
R_1	−12.75	−8.51	−6.38	−4.21	0.10	0.05
V_1	−23.49	−16.50	−12.62	−8.85	−1.29	0.03
R_2	−11.94	−8.64	−6.92	−5.12	−1.55	0.01
V_2	−20.37	−13.42	−10.02	−6.42	0.17	0.05

the posterior distributions of the ω_i are shown in Table 9.4, along with Bayesian p-values for testing each null hypothesis $\omega_i = 1$ against the two-sided alternative $\omega_i \neq 1$. Based on the posterior medians, we estimate that children in moderate-risk families are about 4.5 times as likely (on the odds scale) to display adverse symptoms than children in low-risk families.

Risk and comprehension scores

The association between risk and comprehension is summarized by the coefficients of the linear term for G in the regression model for R_1, V_1, R_2 and V_2. Boxplots of the simulated regression coefficients from DABIPF are displayed in Figure 9.5. For each coefficient, the majority of the simulated values lie well below zero, providing evidence that increasing risk is associated with decreasing reading and verbal comprehension. Simulated posterior percentiles for the four coefficients are given in Table 9.5, along with a two-tailed Bayesian p-value for testing the null hypothesis that each coefficient is zero. All four effects are 'statistically significant.' From the medians, we estimate that increasing risk by one category (low to moderate or moderate to high) is associated with a drop of 6–7 points in reading comprehension and 10–13 points in verbal comprehension for each child.

9.5.2 Foreign Language Attitude Scale

In Section 6.3, we examined data pertaining to the Foreign Language Attitude Scale (FLAS), an instrument designed to predict achievement in the study of foreign languages. Of the twelve variables in the dataset, five are categorical and seven are continuous. The analyses in Chapter 6 relied on multiple imputations created under a multivariate normal model. Prior to imputation, we recoded some of the categorical variables to make the normal model appear more reasonable. In the process of recoding, however, some potentially useful detail was lost. For example, the final grade variable GRD was collapsed from five categories to only two. Now, using the general location model, we will re-impute the missing data without altering any of the categorical variables.

The imputation model

For imputation purposes, we fitted a restricted version of the general location model to the twelve variables listed in Table 6.5. The categorical variables LAN, AGE, PRI, SEX and GRD define a five-dimensional contingency table with $4 \times 5 \times 5 \times 2 \times 5 = 1000$ cells. This table was described by a loglinear model with all main effects and two-variable associations. The seven continuous variables were then described by a regression with main effects for each categorical variable. The design matrix, which had 1000 rows and eight columns, included a constant term for the intercept, three dummy indicators for LAN, a dummy indicator for SEX and linear contrasts for AGE, PRI and GRD. The coding scheme for the design matrix is shown in Table 9.6.

Like the multivariate normal distribution, this model allows simple associations between any two variables. Imputations generated under the model will preserve simple marginal and conditional associations, but higher-order effects such as interactions will not be

Table 9.6. *Columns of design matrix in imputation model, foreign language achievement study data*

Variable	Description
INT	constant term for intercept (1)
LAN_2	Spanish indicator (1=Spanish, 0=other language)
LAN_3	German indicator (1=German, 0=other language)
LAN_4	Russian indicator (1=Russian, 0=other language)
AGE_L	linear contrast for age (-2=less than 20, -1=20–21, 0=22–23, 1=24–25, 2=26+)
PRI_L	linear contrast for prior courses (-2=none,-1=1, 0=2, 1=3, 2=4+)
SEX_2	female indicator (1=female, 0=male)
GRD_L	linear contrast for grade (-2=F, -1=D, 0=C, 1=B, 2=A)

reflected in the imputed values. If the post-imputation analyses involve only simple associations (e.g. regressions with main effects but no interactions) then this imputation model may be expected to perform well. More elaborate analyses involving interactions, however, would require a more elaborate imputation model.

Prior distributions

Recall from Section 6.3 that certain parameters of the normal model were inestimable, because values of GRD were missing for all students enrolled in Russian (LAN=4). In the new imputation model, some aspects of the association between GRD and LAN are again inestimable for the same reason. Furthermore, the sparseness of the contingency table (recall that there are 1000 cells but only $n = 279$ observations) results in ML estimates on the boundary of the parameter space. These difficulties can be addressed by specifying a proper prior distribution for the cell probabilities.

In previous examples involving sparse tables, we applied flattening priors, Dirichlet or constrained Dirichlet distributions with hyperparameters set to a small positive constant. Flattening priors smooth the estimated cell probabilities toward a uniform table. This type of smoothing may be undesirable in this application, because some of the categorical variables (AGE and GRD, in particular) have categories that are quite rare; flattening priors could distort the marginal distributions for these variables, leading to an over-representation of rare categories in the imputed values. Another possibility is a data-dependent prior that smooths the estimates toward a table of mutual independence among the variables, but leaves the marginal distribution of each variable unchanged (Section 7.2.5). To generate multiple imputations, we ran DABIPF under two different priors: (a) a data-dependent prior of this type, with hyperparameters scaled to add to 50; and (b) the Jeffreys prior with all hyperparameters equal to 1/2. The latter may arguably result in oversmoothing; we include it primarily to assess the sensitivity of our results to the choice of prior.

Generating the imputations

Under each prior, we generated $m = 10$ imputations by running a single chain of DABIPF, allowing 250 cycles between imputations. To obtain a starting value of θ, we first ran the ECM algorithm, setting hyperparameters to 1.05 to ensure a mode in the interior of the parameter space. The continuous variables were modeled and imputed on their original scales without transformation. The imputed values for these variables hardly ever strayed outside their natural ranges. For example, only two of the $10 \times 34 = 340$ values of CGPA imputed in the first DABIPF run fell above the maximum of 4.0. Because these 'impossible' imputations occurred so rarely, we simply allowed them to remain in the imputed data rather than editing or re-drawing them.

A proportional-odds model

In keeping with the purpose of this study, a model was fitted to predict final grade GRD from the other eleven variables. Because GRD is an ordinal scale (0=F, 1=D, 2=C, 3=B, 4=A), we used a logistic model for ordinal responses known as the proportional-odds model (McCullagh, 1980; Agresti, 1990). For any subject i, let π_{ij} denote the probability of the event GRD $\geq j$, and let x_i be a vector of covariates. The proportional-odds model is

$$\log \frac{\pi_{ij}}{1 - \pi_{ij}} = \alpha_j + x_i^T \beta, \quad j = 1, 2, 3, 4.$$

In other words, the log-odds of falling above each of the four GRD cut-points are simultaneously modeled as parallel linear functions with common slopes β and intercepts $\alpha_1 \geq \alpha_2 \geq \alpha_3 \geq \alpha_4$. Routines for maximum-likelihood estimation in the proportional-odds

Table 9.7. *Estimates, standard errors, p-values and percent missing information for coefficients in the proportional-odds model, from $m = 10$ multiple imputations under (a) data-dependent and (b) Jeffreys priors*

variable	(a) Data-dependent				(b) Jeffreys			
	est.	SE	p	mis.	est.	SE	p	mis.
INT$_1$	−6.69	2.07	.00	35	−8.38	1.86	.00	22
INT$_2$	−9.00	2.13	.00	42	−10.2	1.87	.00	20
INT$_3$	−11.3	2.19	.00	42	−12.3	1.92	.00	19
INT$_4$	−13.7	2.23	.00	38	−14.6	2.00	.00	19
LAN$_2$	−.203	.399	.61	16	−.113	.398	.77	16
LAN$_3$	.684	.378	.07	15	.708	.371	.06	13
LAN$_4$	−.857	1.08	.44	76	−2.70	1.06	.02	75
AGE$_L$	.381	.201	.06	25	.213	.266	.43	65
PRI$_L$	.344	.109	.00	32	.371	.116	.00	40
SEX$_2$	.336	.352	.34	22	.318	.368	.39	30
FLAS × 10	.452	.128	.00	35	.456	.132	.00	38
MLAT	.104	.046	.03	60	.130	.041	.00	46
SATV × 100	−.290	.265	.28	31	−.223	.296	.45	48
SATM × 100	.029	.207	.89	17	.165	.197	.40	10
ENG × 10	−.027	.195	.89	44	−.139	.185	.46	37
HGPA	2.21	.348	.00	29	2.23	.317	.00	16
CGPA	.912	.435	.04	31	.752	.422	.08	28

model are available in several popular statistical software packages, including SAS (SAS Institute Inc., 1990) and BMDP (BMDP Statistical Software, Inc., 1992).

The covariates in our proportional-odds model included all seven of the continuous variables in the dataset. In addition, we included three dummy indicators for LAN, a dummy indicator for SEX and linear contrasts for AGE and PRI, coded as shown in Table 9.6. For each imputed dataset, we calculated ML estimates using software developed by Harrell (1990) for the statistical system S (Becker, Chambers and Wilks, 1988). The estimates, along with standard errors based on score statistics, were then combined using Rubin's rules for scalar estimands (Section 4.3.2). Estimated coefficients and standard errors are displayed in Table 9.7, along with percent missing information and two-tailed p-values for testing the null hypothesis that each coefficient is zero.

Results using a data-dependent prior, shown in Table 9.7 (a), are fairly consistent with our findings in Section 6.3 where we fitted a simple logit model to the dichotomized version of GRD. The only substantial difference is that under the proportional-odds model, PRI has a significant effect on GRD but SEX does not; under the dichotomous model, SEX had a significant effect but PRI did not. Results under the Jeffreys prior, shown in Table 9.7 (b), are similar to those from the data-dependent prior, with the following two exceptions: first, the linear effect of AGE is no longer significant; second, the coefficient of the dummy indicator LAN_4 is now highly significant. The latter is rather curious, because we know that the data provide essentially no information about the effect of LAN_4 on GRD given the other variables. This 'statistically significant' relationship appears to be a figment of the Jeffreys prior, which smooths the data quite heavily. The high fraction of missing information for this coefficient, along with its sensitivity to the choice of prior, should alert us to use extreme caution when trying to make any inferences regarding grades for the LAN = 4 group.

Partial correlation coefficients

Apart from determining which predictors are significantly related to GRD, it is also useful to consider the practical importance of the estimated effects. In many areas of social science, associations are expressed and compared in terms of simple or partial correlation coefficients. In linear regression, a partial correlation measures the expected change in the response variable (expressed in standard units) associated with a one-unit increase in a predictor (also in standard units) when all other predictors are held constant. A squared partial correlation measures the proportion of variance in the response variable 'explained by' the predictor, after accounting for the measureable effects of all other predictors. Even if the classical regression model does not hold, e.g. when the response is ordinal, the partial correlation still serves as a heuristically useful benchmark for gauging the practical importance of an association.

A partial correlation can be calculated from the usual t-statistic used for testing the significance of a regression coefficient. Let T denote a t-statistic (the estimated coefficient divided by its standard error) and ν its degrees of freedom. The estimated partial correlation is

$$r = \pm\sqrt{\frac{T^2}{T^2 + \nu}},$$

where the sign is chosen to be consistent with that of T. Under an assumption of multivariate normality, r is approximately nor-

Table 9.8. *Estimated partial correlation coefficients, 95% intervals and percent missing information from m = 10 multiple imputations under (a) data-dependent and (b) Jeffreys priors*

variable	(a) Data-dependent				(b) Jeffreys			
	est.	low	high	mis.	est.	low	high	mis.
LAN$_2$	−.08	−.21	.05	14	−.08	−.20	.05	14
LAN$_3$	.07	−.05	.20	12	.07	−.06	.20	11
LAN$_4$	−.10	−.34	.15	76	−.33	−.54	−.07	78
AGE$_L$	.11	−.03	.24	24	.04	−.15	.23	60
PRI$_L$	.24	.11	.37	20	.26	.11	.40	36
SEX$_2$	.04	−.10	.17	21	.03	−.12	.18	33
FLAS	.28	.14	.40	28	.29	.14	.42	40
MLAT	.18	−.01	.36	60	.22	.06	.36	40
SATV	−.06	−.21	.08	33	−.05	−.22	.13	51
SATM	.02	−.11	.15	15	.06	−.07	.19	15
ENG	−.03	−.18	.12	37	−.08	−.23	.07	36
HGPA	.45	.34	.55	20	.46	.35	.56	18
CGPA	.16	.02	.30	32	.14	.00	.27	21

mally distributed about the population coefficient ρ. An even better approximation is provided by Fisher's (1921) transformation $\tan^{-1}(r)$, which in large samples is essentially normally distributed about $\tan^{-1}(\rho)$ with variance $1/(\nu - 1)$ (Anderson, 1984).

For each imputed dataset, we regressed GRD on the same set of predictors used in the proportional-odds model. Using Rubin's rules, we calculated estimates and 95% intervals for $\tan^{-1}(\rho)$, and then transformed the results back to the correlation scale. The resulting point and interval estimates are shown in Table 9.8. These figures should be interpreted somewhat loosely, because the assumptions underlying the classical regression model and the normal approximation to $\tanh^{-1}(r)$ clearly do not hold. Yet it is apparent that FLAS, the predictor of primary interest, has substantial validity for predicting achievement in the study of foreign languages. Except for HGPA, FLAS has the highest partial correlation with GRD, higher even than the well established instrument MLAT.

9.5.3 National Health and Nutrition Examination Survey

The largest and most notable application of these methods to date has been to the Third National Health and Nutrition Examination

Survey (NHANES III). This survey, conducted by the National Center for Health Statistics, provides basic information on health and nutritional status for the civilian noninstitutionalized U.S. population. NHANES III is a complex, multistage area sample with oversampling of young children, the elderly, Mexican Americans and African Americans. Details of the design are given by Ezzati *et al.* (1992). Data were collected over six years (1988 94) with a total sample size of 39 695. The data collection occurred in two stages: (a) personal interviews with subjects at home, and (b) detailed physical examinations of subjects in Mobile Examination Centers (MECs). Because of the inconvenience associated with going to a MEC and completing the exam, nonresponse rates at the examination phase were understandably high; many key survey variables had missingness rates of 30% or more.

In 1992, NCHS initiated a research project to investigate alternative missing-data procedures for NHANES III, including multiple imputation. This project will culminate in the public release of a multiply-imputed research dataset, currently scheduled for 1997. The dataset will contain five imputations of more than 60 variables. Here we briefly summarize the imputation model and the results of an extensive simulation study to assess the performance of the method. Complete details are given by Schafer *et al.* (1996) and their references.

The imputation model

The imputation model was designed to produce imputations appropriate for a wide variety of analyses. Data from NHANES are used to estimate important health-related quantities at the national level, e.g. rates of obesity by age and sex. These estimates, produced and reported by NCHS, are based on classical methods of survey inference (Cochran, 1977) and are designed to be approximately unbiased over repetitions of the sampling procedure. Standard errors are calculated using special variance-estimation techniques appropriate for data from complex samples (Wolter, 1985). To be compatible with these procedures, an imputation model must be sensitive to major features of the sample design. Outside NCHS, the data are also subjected to secondary analysis by researchers in many health-related fields. For example, researchers might fit linear or logistic regression models to NHANES data to investigate relationships among health outcomes and potential risk factors. For this reason, the imputation model needed to preserve important marginal and conditional associations among variables.

We created multiple imputations under a general location model that included over 30 variables. Because individuals' probabilities of selection varied by age group, gender and race/ethnicity, the distributions of other survey variables had to be allowed to vary across the levels of these three; otherwise, biases could be introduced into many important estimators, both nationally and within demographic subclasses. The imputation model was also designed to reflect potential variation in characteristics across primary sampling units (PSUs), the clusters that enter into the NCHS procedures for variance estimation; without these effects, the quality of the standard errors calculated from the resulting imputed datasets could be impaired.

The categorical part of the general location model used a four-way classification by age, gender, race/ethnicity and PSU. The remaining variables were modeled by a multivariate linear regression with full three-way interactions for age, gender and race/ethnicity, plus main effects for PSUs. Most of the response variables in this regression were continuous, but a few were binary or ordinal. Multiple imputations were generated using the DABIPF algorithm of Section 9.4.4, and the imputed values for the binary and ordinal variables were rounded off to the nearest category. Preliminary analyses of the imputed data suggested that for most purposes, $m = 5$ imputations would be sufficient to obtain accurate and efficient inferences.

A simulation study

Recognizing that this imputation procedure was based upon a probability model that was, at best, only approximately true, we carried out an extensive simulation experiment. The goal of this simulation was to evaluate the performance of the imputation procedure from a purely frequentist perspective, without reference to any particular probability model. For example, we wanted to learn whether 95% interval estimates in typical applications would really cover the quantity of interest 95% of the time over repetitions of the sampling and imputation procedure. To this end, we constructed an artificial population of 31 847 persons by pooling data from four NCHS examination surveys conducted since 1971. This artificial population was weighted to resemble the projected U.S. population in the year 2000 in terms of race/ethnicity and geography. From this population, we drew stratified random samples of 6000 persons

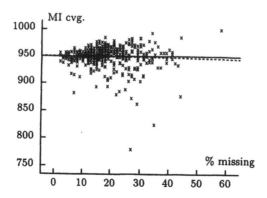

Figure 9.6. *Simulated coverage of 95% multiple-imputation (MI) intervals by average percent missing information for 448 means.*

using a sampling plan resembling that of NHANES III. Missing values were imposed on each sample using a random, ignorable mechanism to mimic the rates and patterns of nonresponse observed in NHANES III. The missing data were then imputed five times under a general location model, and multiple-imputation point and interval estimates were calculated for a variety of estimands (means and proportions, subdomain means, quantiles, and conditional log-odds ratios) using methods appropriate for stratified random samples. The entire sampling, imputation and estimation procedure was repeated 1000 times.

Here we briefly summarize our results for means. We examined means for ten exam variables for the entire population and within demographic categories defined by age, race/ethnicity and gender. Among these 448 means, the average simulated coverage of the 95% intervals over 1000 repetitions was 949.3, not significantly different from 950. Individually, however, 81 of the 448 means (18%) had coverage significantly different from 950 at the 0.05 level. The coverages of the multiple-imputation (MI) intervals are shown in Figure 9.6, plotted against the average estimated percent missing information for the respective estimands. In this plot, the least-squares fit (dashed line) is nearly indistinguishable from a horizontal line through 950 (solid); there is no overall tendency for the actual coverage to increase or decrease with the fraction of missing information. There is, however, some tendency for the coverage to vary more as the rate of missing information goes up.

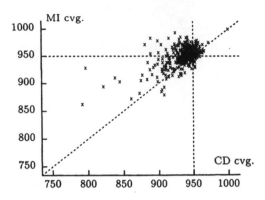

Figure 9.7. *Simulated coverage of 95% multiple-imputation (MI) intervals versus complete data (CD) intervals, with points (507, 824), (608, 799) and (479, 876) not shown.*

Further analysis revealed that, among the intervals whose coverage departed substantially from 95%, the departures could be largely traced to failure in the normal approximation for the inference without missing data. In Figure 9.7, the simulated coverage of each MI interval is plotted against the coverage of the corresponding normal-based interval (the point estimate plus or minus 1.96 standard errors) that one would have used if no data were missing. The two coverages are strongly correlated. Somewhat surprisingly, for the estimands for which the complete-data (CD) interval exhibited gross undercoverage (and especially the three pathological cases that fell outside the plotting region) the MI intervals performed substantially better than their CD counterparts. On the other hand, there were no estimands for which CD did well but MI did poorly. Results for other types of estimands revealed similar trends: the MI intervals tended to perform very well, except where difficulties were observed in the corresponding CD intervals. Further discussion of this simulation study, including its limitations, are given by Schafer *et al.* (1996).

Further remarks

In this application, it was feasible to add PSU to the general location model because there were relatively few PSUs and a large number of subjects within each PSU; we were able to include dummy indicators for PSU in the design matrix without experiencing problems of inestimability. In other surveys, the number of clusters may be too large to adopt such an approach. In those settings, it may be possible to produce multiple imputations under hierarchical or random-effects models that impose probability distributions on the cluster-specific parameters. Estimation and imputation algorithms for random-effects models can be developed by extending the techniques of this chapter, but they are beyond the scope of this book. For an example of imputation under a random-effects model for multivariate categorical data, see Schafer (1995).

CHAPTER 10

Further topics

10.1 Introduction

The basic computational methods discussed in this book, the EM algorithm and its extensions, Markov chain Monte Carlo and multiple imputation, provide a valuable and flexible toolkit for statistical inference with incomplete data. The theory surrounding these methods, and their application to missing data and related problems, are among the most rapidly developing areas of modern statistical science. This chapter describes some ongoing work by statisticians relating to missing data in multivariate settings and lists some promising areas of future research and application.

10.2 Extensions of the normal model

10.2.1 Restricted covariance structures

The methods of Chapters 5–6 based on the multivariate normal distribution made no assumptions about the covariance matrix Σ other than positive definiteness. This generality may be attractive when the number of observations is large enough to support the estimation of all variances and pairwise covariances. In other settings, however, the estimation of an unstructured covariance matrix may be undesirable or perhaps impossible with the data at hand. When the variables represent repeated measurements on a sample of units over time, it is often helpful to assume that the covariance matrix follows a simple pattern such as compound symmetry or a first-order autoregressive structure. Statistical methods for repeated measures are described by Lindsey (1993) and Diggle, Liang and Zeger (1994). Jennrich and Schluchter (1986) and Schluchter (1988) present methods for maximum-likelihood estimation in normal repeated-measures models with incomplete data; these methods have been widely used since their implementation in BMDP 5V (BMDP Statistical Software, Inc., 1992). To the author's knowledge, however, there are no general algorithms or software currently available that apply Markov chain Monte Carlo to the same general class of repeated-measures models, either with complete or incomplete data. Markov chain Monte Carlo methods for repeated measures are discussed to varying degrees of generality by Lange, Carlin and Gelfand (1992); Clayton (1996); and Carlin (1996). Much of this work on repeated measures falls within the framework of general linear mixed models; see Section 10.3.1 below.

Restricted covariance structures are also central to the analysis of graphical models (Whittaker, 1990; Cox and Wermuth, 1996; Lauritzen, 1996). EM and Markov chain Monte Carlo can be highly useful for fitting certain types of graphical models, whether the data are complete or partially missing.

10.2.2 Heavy-tailed distributions

In practice, multivariate data rarely conform to normality assumptions. Simple transformations may be helpful in reducing skewness but are often inadequate to compensate for heavier-than-normal tails. Inferences based on a multivariate normal model may be unduly influenced by heavy tails and outliers. Whether the goal is to immediately draw inferences about parameters or to impute data for future analyses, it is sometimes worthwhile to explicitly apply a multivariate model with heavier-than-normal tails, e.g. a contaminated normal or multivariate t-distribution. Little and Rubin (1987) discuss EM algorithms for fitting these models to complete or incomplete data, but those methods require the user to specify fixed values for the contamination rate in the case of the contaminated normal, and the degrees of freedom in the case of the multivariate t. Algorithms that allow these parameters to be freely estimated are discussed by Lange, Little and Taylor (1989) and Liu and Rubin (1996).

10.2.3 Interactions

The standard multivariate normal model assumes that each variable can be predicted from the others by an additive linear regression; interactions and nonlinear (e.g. quadratic or higher-order polynomial) relationships are not allowed. When interactions are present in a dataset, it could be a serious mistake to impute missing values under the usual multivariate normal model, particularly if those interactions are going to be the focus of subsequent analyses.

In certain cases, interactions can be preserved within the framework of models described in Chapters 5–9. If variables Y_1 and Y_2 are completely observed, then terms such as Y_1^2 or $Y_1 Y_2$ can be included in a multivariate normal imputation model without adverse consequences; misspecification of the marginal distribution for (Y_1, Y_2) will be of no consequence because these variables will never be imputed. If Y_1 and Y_2 are partially missing, and if they are categorical or can be categorized without serious loss of information, then an interaction of $Y_1 Y_2$ on another variable can be explicitly added to a loglinear or general location model. If Y_1 and Y_2 are partially missing and must be regarded as continuous, however, there are no readily available models or imputation algorithms that can preserve a $Y_1 Y_2$ interaction. Interactions and, more generally, nonlinear relationships among continuous variables are an important area for future work.

10.2.4 Semicontinuous variables

Semicontinuous variables have a proportion of responses equal to a single value (typically zero), and a continuous distribution among the remaining responses. Such data are common in a wide variety of contexts. Variables in economic surveys pertaining to income or expenditures tend to be semicontinuous, because many individuals will have no income or expenditures of a certain type in a given year. In studies of drug or alcohol use, many subjects will report no use during the study period. In many areas of substantive research, it has become increasingly common to model semicontinuous variables in two stages: (a) a dichotomous regression (e.g. a logit or probit model) for predicting whether the response is zero or not zero, and (b) a continuous regression model for predicting the level of response among the cases whose responses are nonzero (Manning et al., 1987). The two regression models need not involve the same set of covariates. It is even conceivable that a covariate whose coefficient is positive in (a) could have a negative coefficient in (b) or vice-versa.

When missing values occur on semicontinuous variables, one should apply missing-data methods that are explicitly designed for them. Ad hoc approaches (e.g. imputing the variables as though they were normally distributed, and then rounding off the negative imputed values to zero) are unlikely to work well. More principled methods can be developed by extending the general location model of Chapter 9. For a semicontinuous variable Y_j, define a binary indicator W_j that takes the value 1 if $Y_j = 0$ and 2 if $Y_j \neq 0$. Then define a continuous variable Z_j that is equal to Y_j if $W_j = 2$ and irrelevant (i.e. always missing) if $W_j = 1$. The regression coefficient relating W_j to Z_j would have to be omitted from the model, because the data provide no information about the conditional mean of Z_j given that $W_j = 1$. Omitting the effect of W_j on Z_j, but retaining the effects of W_j on other continuous variables, is known in the econometric literature as *seemingly unrelated regressions* (Press, 1982). Estimation techniques for seemingly unrelated regressions can be worked into the model-fitting algorithms of Chapter 9.

10.3 Random-effects models

An important and highly useful set of models for data analysis is the class of *general linear mixed models* (Laird and Ware, 1982). These models have the form

$$y_i = X_i\beta + Z_i b_i + \epsilon_i$$

for units $i = 1, \ldots, n$, where y_i is a response vector whose length may vary among units, β is a vector of 'fixed effects', $b_i \sim N(0, \Lambda)$ is a vector of 'random effects' for unit i, $\epsilon_i \sim N(0, \sigma^2 I)$ is a vector of residual errors and X_i and Z_i are matrices of covariates. These models have often been fitted by EM-type algorithms (Laird, Lange and Stram, 1987; Bryk and Raudenbush, 1992). Markov chain Monte Carlo methods have been applied as well; these can readily be extended to accommodate multiple levels of nested and crossed random effects (Gelfand *et al.*, 1990; Gelman *et al*, 1995; Clayton, 1996; Carlin, 1996). Extensions to nonnormal responses within the exponential family, called *generalized linear mixed models*, are described by Zeger and Karim (1991) and Clayton (1996). When applied naively, these iterative algorithms may exhibit notoriously slow convergence; methods for speeding convergence are discussed by Liu and Rubin (1995) and in several chapters of Gilks, Richardson and Spiegelhalter (1996). Non-Markov chain simulation methods for multivariate normal random-effects models are described by Everson and Morris (1996). Most of these algorithms are readily extended to accommodate ignorably missing values in y_i (Liu, Taylor and Belin, 1995). Missing values in X_i and Z_i are more problematic, however, requiring us to impose a probability model on the covariates; handling this in general may require us to incorporate random effects into models for mixed continuous and categorical data.

10.4 Models for complex survey data

Random-effects models for normal and nonnormal variables are increasingly being applied to data from complex surveys. Multistage cluster samples are quite naturally described by random effects for each stage of sampling. Models can be helpful for estimating quantities for *small areas*, domains for which the sample size is not large enough to yield stable estimates using a purely design-based approach; see Ghosh and Rao (1994) and their references. Another important use of models is variance estimation (Malec and Sedransk, 1985, 1995; Aitken and Longford, 1986; Battese, Harter and Fuller, 1988). In certain cases, model-based variance estimates can be substantially more efficient than those based on the jackknife and other competing design-based methods (Longford, 1992). Whether the estimation techniques ultimately applied to survey data are model-based or design-based, missing values should be handled by techniques that reflect important features of the sample design. Random-effects models may be very helpful for creating imputations of missing values with appropriate levels of intra-cluster correlation.

Imputation in sample surveys has traditionally been confined to problems of *item nonresponse*, in which the survey data for a sampled unit are only partially missing. A brief overview of traditional imputation methods in surveys is given by Little and Rubin (1987); for detailed presentations, see the volumes by Madow, Nisselson and Olkin (1983); Madow and Olkin (1983); and Madow, Olkin and Rubin (1983). The model-based imputation methods described in this book, and their extensions to more complex models suitable for data from complex surveys, may conceivably lead to an expanded role for imputation in the future. When estimating quantities for well-defined finite populations (particularly when the sample constitutes a non-trivial portion of the population) it can be advantageous to regard the non-sampled units as 'missing data', and use imputation as the primary estimation technique. This method, known as *mass imputation*, is described by Kaufman and Scheuren (1996). Multiple imputations of the non-sampled units could provide model-based variance estimates appropriate for the finite-population inference. Mass imputation for nonresponse in the U.S. Census is described by Schafer (1995). Models for multivariate data from complex surveys can (and undoubtedly should) be quite complex, and more work needs to be done to formulate flexible models and algorithms applicable to a variety of survey datasets.

10.5 Nonignorable methods

The assumption of ignorable nonresponse (Chapter 2) is computationally very convenient because it allows us to conduct inferences without explicitly specifying a missingness mechanism. In many situations, however, ignorability is questionable or implausible, and it would be worthwhile to investigate nonignorable alternatives. Brief discussion and some references on nonignorable alternatives were given in Section 2.5.3. Broadly speaking, the literature on nonignorable methods has been rather sporadic, with extended discussion of special cases but relatively few overall themes. In principle, the same computational tools used throughout this book, EM-type algorithms and Markov chain Monte Carlo, could be used to summarize likelihood functions and posterior distributions that do not ignore the missingness mechanism. The major barriers are no longer computational but conceptual; models for nonignorable response appropriate for wide classes of data (especially multivariate data) have not been proposed. Construction and evaluation of general models for nonignorable nonresponse are an important area for future study.

10.6 Mixture models and latent variables

Mixture models have a long history of application in a wide variety of contexts. Models applied to data in the social sciences are often posed in terms of latent variables—unobservable quantities (e.g. intelligence, assertiveness) that explain relationships among the variables that are actually seen (e.g. responses to questionnaire or test items). Latent class models attempt to explain the structure of multidimensional contigency tables by means of an unobserved categorical variable (Goodman, 1974; Clogg and Goodman, 1984). Factor analysis and structural equations models describe relationships among latent and observed continuous variables (Jöreskog and Sörbom, 1988; Bentler, 1989; Bollen, 1989); extensions to discrete data have also been considered (Muthén, 1984). Models for finite mixtures of continuous variables are common in biometry and the natural sciences (Titterington, Smith and Makov, 1985).

In some respects, parametric mixture models lend themselves well to the algorithms described in this book. EM algorithms have been used routinely to fit latent class and factor models (Rubin and Thayer, 1982, 1983; Clogg and Goodman, 1984). Markov chain Monte Carlo methods for parametric mixtures are described by Gelman *et al.* (1995) and in several chapters of Gilks, Richardson and Spiegelhalter (1996). EM and simulation methods enjoy some advantages over other types of model-fitting procedures. The algorithms can be extended to handle missing data in a straightforward manner. They can be simpler to implement and computationally more stable than gradient methods such as Newton-Raphson. In many cases, however, the convergence of EM and Markov chain Monte Carlo methods can be painfully slow and difficult to detect. Problems of multimodality and inestimability may complicate the statistical inference. More work needs to be done to develop algorithms with better convergence properties applicable to wide classes of latent-variable problems.

10.7 Coarsened data and outlier models

In this book we have focused on methods for handling missing values in rectangular data matrices. These methods may also be applied more generally to problems of *coarsened data*, including observations that are grouped, censored, rounded and truncated (Heitjan, 1989, 1994; Heitjan and Rubin, 1990, 1991). EM and similar computational techniques may be applied to censored data in survival analysis (Cox and Oakes, 1984). Censored observations in a variety of contexts may be handled by multiple imputation (Wei and Tanner, 1991; Dorey, Little and Schenker, 1993).

Another issue closely related to missing data is that of outlier detection and modeling. In many statistical analyses, outliers are merely an indication of model failure; a probability model that adequately describes the majority of the observations simply does not hold for a few. In these situations, it may be more realistic to model the data as a mixture (see above). In other cases, however, outliers represent genuine mistakes that mask the underlying 'true' values. In surveys, for example, outliers may arise from misreporting by sampled individuals or data collectors, or by occasional errors in data processing. If reliable followup data are available for at least a subset of units, the problem of response errors can be recast as a simple missing-data problem; see the example in Section 7.4.3 and 8.6.2. When no followup data are available, the problem may be viewed in stages: (a) For each element y_{ij} of the data matrix, there is an unobserved indicator R_{ij} equal to 1 if y_{ij} is reliable and 2 if y_{ij} is erroneous. (b) For each y_{ij}, there is an corresponding 'true' value y_{ij}^* equal to y_{ij} if $R_{ij} = 1$ and missing if $R_{ij} = 2$. Adopting a Bayesian perspective, one could propose a model for the true data $Y^* = \{y_{ij}^*\}$ and a probability mechanism for $R = \{R_{ij}\}$ given Y^*, and proceed to draw inferences about the parameters of the true-data model given the observed data $Y = \{y_{ij}\}$. Alternatively, one could multiply impute versions of the underlying true dataset Y^*. Some Bayesian approaches to problems of outliers and response errors using Markov chain Monte Carlo are described by Verdinelli and Wasserman (1991); Justel and Peña (1996); and Richardson (1996).

10.8 Diagnostics

Despite this book's heavy reliance upon parametric modeling, relatively little has been said about model checking and diagnostics. For models that involve constraints on the natural parameter space, e.g. the loglinear models of Chapter 8 and the restricted general location models of Chapter 9, the deviance statistic may provide some overall index of the quality of fit. In many situations, however, the asymptotic chisquare approximation (Section 3.2.4) will not produce an accurate p-value for testing the current model against the saturated alternative. Regardless of whether the chisquare approximation works well, it is important to consider whether the current model realistically describes the given data, and to diagnose relevant aspects of model failure. The method of *posterior predictive checks* (Rubin, 1984; Gelman *et al.*, 1995; Gelman and Meng, 1996) combines the framework of Bayesian modeling with frequentist calculations of model adequacy. Posterior predictive checks are a natural extension of parameter simulation and imputation procedures; to the author's knowledge, these have not yet been applied to incomplete-data problems. Another useful set of diagnostic tools that can be readily integrated into the algorithms of this book are the Bayesian case-influence statistics described by Bradlow and Zaslavsky (1996).

Data examples

Table A.1. *Data from foreign language achievement study (Y_1=LAN, Y_2=AGE, Y_3=PRI, Y_4=SEX, Y_5=FLAS, Y_6=MLAT, Y_7=SATV, Y_8=SATM, Y_9=ENG, Y_{10}=HGPA, Y_{11}=CGPA, Y_{12}=GRD)*

	Y_1	Y_2	Y_3	Y_4	Y_5	Y_6	Y_7	Y_8	Y_9	Y_{10}	Y_{11}	Y_{12}
1	1	2	4	1	74	32	540	660	58	3.77	3.75	4
2	3	1	3	1	69	28	610	760	75	2.18	3.81	4
3	3	2	1	2	81	28	610	560	61	3.19	3.73	4
4	3	1	5	2	89	13	430	470	33	2.21	3.54	3
5	4	1	4	1	56	26	630	630	78	3.59	4.00	—
6	2	2	4	2	95	22	440	580	48	3.25	3.20	4
7	2	—	—	1	71	—	—	—	—	2.46	—	—
8	4	1	5	2	95	—	560	540	55	2.00	2.77	—
9	2	2	3	2	87	23	500	570	41	2.67	3.52	4
10	2	2	2	1	28	10	360	500	—	2.23	2.69	—
11	1	2	1	1	62	20	560	610	54	3.31	3.93	3
12	4	1	5	2	86	—	460	550	53	3.20	3.41	—
13	2	2	4	2	78	23	470	400	50	2.93	3.93	3
14	2	1	4	2	99	26	600	430	61	2.17	2.60	3
15	1	—	—	1	71	13	—	—	—	2.69	—	2
16	4	1	5	1	66	23	550	590	56	3.74	3.43	—
17	2	1	5	2	76	20	—	—	—	2.56	—	—
18	3	2	5	1	89	25	721	581	79	2.92	3.57	4
19	1	1	1	2	94	24	490	520	53	2.38	2.93	2
20	3	3	5	1	93	29	430	510	38	3.07	3.75	4
21	2	1	4	2	102	24	380	490	51	3.35	3.03	4
22	3	—	—	2	83	—	500	690	71	2.71	3.06	3
23	3	2	1	2	89	23	550	620	65	2.86	4.00	4
24	2	2	1	1	57	19	520	580	38	2.38	3.21	2
25	3	2	5	2	100	16	490	440	54	2.32	3.06	4
26	3	5	2	1	79	20	—	—	—	3.39	—	3

Table A.1. *(continued)*

	Y_1	Y_2	Y_3	Y_4	Y_5	Y_6	Y_7	Y_8	Y_9	Y_{10}	Y_{11}	Y_{12}
27	2	1	5	2	90	24	480	560	64	2.15	3.38	3
28	2	1	5	1	74	12	430	610	47	2.45	3.37	3
29	2	1	5	2	93	35	480	600	71	2.81	3.70	4
30	1	1	1	1	102	23	590	680	—	3.60	2.97	4
31	3	1	1	2	83	19	400	630	46	2.53	3.23	3
32	1	1	3	2	97	9	310	460	40	2.47	3.31	—
33	2	1	1	2	89	14	390	340	29	1.63	3.00	—
34	1	1	1	2	86	32	460	520	40	3.13	3.57	3
35	1	3	1	1	94	—	570	690	55	2.32	3.33	2
36	2	1	1	2	97	33	460	500	72	3.20	3.75	4
37	2	1	4	2	93	22	390	590	38	1.74	3.07	2
38	1	2	4	2	93	33	540	630	69	3.24	3.69	4
39	3	2	5	1	83	17	470	480	33	2.72	3.23	4
40	3	2	1	2	101	26	510	490	47	3.32	3.36	4
41	2	1	2	2	72	21	430	580	48	3.25	3.74	4
42	3	4	2	1	51	—	—	—	—	2.28	—	1
43	1	2	5	1	48	25	480	720	62	3.34	3.21	3
44	3	1	3	1	87	21	500	460	35	2.69	3.47	2
45	2	2	3	1	96	28	550	650	47	3.41	3.94	4
46	2	2	1	2	38	25	—	—	—	2.68	—	—
47	3	2	4	1	93	30	460	500	76	3.27	3.33	4
48	2	3	3	1	91	—	420	490	40	2.23	2.97	3
49	2	2	2	1	84	—	340	410	38	1.80	2.08	—
50	4	1	5	2	55	21	540	370	57	2.15	3.37	—
51	2	1	1	2	97	24	630	530	50	3.05	2.87	2
52	1	2	1	1	73	23	510	720	51	3.31	2.93	4
53	4	1	1	2	103	27	580	510	63	3.42	3.61	—
54	2	2	2	1	81	13	330	440	27	2.11	2.89	2
55	1	2	5	1	53	—	570	460	58	2.14	2.47	3
56	4	2	5	2	86	19	—	—	—	3.40	—	—
57	4	1	5	2	45	19	420	570	39	2.30	3.06	—
58	2	1	5	1	73	17	490	380	48	2.84	2.63	3
59	2	1	3	2	89	22	470	540	39	3.00	3.87	4
60	3	1	4	1	90	27	500	620	38	3.69	3.38	4
61	1	1	3	2	101	23	500	380	52	2.95	3.56	3
62	2	1	1	1	89	27	600	620	68	3.27	3.81	4
63	1	1	5	2	79	—	530	570	55	2.89	2.93	3
64	2	4	3	1	79	—	540	410	34	2.32	2.53	2
65	2	2	3	1	100	16	500	690	37	2.52	2.72	2
66	2	2	3	1	68	17	—	—	—	2.56	—	1
67	2	1	5	2	80	15	360	530	43	2.07	2.59	3

Table A.1. *(continued)*

	Y_1	Y_2	Y_3	Y_4	Y_5	Y_6	Y_7	Y_8	Y_9	Y_{10}	Y_{11}	Y_{12}
68	3	2	3	1	74	27	480	580	44	2.34	3.29	3
69	1	4	5	1	93	22	—	—	—	3.80	—	4
70	3	2	3	1	89	20	—	—	—	2.25	—	2
71	3	1	2	2	83	28	410	520	44	2.61	3.66	4
72	1	1	1	2	70	39	600	680	79	1.45	3.36	2
73	1	1	4	2	82	—	640	430	80	2.09	3.21	2
74	3	1	5	2	91	29	430	610	64	2.05	3.81	4
75	3	1	4	2	86	37	540	620	59	3.70	3.94	4
76	2	1	4	2	98	18	440	560	55	2.14	3.19	3
77	3	1	1	2	70	37	510	640	80	3.59	3.97	4
78	3	—	—	2	98	—	400	530	49	2.41	3.03	—
79	3	2	1	1	80	34	520	540	55	3.39	3.15	4
80	3	2	4	1	58	17	550	620	40	3.40	3.63	3
81	1	2	3	1	76	—	570	520	30	2.89	2.30	4
82	1	1	3	2	97	—	450	370	61	2.52	3.20	4
83	3	2	1	1	97	23	550	530	82	2.79	2.81	4
84	2	1	5	1	65	29	500	670	59	2.77	3.79	3
85	3	1	5	2	75	38	550	620	66	3.53	4.00	4
86	3	1	5	2	82	27	500	590	55	2.41	2.83	3
87	2	1	3	1	81	—	—	—	—	2.68	—	3
88	3	2	3	2	75	25	480	570	40	2.83	3.74	4
89	1	2	5	1	94	26	460	540	38	2.60	3.81	3
90	2	2	3	1	63	22	440	630	39	3.67	3.71	4
91	4	1	5	1	90	—	360	490	44	3.35	2.93	—
92	2	1	5	2	99	28	360	450	43	2.52	3.83	3
93	3	2	5	2	78	22	560	600	57	3.02	3.84	4
94	2	2	5	2	88	32	460	520	55	3.46	3.43	4
95	3	1	4	2	66	32	500	470	62	3.44	3.93	4
96	3	2	1	1	87	23	350	610	40	2.13	2.57	1
97	3	1	5	1	91	—	650	530	80	2.53	3.12	4
98	3	2	5	2	80	21	600	550	68	2.65	3.13	4
99	3	1	1	1	72	—	580	710	61	3.56	3.81	4
100	2	4	1	2	43	19	—	—	—	1.68	—	2
101	2	2	5	1	62	—	570	730	53	3.40	3.94	3
102	3	1	1	1	81	24	640	640	66	1.27	2.64	1
103	1	1	1	2	83	29	450	590	70	3.38	3.42	2
104	2	2	2	1	77	16	350	320	19	2.41	2.71	3
105	3	1	4	1	90	22	550	580	49	2.12	3.44	3
106	2	2	3	1	71	15	410	430	37	2.60	2.00	—
107	1	1	1	1	90	36	510	620	55	1.74	3.47	3
108	3	1	4	1	86	36	520	760	72	3.33	3.33	4

Table A.1. *(continued)*

	Y_1	Y_2	Y_3	Y_4	Y_5	Y_6	Y_7	Y_8	Y_9	Y_{10}	Y_{11}	Y_{12}
109	2	1	1	1	54	23	480	590	48	2.04	3.07	1
110	1	2	5	2	75	32	390	690	36	1.98	3.41	4
111	3	—	—	2	90	30	420	530	57	2.48	3.73	4
112	2	1	5	2	87	16	470	560	40	1.26	3.13	1
113	3	1	1	2	89	—	390	450	46	2.04	2.41	—
114	3	2	1	1	70	22	280	510	31	2.03	3.00	2
115	2	2	5	1	74	20	340	450	27	2.56	3.00	4
116	1	1	5	2	79	—	540	580	60	3.03	3.73	3
117	3	1	5	2	84	—	560	580	67	1.63	3.18	4
118	4	1	3	1	78	20	440	500	28	2.05	2.67	—
119	3	1	1	1	90	—	600	630	88	1.57	3.13	2
120	1	2	1	1	56	27	510	610	46	2.94	3.54	4
121	1	—	—	2	92	18	—	—	—	2.09	—	3
122	3	3	2	2	103	19	350	380	32	3.77	2.58	4
123	2	2	1	1	94	26	—	—	—	—	—	3
124	3	2	3	2	89	19	480	480	62	3.56	4.00	4
125	3	2	1	1	72	34	690	710	77	2.87	3.50	3
126	3	1	4	1	84	25	530	650	63	3.73	3.63	4
127	3	1	1	1	85	27	450	670	39	3.82	3.67	4
128	1	2	3	1	84	18	450	700	58	2.25	2.91	4
129	3	1	5	1	81	26	490	520	56	2.80	2.68	2
130	1	2	1	1	93	15	—	—	—	2.11	—	2
131	3	1	1	1	94	33	620	650	91	3.18	3.62	3
132	3	2	3	1	73	27	430	660	44	3.46	3.06	4
133	3	1	5	2	84	37	520	640	59	2.82	4.00	4
134	3	1	5	2	96	31	590	570	68	3.25	2.91	4
135	3	5	1	2	98	33	—	—	—	2.50	—	4
136	1	1	5	2	97	27	—	—	—	3.03	—	3
137	3	2	4	2	65	—	550	590	71	3.54	3.94	—
138	3	2	1	1	89	29	510	540	54	3.22	4.00	4
139	1	2	3	1	79	22	380	610	46	2.10	3.27	3
140	1	1	4	2	53	25	540	620	62	2.86	3.56	2
141	3	2	3	2	84	20	450	570	39	3.34	2.62	4
142	3	2	5	2	76	—	490	570	46	2.68	3.19	3
143	3	1	5	2	106	25	610	570	71	3.59	3.50	4
144	4	2	3	1	78	—	500	570	57	2.09	2.90	—
145	1	3	5	1	68	19	—	—	—	2.44	—	3
146	3	2	1	2	97	26	530	650	48	2.52	3.80	4
147	3	1	2	1	76	—	500	600	45	3.10	3.71	4
148	3	2	3	1	73	21	410	590	41	2.54	2.88	4
149	3	1	3	1	91	22	570	530	66	2.72	3.20	3

Table A.1. *(continued)*

	Y_1	Y_2	Y_3	Y_4	Y_5	Y_6	Y_7	Y_8	Y_9	Y_{10}	Y_{11}	Y_{12}
150	2	2	5	1	80	22	420	450	37	2.97	3.47	4
151	3	2	1	1	90	36	550	800	83	3.85	3.97	4
152	2	4	2	1	73	—	—	—	—	2.16	—	—
153	1	2	5	1	83	14	310	610	22	1.84	2.79	3
154	1	1	5	2	87	24	480	520	44	2.58	2.93	3
155	3	2	3	2	92	23	—	—	—	2.67	—	4
156	3	4	3	1	76	28	560	580	74	3.20	2.84	4
157	3	1	1	2	78	27	540	580	59	2.81	3.59	4
158	3	1	1	1	68	28	510	540	43	3.00	2.12	—
159	3	1	5	2	104	30	580	570	77	2.45	3.64	4
160	2	2	5	1	44	28	460	770	48	3.86	4.00	4
161	3	2	5	1	94	—	360	530	39	2.82	3.03	4
162	2	2	3	1	58	15	510	520	36	2.61	2.73	2
163	2	1	3	2	66	29	590	610	57	3.03	3.75	4
164	2	1	5	1	81	25	490	550	67	2.50	3.29	4
165	1	1	3	1	76	24	630	610	66	3.14	3.59	4
166	2	2	3	1	35	—	510	490	54	3.32	3.28	4
167	2	2	5	2	104	—	460	470	52	2.25	3.27	4
168	3	2	1	2	84	—	410	550	39	3.22	2.56	4
169	1	2	5	2	92	35	600	630	67	3.24	3.81	4
170	3	2	3	2	91	19	480	520	44	2.16	3.87	4
171	3	2	5	1	67	18	—	—	—	1.71	—	3
172	3	1	1	1	82	28	540	540	50	3.55	3.47	4
173	3	3	1	1	81	32	560	650	82	3.47	3.24	4
174	2	3	1	1	69	20	550	510	51	2.76	3.17	2
175	1	2	1	2	77	23	440	480	48	2.82	3.07	3
176	2	5	1	1	93	18	—	—	—	2.50	—	2
177	3	1	5	1	87	16	350	560	36	1.33	2.34	2
178	3	1	1	2	101	40	740	730	113	3.95	4.00	4
179	4	1	4	2	93	—	520	540	59	2.96	3.50	—
180	2	2	5	1	45	28	510	480	50	2.75	3.21	3
181	3	2	4	1	91	26	560	620	60	2.52	3.11	4
182	1	1	5	2	93	19	—	—	—	1.57	—	2
183	3	1	1	1	84	30	590	620	49	1.64	3.38	3
184	1	1	1	1	99	26	550	600	55	3.33	3.26	—
185	1	1	5	2	93	19	—	—	—	1.57	—	2
186	2	2	4	1	83	28	570	650	58	2.67	3.57	4
187	1	2	3	1	89	19	610	500	74	2.25	2.67	3
188	3	2	5	1	76	—	520	540	44	2.36	2.67	—
189	4	—	—	1	96	26	340	440	51	2.56	2.60	—
190	3	2	1	1	88	20	510	610	54	3.36	2.43	4

Table A.1. *(continued)*

	Y_1	Y_2	Y_3	Y_4	Y_5	Y_6	Y_7	Y_8	Y_9	Y_{10}	Y_{11}	Y_{12}
191	2	2	4	2	89	26	450	610	40	2.79	3.13	4
192	3	2	3	1	79	26	—	—	—	2.67	—	—
193	3	1	4	2	91	19	540	450	55	2.50	3.19	4
194	3	2	1	2	96	28	410	500	43	2.73	3.27	—
195	3	4	1	1	65	23	500	520	42	3.14	2.17	3
196	1	1	5	2	109	24	470	540	64	3.23	3.61	4
197	1	2	3	2	90	24	490	490	45	2.07	3.45	3
198	3	1	1	2	82	38	580	720	82	3.67	3.93	4
199	4	1	5	2	69	16	460	490	30	2.16	3.29	—
200	2	5	3	1	92	18	—	—	—	3.57	—	4
201	1	2	5	1	102	21	460	540	50	3.24	3.75	4
202	1	2	1	1	70	27	430	550	48	2.76	3.07	4
203	1	1	5	2	96	30	460	610	63	2.72	3.38	3
204	1	2	3	1	84	28	570	760	62	2.66	3.13	4
205	3	3	3	1	72	32	710	740	88	3.78	4.00	3
206	3	2	4	2	87	29	570	690	61	3.71	3.81	4
207	3	2	4	1	93	23	510	640	44	3.28	3.76	4
208	1	1	5	1	79	18	420	650	33	1.93	2.29	3
209	3	1	1	2	103	—	640	610	83	2.73	2.56	—
210	3	1	5	2	90	40	600	610	74	3.97	3.81	4
211	2	1	5	2	77	—	530	540	61	3.03	3.20	—
212	3	1	5	2	65	27	500	510	46	2.00	3.27	4
213	1	4	1	2	92	16	—	—	—	3.13	—	4
214	4	1	5	2	104	—	480	500	40	2.46	3.56	—
215	1	2	1	1	81	25	560	530	57	3.18	3.05	4
216	4	1	5	1	87	29	360	630	31	2.78	3.06	—
217	3	1	1	2	60	25	470	630	46	3.37	3.87	4
218	1	2	4	—	99	13	600	520	57	2.94	2.79	—
219	3	1	3	1	80	16	300	530	39	2.71	2.93	3
220	1	3	5	1	67	22	570	600	54	2.75	3.06	3
221	2	1	5	1	91	32	480	570	74	2.86	3.93	4
222	3	1	5	1	81	—	710	750	55	1.41	3.10	3
223	2	2	3	2	77	17	310	400	40	0.50	2.21	1
224	2	2	3	1	72	22	440	400	29	2.77	3.13	3
225	2	2	5	2	92	—	500	530	46	3.30	3.66	4
226	1	2	1	1	58	13	400	450	35	1.94	3.07	—
227	3	1	3	1	72	26	570	550	60	2.08	2.80	2
228	4	1	4	1	84	—	490	590	60	3.22	2.73	—
229	1	2	4	1	85	17	—	—	—	1.23	—	3
230	1	2	5	2	99	23	710	450	68	2.75	3.73	4
231	1	1	5	2	80	27	590	490	66	3.20	3.47	4

Table A.1. *(continued)*

	Y_1	Y_2	Y_3	Y_4	Y_5	Y_6	Y_7	Y_8	Y_9	Y_{10}	Y_{11}	Y_{12}
232	3	2	3	1	78	32	540	540	58	2.47	2.93	4
233	1	1	1	1	105	33	480	580	48	3.38	3.12	4
234	3	1	1	1	78	26	520	630	41	2.86	3.63	—
235	2	3	3	1	69	20	500	630	56	3.07	3.21	4
236	3	3	3	1	66	17	—	—	—	2.18	—	1
237	3	2	5	1	61	24	—	—	—	2.50	—	2
238	2	2	2	1	70	23	460	520	40	2.07	3.64	0
239	2	2	4	1	102	17	—	—	—	2.07	—	—
240	3	1	2	1	89	19	590	630	71	2.65	2.67	3
241	3	2	3	2	94	23	590	560	63	2.77	3.80	4
242	3	2	3	2	102	34	610	540	61	3.12	2.97	4
243	4	1	5	2	91	—	480	510	51	3.87	3.81	—
244	2	1	3	1	89	25	500	570	65	3.43	4.00	4
245	2	2	3	2	86	9	400	500	39	3.09	2.64	2
246	3	2	2	2	84	24	—	—	—	3.32	—	4
247	3	1	5	2	101	25	490	500	38	3.48	3.83	4
248	1	3	1	2	110	36	790	640	106	3.81	4.00	4
249	1	1	1	1	88	24	490	650	37	3.21	3.73	3
250	2	2	2	2	83	—	500	490	52	2.80	3.86	4
251	1	—	—	2	108	31	480	630	55	2.86	3.20	4
252	2	2	3	1	92	31	530	630	62	3.38	3.78	4
253	3	2	5	2	89	32	660	550	86	3.31	3.67	4
254	2	1	3	2	91	26	470	620	54	2.06	3.53	3
255	2	5	1	1	88	13	—	—	—	1.86	—	—
256	3	1	3	1	81	27	480	550	62	2.60	3.81	4
257	4	5	3	1	59	22	—	—	—	2.97	—	—
258	1	2	5	2	72	29	420	510	47	2.24	3.40	4
259	2	2	5	2	81	20	360	560	42	3.11	4.00	4
260	4	2	3	2	80	24	300	340	—	1.94	2.38	—
261	2	2	5	2	78	34	680	650	67	3.60	4.00	4
262	2	2	2	1	78	—	450	460	43	1.88	2.12	3
263	1	—	—	1	104	28	340	520	40	2.00	3.21	3
264	3	1	5	1	79	21	410	610	43	2.61	3.81	3
265	3	3	5	1	77	18	620	520	52	2.78	2.38	3
266	1	3	5	1	84	29	610	690	71	2.78	3.26	4
267	3	2	4	2	76	30	550	660	75	3.99	3.94	—
268	3	—	—	1	92	—	600	660	89	2.65	3.14	3
269	2	1	5	1	92	—	460	560	37	2.10	3.23	—
270	1	1	5	2	94	—	210	470	26	2.80	3.29	4
271	3	1	1	2	76	17	600	470	76	2.38	2.67	1
272	1	—	—	2	89	—	530	500	48	2.55	3.57	3

Table A.1. *(continued)*

	Y_1	Y_2	Y_3	Y_4	Y_5	Y_6	Y_7	Y_8	Y_9	Y_{10}	Y_{11}	Y_{12}
273	2	1	1	2	102	30	470	560	50	3.04	3.33	4
274	3	1	5	1	72	—	440	620	47	2.80	3.71	4
275	2	2	5	1	94	26	670	730	86	3.66	4.00	4
276	1	2	4	1	99	22	480	560	46	2.07	2.79	3
277	1	2	1	1	78	24	560	730	63	3.41	3.52	4
278	3	1	5	1	71	21	680	660	65	2.44	2.79	2
279	2	1	1	1	72	17	490	370	38	2.50	3.38	—

Source: Dr. Mark Raymond

Storage of categorical data

The algorithms for categorical data in Chapters 7–9 involve the manipulation of contingency tables of varying dimensions. This appendix shows how the data needed for these algorithms can be stored and accessed in an efficient manner.

Consider first the problem of storing a table that cross-classifies units by variables $Y_1, Y_2, \ldots, Y_p$, where Y_j takes values $1, 2, \ldots, d_j$. The total number of cells in this table is $D = \prod_{j=1}^{p} d_j$. For a single dataset, one could simply allocate a p-dimensional array of size $d_1 \times d_2 \times \cdots \times d_p$. In writing general-purpose software to handle a variety of datasets, however, the programming may become difficult if we adopt this approach, because the dimensions will vary from application to application. It will be more convenient to store the table as a one-dimensional array, indexing the cells by a single subscript $d = 1, 2, \ldots, D$. For simplicity, let us adopt a storage order that is *anti-lexicographical*, meaning that the first subscript y_1 will vary the fastest, the second subscript y_2 will vary the second fastest, and so on. The correspondence between a generic response pattern $y = (y_1, y_2, \ldots, y_p)$ and its linear position d in anti-lexicographical storage is shown in Table 7.1. The value of d can be calculated from y by the relationship

$$d = 1 + \sum_{j=1}^{p} \left[(y_j - 1) \prod_{k=1}^{j-1} d_k \right]. \tag{B.1}$$

Now consider what happens when some variables are missing for some units. As described in Section 7.3, the data can no longer be summarized by a single contingency table with D cells. Rather, we must retain the potentially smaller table $z^{(s)}$ for each missingness pattern $s = 1, 2, \ldots, S$ which classifies the units by only those variables seen in that pattern. Let $\mathcal{O}(s)$ and $\mathcal{M}(s)$ denote the subsets of $\{1, 2, \ldots, p\}$ corresponding to variables that are observed and

Table B.1. *Linear position d of cell y* $= (y_1, y_2, \ldots, y_p)$ *when stored in anti-lexicographical order*

y_1	y_2	$\cdots$	y_p	d
1	1	$\cdots$	1	1
2	1	$\cdots$	1	2
$\vdots$	$\vdots$		$\vdots$	$\vdots$
d_1	1	$\cdots$	1	d_1
1	2	$\cdots$	1	$d_1 + 1$
2	2	$\cdots$	1	$d_1 + 2$
$\vdots$	$\vdots$		$\vdots$	$\vdots$
d_1	d_2	$\cdots$	d_p	D

missing, respectively, in pattern s. The observed table $z^{(s)}$ has a total of

$$D^{(s)} = \prod_{j \in \mathcal{O}(s)} d_j$$

cells, but in practice many of these cells may be empty.

Both the E-step of the EM algorithm and the I-step of data augmentation involve an allocation of the nonzero cell counts in each $z^{(s)}$ to the cells of the full p-dimensional table. Notice that for any missingness pattern s, the linear position d given by (B.1) can be expressed as the sum of an observed part and a missing part,

$$d = 1 + d_{obs} + d_{mis},$$

where

$$d_{obs} = \sum_{j \in \mathcal{O}(s)} \left[(y_j - 1) \prod_{k=1}^{j-1} d_k \right]$$

and

$$d_{mis} = \sum_{j \in \mathcal{M}(s)} \left[(y_j - 1) \prod_{k=1}^{j-1} d_k \right].$$

By holding d_{obs} constant and stepping d_{mis} through all possible values of y_j, $j \in \mathcal{M}(s)$, we can cycle through all cells of the p-way table that contribute to a marginal count in $z^{(s)}$. For EM and data augmentation, therefore, it is sufficient to store only the nonzero elements of each $z^{(s)}$ and their corresponding values of d_{mis}.

A similar decomposition of (B.1) can be used in general-purpose implementations of the IPF and Bayesian IPF algorithms described in Chapter 8. Instead of decomposing d into observed and missing parts, we partition it according to the variables included or excluded by a particular sufficient configuration C (Section 8.3.2). By fixing the part of d corresponding to C and varying the part corresponding to the complement of C, we can easily step through all the cells of the complete-data table that contribute to a particular marginal count, and perform the proportionate adjustments required for IPF or Bayesian IPF.

APPENDIX C

Software

All of the algorithms described in this book have been implemented for general use as functions in the statistical languages S and Splus (Becker, Chambers and Wilks, 1988). These functions, written with a combination of S and Fortran-77, may be obtained by anyone free of charge. Three packages are available:

1. NORM: algorithms based on the multivariate normal model, described in Chapters 5–6.

2. CAT: algorithms for multivariate categorical data based on the saturated multinomial model and loglinear models, as described in Chapters 7–8.

3. MIX: algorithms for mixed continuous and categorical data based on the general location model, as described in Chapter 9.

The packages, including source code and full documentation, may be downloaded from the ftp server at the Department of Statistics, The Pennsylvania State University. To obtain copies via the World Wide Web, connect to

`http://www.stat.psu.edu/~jls/`

and follow the on-line instructions.

References

Agresti, A. (1984) *Analysis of Ordinal Categorical Data.* J. Wiley & Sons, New York.

Agresti, A. (1990) *Categorical Data Analysis.* J. Wiley & Sons, New York.

Aitkin, M.A. and Longford, N.T. (1986) Statistical modelling issues in school effectiveness studies. *Journal of the Royal Statistical Society Series A,* **149,** 1–43.

Amemiya, T. (1984) Tobit models: a survey. *Journal of Econometrics,* **24,** 3–61.

Anderson, R.L. (1942) Distribution of the serial correlation coefficient. *Annals of Mathematical Statistics,* **13,** 1–13.

Anderson, T.W. (1957) Maximum likelihood estimates for the multivariate normal distribution when some observations are missing, *Journal of the American Statistical Association,* **52,** 200–203.

Anderson, T.W. (1984) *An Introduction to Multivariate Statistical Analysis* (Second edition). J. Wiley & Sons, New York.

Arnold, S.F. (1993) Gibbs sampling. *Handbook of Statistics, Volume 9: Computational Statistics* (ed. C.R. Rao), Elsevier Science Publishers, New York.

Baker, S.G. (1994) Regression analysis of grouped survival data with incomplete covariates. *Biometrics,* **50,** 1102–1116.

Baker, S.G. and Laird, N.M. (1988) Regression analysis for categorical variables with outcome subject to nonignorable nonresponse. *Journal of the American Statistical Association,* **83,** 62–69, correction 1232.

Bartlett, M.S. (1946) On the theoretical specification of sampling properties of autocorrelated time series. *Journal of the Royal Statistical Society Series B,* **8,** 27–41, correction **10,** 1.

Battese, G.E., Harter, R.M. and Fuller, W.A. (1988) An error-components model for prediction of county crop areas using survey and satellite data. *Journal of the American Statistical Association,* **83,** 23–36.

Beale, E.M.L. and Little, R.J.A. (1975) Missing data in multivariate analysis. *Journal of the Royal Statistical Society Series B,* **37,** 129–145.

Beaton, A.E. (1964) The use of special matrix operations in statistical calculus. Research Bulletin RB-64-51, Educational Testing Service, Princeton, NJ.

Becker, R.A., Chambers, J.M. and Wilks, A.R. (1988) *The New S Language: A programming environment for data analysis and graphics.* Wadsworth and Brooks/Cole Advanced Books and Software, Pacific Grove, CA.

Belin, T.R. and Diffendal, G.J. (1991) Results from the handling of unresolved enumeration status, missing characteristic data, and noninterviews in the 1990 Post-Enumeration Survey. STSD Decennial Census Memorandum Series V-112, Bureau of the Census, Washington DC.

Bentler, P.M. (1989) *Theory and implementation of EQS, a structural equations program.* BMDP Statistical Software Inc, Los Angeles.

Berger, J.O. (1985) *Statistical Decision Theory and Bayesian Analysis* (Second edition). Springer-Verlag, New York.

Besag, J. (1974) Spatial interaction and the statistical analysis of lattice systems (with discussion). *Journal of the Royal Statistical Society Series B*, **36**, 192–236.

Besag, J. (1986) On the statistical analysis of dirty pictures. *Journal of the Royal Statistical Society Series B*, **48**, 259–279.

Binder, D.A. and Sun, W. (1996) Frequency valid multiple imputation for surveys with a complex design. *Proceedings of the Survey Research Methods Section of the American Statistical Association*, to appear.

Birch, M.W. (1963) Maximum likelihood in three-way contingency tables. *Journal of the Royal Statistical Society Series B*, **25**, 220–233.

Bishop, Y.M.M., Fienberg, S.E. and Holland, P.W. (1975) *Discrete Multivariate Analysis: Theory and Practice.* MIT Press, Cambridge, MA.

Blenkner, M., Bloom, M. and Nielsen, M. (1971) A research and demonstration project of protective services. *Social Casework*, **52**, 483–499.

BMDP Statistical Software, Inc. (1992) *BMDP Statistical Software Manual* (ed. W.J. Dixon). University of California Press, Los Angeles.

Bollen, K.A. (1989) *Structural Equations with Latent Variables.* J. Wiley & Sons, New York.

Box, G.E.P. and Cox, D.R. (1964) An analysis of transformations (with discussion). *Journal of the Royal Statistical Society Series B*, **26**, 211–252.

Box, G.E.P. and Jenkins, G.M. (1976) *Time Series Analysis: Forecasting and Control* (Revised edition).. Prentice Hall, Englewood Cliffs, NJ.

Box, G.E.P. and Tiao, G.C. (1992) *Bayesian Inference in Statistical Analysis* (Wiley Classics Library Edition). J. Wiley & Sons, New York.

Bradlow, E. and Zaslavsky, A.M. (1996) Case influence analysis in Bayesian inference. *Proceedings of the Bayesian Statistics Section of the American Statistical Association*, to appear.

Brown, M.B. and Bromberg, J. (1984) An efficient two-stage procedure for generating random variates from the multinomial distribution. *American Statistician*, **38**, 216–219.

Brownstone, D. (1991) Multiple imputations for linear regression models. Technical Report MBS 91-37, Department of Mathematical Behavioral Sciences, University of California at Irvine.

Bryk, A. and Raudenbush, S. (1992) *Hierarchical Linear Models: Applications and Data Analysis Methods.* Sage Publications, Newbury Park, CA.

Carlin, B.P. (1996) Hierarchical longitudinal modelling. *Markov Chain Monte Carlo in Practice* (eds W.R. Gilks, S. Richardson and D.J. Spiegelhalter), 303–319. Chapman & Hall, London.

Casella, G. and George, E.I. (1992) Explaining the Gibbs sampler. *The American Statistician*, **46**, 167–174.

Chen, T.T. (1989) A review of methods for misclassified categorical data in epidemiology. *Statistics in Medicine*, **8**, 1095–1106.

Chen, T.T. and Fienberg, S.E. (1974) Two-dimensional contingency tables with both completely and partially cross-classified data. *Biometrics*, **32**, 133–144.

Clayton, D.G. (1996) Generalized linear mixed models. *Markov Chain Monte Carlo in Practice* (eds W.R. Gilks, S. Richardson and D.J. Spiegelhalter), 275–301. Chapman & Hall, London.

Clogg, C.C. and Goodman, L.A. (1984) Latent structure analysis of a set of multidimensional contingency tables. *Journal of the American Statistical Association*, **79**, 762–771.

Clogg, C.C. and Shihadeh, E.S. (1994) *Statistical Models for Ordinal Variables.* Sage Publications, Newbury Park, CA.

Clogg, C.C. and von Eye, A., eds (1994) *Latent Variables Analysis.* Sage Publications, Thousand Oaks, CA.

Clogg, C.C., Rubin, D.B., Schenker, N., Schultz, B., and Weidman, L. (1991) Multiple imputation of industry and occupation codes in census public-use samples using Bayesian logistic regression. *Journal of the American Statistical Association*, **86**, 68–78.

Cochran, W.J. (1977) *Sampling Techniques* (Second edition). J. Wiley & Sons, New York.

Conaway, M.R. (1992) The analysis of repeated categorical measurements subject to nonignorable nonresponse. *Journal of the American Statistical Association*, **87**, 817–824.

Conaway, M.R. (1994) Causal nonresponse models for repeated categorical measurements. *Biometrics*, **50**, 1102–1116.

Cox, D.R. and Hinkley, D.V. (1974) *Theoretical Statistics.* Chapman & Hall, London.

Cox, D.R. and Oakes, D. (1984) *Analysis of Survival Data.* Chapman & Hall, London.

Cox, D.R. and Wermuth, N. (1996) *Multivariate dependencies.* Chapman & Hall, London.

David, M., Little, R.J.A., Samuhel, M.E. and Triest, R.K. (1986) Alternative methods for CPS income imputation. *Journal of the American Statistical Association*, **81**, 29–41.

DeGroot, M.H. (1970) *Optimal Statistical Decisions.* McGraw-Hill, New York.

Deming, W.E. and Stephan, F.F. (1940) On a least squares adjustment of a sampled frequency table when the expected marginal totals are known. *Annals of Mathematical Statistics*, **11**, 427–444.

Dempster, A.P. (1969a) Upper and lower probability inferences for families of hypotheses with monotone density ratios. *Annals of Mathematical Statistics*, **40**, 953–969.

Dempster, A.P. (1969b) *Elements of Continuous Multivariate Analysis.* Addison-Wesley, Reading, MA.

Dempster, A.P., Laird, N.M. and Rubin, D.B. (1977) Maximum likelihood estimation from incomplete data via the EM algorithm (with discussion). *Journal of the Royal Statistical Society Series B*, **39**, 1–38.

Devroye, L. (1987) *A Course in Density Estimation.* Birkhauser, Boston.

Diggle, P.J. and Kenward, M.G. (1994) Informative drop-out in longitudinal data analysis (with discussion). *Applied Statistics*, **43**, 49–73.

Diggle, P.J., Liang, K. and Zeger, S.L. (1994) *Analysis of Longitudinal Data.* Clarendon Press, Oxford.

Dodge, Y. (1985) *Analysis of Experiments with Missing Data.* J. Wiley & Sons, New York.

Dorey, F.J., Little, R.J.A., and Schenker, N. (1993) Multiple imputation for threshold-crossing data with interval censoring. *Statistics in Medicine*, **12**, 1589–1603.

Draper, N.R. and Smith, H. (1981) *Applied Regression Analysis.* (Second Edition), J. Wiley & Sons, New York.

Efron, B. (1994) Missing data, imputation, and the bootstrap (with discussion). *Journal of the American Statistical Association*, **89**, 463–479.

Efron, B. and Tibshirani, R.J. (1993) *An Introduction to the Bootstrap.* Chapman & Hall, New York.

Emerson, J.D. (1991) Introduction to Transformation. *Fundamentals of Exploratory Analysis of Variance* (eds D.C. Hoaglin, F. Mosteller and J.W. Tukey), 365–400. J. Wiley & Sons, New York.

Everson, P.J. and Morris, C.N. (1996) Inference for multivariate normal hierarchical models. Technical report, Department of Statistics, Harvard University, Cambridge, MA.

Ezzati, T., Massey, J., Waksberg, J., Chu, A. and Maurer, K. (1992) Sample design: Third National Health and Nutrition Examination Survey. *Vital Health Statistics*, Series 2, No. 113, National Center for Health Statistics, Hyattsville, MD.

Ezatti-Rice, T.M., Johnson, W., Khare, M., Little, R.J.A., Rubin, D.B. and Schafer, J.L. (1995) A simulation study to evaluate the performance of model-based multiple imputations in NCHS health examination surveys. *Proceedings of the Annual Research Conference*, 257–266, Bureau of the Census, Washington, DC.

Fay, R.E. (1986) Causal models for patterns of nonresponse. *Journal of the American Statistical Association*, **81**, 354–365.

Fay, R.E. (1992) When are inferences from multiple imputation valid? *Proceedings of the Survey Research Methods Section of the American Statistical Association*, 227–232.

Fienberg, S.E. and Holland, P.W. (1970) Methods for eliminating zero counts in contingency tables. *Random Counts on Models and Structures* (ed. G.P. Patil), Pennsylvania State University Press, University Park, PA.

Fienberg, S.E. and Holland, P.W. (1973) Simultaneous estimation of multinomial cell probabilities. *Journal of the American Statistical Association*, **68**, 683–691.

Fischer, J. (1973) Is casework effective? A review. *Social Work*, **18**, 5–20.

Fisher, R.A. (1921) On the probable error of a correlation coefficient... Reprinted in *Collected Papers of R.A. Fisher*, Vol. I (1971) (ed. J.H. Bennet). University of Adelaide Press, Adelaide, South Australia.

Francisco, C.A. and Fuller, W.A. (1991) Quantile estimation with a complex survey design. *Annals of Statistics*, **19**, 454–469.

Fuchs, C. (1982) Maximum likelihood estimation and model selection in contingency tables with missing data. *Journal of the American Statistical Association*, **77**, 270–278.

Gelfand, A.E. and Smith, A.F.M. (1990) Sampling-based approaches to calculating marginal densities. *Journal of the American Statistical Association*, **85**, 398–409.

Gelfand, A.E., Hills, S.E., Racine-Poon, A. and Smith, A.F.M. (1990) Illustration of Bayesian inference in normal data models using Gibbs sampling. *Journal of the American Statistical Association*, **85**, 972–985.

Gelman, A. (1992) Iterative and non-iterative simulation algorithms. *Computing Science and Statistics: Proceedings of the 24th Symposium on the Interface*, 433–438. Interface Foundation of North America, Fairfax, VA.

Gelman, A. and Meng, X.L. (1996) Model checking and model improvement. *Markov Chain Monte Carlo in Practice* (eds W.R. Gilks, S. Richardson and D.J. Spiegelhalter), 189–201. Chapman & Hall, London.

Gelman, A. and Rubin, D.B. (1992a) Inference from iterative simulation using multiple sequences (with discussion). *Statistical Science*, **7**, 457–472.

Gelman, A. and Rubin, D.B. (1992b) A single series from the Gibbs sampler provides a false sense of security. *Bayesian Statistics* (eds J.M. Bernardo, J.O. Bergen, A.P. Dawid and A.F.M. Smith), 627–633.

Oxford University Press.

Gelman, A., Rubin, D.B., Carlin, J. and Stern, H. (1995) *Bayesian Data Analysis*. Chapman & Hall, London.

Geman, D. and Geman, S. (1984) Stochastic relaxation, Gibbs distributions, and the Bayesian reconstruction of images. *IEEE Transactions on Pattern Analysis and Machine Intelligence*, 6, 721–741.

Geweke, J. (1992) Evaluating the accuracy of sampling-based approaches to the calculation of posterior moments (with discussion). *Bayesian Statistics* (eds. J.M. Bernardo, J.O. Bergen, A.P. Dawid and A.F.M. Smith), 169–193. Oxford University Press.

Geyer, C. (1992) Practical Markov chain Monte Carlo (with discussion). *Statistical Science*, 7, 473–483.

Ghosh, M. and Rao, J.N.K. (1994) Small area estimation: an appraisal (with discussion). *Statistical Science*, 9, 55–93.

Gilks, W.R., Richardson, S. and Spiegelhalter, D.J., eds (1996) *Markov-Chain Monte Carlo in Practice*. Chapman & Hall, London.

Gilks, W.R., Clayton, D.G., Spiegelhalter, D.J., Best, N.G., McNeil, A.J., Sharples, L.D. and Kirby, A.J. (1993) Modelling complexity: applications of Gibbs sampling in medicine. *Journal of the Royal Statistical Society Series B*, 55, 39–52.

Glynn, R.J., Laird, N.M., and Rubin, D.B. (1993) Multiple imputation in mixture models for nonignorable nonresponse with followups. *Journal of the American Statistical Association*, 88, 984–993.

Good, I.J. (1956) On the estimation of small frequencies in contingency tables. *Journal of the Royal Statistical Society Series B*, 18, 113–124,

Good, I.J. (1967) A Bayesian significance test for multinomial distributions (with discussion). *Journal of the Royal Statistical Society Series B*, 29, 399–431.

Goodman, L.A. (1970) The multivariate analysis of qualitative data: interactions among multiple classifications. *Journal of the American Statistical Association*, 65, 226–256.

Goodman, L.A. (1974) Exploratory latent structure analysis using both identifiable and unidentifiable models. *Biometrika*, 61, 215–231.

Graham, J.W., Hofer, S.M. and Piccinin, A.M. (1994) Analysis with missing data in drug prevention research. *Advances in Data Analysis for Prevention Intervention Research* (eds L.M. Collins and L.A. Seitz), 13–63. National Institute on Drug Abuse.

Greenlees, J.S., Reece, W.S. and Zieschang, K.D. (1982) Imputation of missing values when the probability of response depends on the value being imputed. *Journal of the American Statistical Association*, 77, 251–261.

Haberman, S.J. (1977) Log-linear models and frequency tables with small expected cell counts. *Annals of Statistics*, 5, 1148–1169.

Hansen, M.H. and Hurwitz, W.N. (1946) The problem of nonresponse in surveys. *Journal of the American Statistical Association*, 41, 517–529.

Harrell, F. (1990) Logist: function to fit binary and ordinal logistic regression models using maximum likelihood. Available from the S archive at StatLib (http://lib.stat.cmu.edu/S/).

Hastings, W.K. (1970) Monte Carlo sampling methods using Markov chains and their applications. *Biometrika*, **57**, 97–109.

Heckman, J. (1976) The common structure of statistical models of truncation, sample selection and limited dependent variables, and a simple estimator for such models. *Annals of Economic and Social Measurement*, **5**, 475–492.

Heitjan, D.F. (1989) Inference from grouped continuous data: a review (with discussion). *Statistical Science*, **4**, 164–183.

Heitjan, D.F. (1994) Ignorability in general incomplete-data models. *Biometrika*, **81**, 701–708.

Heitjan, D.F. and Rubin, D.B. (1990) Inference from coarse data via multiple imputation with application to age heaping. *Journal of the American Statistical Association*, **85**, 304–314.

Heitjan, D.F. and Rubin, D.B. (1991) Ignorability and coarse data. *Annals of Statistics*, **19**, 2244–2253.

Hill, J.R. (1987) Comment on "Empirical Bayes confidence intervals based on bootstrap samples" by N.M. Laird and T.A. Louis. *Journal of the American Statistical Association*, **82**, 752–754.

Hochberg, Y. (1977) On the use of double sampling schemes in analyzing categorical data with misclassification errors. *Journal of the American Statistical Association*, **72**, 914–921.

Jennrich, R.I. and Schluchter, M.D. (1986) Unbalanced repeated-measures models with structured covariance matrices. *Biometrics*, **38**, 967–974.

Johnson, R.A. and Wichern, D.W. (1992) *Applied Multivariate Statistical Analysis* (Third edition). Prentice Hall, Englewood Cliffs, NJ.

Jöreskog, K.G. and Sörbom, D. (1988) *LISREL 7: A guide to the program and applications*. SPSS Inc., Chicago.

Justel, A. and Peña, D. (1996) Gibbs sampling will fail in outlier problems with strong masking. *Journal of Computational and Graphical Statistics*, **5**, 176–189.

Kadane, J.B. (1985) Is victimization chronic? A Bayesian analysis of multinomial missing data. *Journal of Econometrics*, **29**, 47–67, correction **35**, 393.

Kaufman, S. and Scheuren, F. (1996) Improved estimation in the Schools and Staffing Survey. *Proceedings of the Survey Research Methods Section of the American Statistical Association*, to appear.

Kennedy, W.J. and Gentle, J.E. (1980) *Statistical Computing*. Marcel Dekker, New York.

Kleijnan, J.P.C. (1974) *Statistical Techniques in Simulation—Part I*. Marcel Dekker, New York.

Knuiman, M.K. and Speed, T.P. (1988) Incorporating prior information into the analysis of contingency tables. *Biometrics*, **44**, 1061–1071.

Kott, P.S. (1992) A note on a counterexample to variance estimation using multiple imputation. Technical report, National Agricultural Statistical Service, Fairfax, VA.

Krzanowski, W.J. (1980) Mixtures of continuous and categorical variables in discriminant analysis. *Biometrics*, **36**, 493–499.

Krzanowski, W.J. (1982) Mixtures of continuous and categorical variables in discriminant analysis: a hypothesis testing approach. *Biometrics*, **38**, 991–1002.

Laird, N.M. (1978) Empirical Bayes methods for two-way contingency tables, *Biometrika*, **65**, 581–590.

Laird, N.M. and Ware, J.H. (1982) Random-effects models for longitudinal data. *Biometrics*, **38**, 963–974.

Laird, N.M., Lange, N. and Stram, D. (1987) Maximum likelihood computations with repeated measures: application of the EM algorithm. *Journal of the American Statistical Association*, **82**, 97–105.

Lange, N., Carlin, B.P. and Gelfand, A.E. (1992) Hierarchical Bayes models for the progression of HIV infection using longitudinal CD4 T-cell numbers (with discussion). *Journal of the American Statistical Association*, **87**, 615–632.

Lange, K.L., Little, R.J.A. and Taylor, J.M.G. (1989) Robust statistical modeling using the t distribution. *Journal of the American Statistical Association*, **84**, 881–896.

Lansky, D. and Casella, G. (1990) Improving the EM algorithm. *Computing Science and Statistics: Proceedings of the 24th Symposium on the Interface*, 420–424. Interface Foundation of North America, Fairfax, VA.

Lauritzen, S.L. (1996) *Graphical Models*. Clarendon Press, Oxford.

Leonard, T. (1975) Bayesian estimation methods for two-way contingency tables. *Journal of the Royal Statistical Society Series B*, **37**, 23–37.

Li, K.H. (1988) Imputation using Markov chains. *Journal of Statistical Computation and Simulation*, **30**, 57–79.

Li, K.H., Raghunathan, T.E. and Rubin, D.B. (1991) Large-sample significance levels from multiply-imputed data using moment-based statistics and an F reference distribution. *Journal of the American Statistical Association*, **86**, 1065–1073.

Li, K.H., Meng, X.L., Raghunathan, T.E. and Rubin, D.B. (1991) Significance levels from repeated p-values with multiply-imputed data. *Statistica Sinica*, **1**, 65–92.

Lindsey, J.K. (1993) *Models for Repeated Measurements*. Clarendon Press, Oxford.

Little, R.J.A. (1988) Approximately calibrated small sample inference about means from bivariate normal data with missing values. *Computational Statistics and Data Analysis*, **7**, 161–178, correction **8**, 210.

Little, R.J.A. (1993) Pattern-mixture models for multivariate incomplete data. *Journal of the American Statistical Association*, **88**, 125–134.

Little, R.J.A. and Rubin, D.B. (1987) *Statistical Analysis with Missing Data*. J. Wiley & Sons, New York.

Little, R.J.A. and Schluchter, M.D. (1985) Maximum likelihood estimation for mixed continuous and categorical data with missing values. *Biometrika*, **72**, 492–512.

Liu, C. (1993) Bartlett's decomposition of the posterior distribution of the covariance for normal monotone ignorable missing data. *Journal of Multivariate Analysis*, **46**, 198–206.

Liu, C. and Liu, J. (1993) Discussion on the meeting on the Gibbs sampler and other Markov chain Monte Carlo methods. *Journal of the Royal Statistical Society Series B*, **55**, 82–83.

Liu, C. and Rubin, D.B. (1995) Application of the ECME algorithm and the Gibbs sampler to general linear mixed models. *Proceedings of the 17th International Biometric Conference*, **1**, 97–107.

Liu, C. and Rubin, D.B. (1996) ML estimation of the multivariate t distribution with unknown degrees of freedom. *Statistica Sinica*, to appear.

Liu, M., Taylor, J.M.G. and Belin, T.R. (1995) Multiple imputation and posterior simulation for multivariate missing data in longitudinal studies. *Computing Science and Statistics: Proceedings of the 27th Symposium on the Interface*, 521–529. Interface Foundation of North America, Fairfax, VA.

Liu, J., Wong, W.H. and Kong, A. (1994) Covariance structure of the Gibbs sampler with applications to the comparisons of estimators and sampling schemes. *Biometrika*, **81**, 27–40.

Liu, J., Wong, W.H. and Kong, A. (1995) Correlation structure and convergence rate of the Gibbs sampler with various scans. *Journal of the Royal Statistical Society Series B*, **57**, 157–169.

Longford, N.T. (1992) Comparison of efficiency of jackknife and variance component estimators of standard errors. Program Statistics Research Technical Report 92-24. Educational Testing Service, Princeton, NJ.

Louis, T.A. (1982) Finding observed information using the EM algorithm. *Journal of the Royal Statistical Society Series B*, **44**, 98–130.

MacEachern, S.N. and Berliner, L.M. (1994) Subsampling the Gibbs sampler. *The American Statistician*, **48**, 188–190.

Madow, W.G. and Olkin, I. (1983) *Incomplete Data in Sample Surveys, Volume 3: Proceedings of the Symposium*. Academic Press, New York.

Madow, W.G., Nisselson, H. and Olkin, I. (1983) *Incomplete Data in Sample Surveys, Volume 1: Report and Case Studies*. Academic Press, New York.

Madow, W.G., Olkin, I. and Rubin, D.B. (1983) *Incomplete Data in Sample Surveys, Volume 2: Theory and Bibliographies*. Academic

Press, New York.

Malec, D. and Sedransk, J. (1985) Bayesian methodology for predictive inference for finite population parameters in multistage cluster sampling. *Journal of the American Statistical Association*, **80**, 897–902.

Malec, D. and Sedransk, J. (1995) Small area estimation for the National Health Interview Survey using hierarchical models. *Seminar on New Directions in Statistical Methodology*, 555–568. Federal Committee on Statistical Methodology, Office of Management and Budget, Washington DC.

Manning, W.G., Newhouse, J.P., Duan, N., Keeler, E.B., Leibowitz, A. and Marquis, M.S. (1987) Health insurance and the demand for medical care: evidence from a randomized experiment. *American Economic Review*, **77**, 251–277.

Mantel, N. and Haenszel, W. (1959) Statistical aspects of the analysis of data from retrospective studies of disease. *Journal of the National Cancer Institute*, **22**, 719–748.

Mardia, K.V., Kent, J.T. and Bibby, J.M. (1979) *Multivariate Analysis.* Academic Press, London.

McCullagh, P. (1980) Regression models for ordinal data (with discussion). *Journal of the Royal Statistical Society Series B*, **42**, 109–142.

McCullagh, P. and Nelder, J.A. (1989) *Generalized Linear Models* (Second edition). Chapman & Hall, London.

McNemar, Q. (1947) Note on the sampling error of the difference between correlation proportions or percentages. *Psychometrika*, **12**, 153–157.

Meng, X.L. (1990) Towards complete results for some incomplete-data problems. Ph.D. thesis, Department of Statistics, Harvard University, Cambridge, MA.

Meng, X.L. (1994) On the rate of convergence of the ECM algorithm. Technical report, Department of Statistics, University of Chicago.

Meng, X.L. (1995) Multiple-imputation inferences with uncongenial sources of input (with discussion). *Statistical Science*, **10**, 538–573.

Meng, X.L. and Pedlow, S. (1992) EM: a bibliographic review with missing articles. *Statistical Computing Section, Proceedings of the American Statistical Association*, 24–27.

Meng, X.L. and Rubin, D.B. (1991a) Using EM to obtain asymptotic variance-covariance matrices: the SEM algorithm. *Journal of the American Statistical Association*, **86**, 899–909.

Meng, X.L. and Rubin, D.B. (1991b) IPF for contingency tables with missing data via the ECM algorithm. *Statistical Computing Section, Proceedings of the American Statistical Association*, 244–247.

Meng, X.L. and Rubin, D.B. (1992a) Recent extensions to the EM algorithm (with discussion). *Bayesian Statistics* (eds J.M. Bernardo, J.O. Bergen, A.P. Dawid and A.F.M. Smith), 307–320. Oxford University Press.

Meng, X.L. and Rubin, D.B. (1992b) Performing likelihood ratio tests with multiply-imputed data sets. *Biometrika*, **79**, 103–111.

Meng, X.L. and Rubin, D.B. (1993) Maximum likelihood estimation via the ECM algorithm: A general framework. *Biometrika*, **80**, 267–278.

Metropolis, N., Rosenbluth, A.W., Rosenbluth, M.N., Teller, A.H. and Teller, E. (1953) Equations of state calculations by fast computing machines. *The Journal of Chemical Physics*, **21**, 1087–1092.

Middleton, R. (1993) Discussion on the meeting on the Gibbs sampler and other Markov chain Monte Carlo methods. *Journal of the Royal Statistical Society Series B*, **55**, 67.

Muirhead, R.J. (1982), *Aspects of Multivariate Statistical Theory*. J. Wiley & Sons, New York.

Murray, G.D. (1977) Comment on "Maximum likelihood estimation from incomplete data via the EM algorithm" by A.P. Dempster, N.M. Laird and D.B. Rubin. *Journal of the Royal Statistical Society Series B*, **39**, 27–28.

Muthén, B. (1984) A general structural equation model with dichotomous, ordered categorical, and continuous latent variable indicators. *Psychometrika*, **49**, 115–132.

National Center for Health Statistics (1994) Plan and operation of the Third National Health and Nutrition Examination Survey. Vital and Health Statistics Series 1, No. 32.

Olkin, I. and Tate, R.F. (1961) Multivariate correlation models with mixed discrete and continuous variables. *Annals of Mathematical Statistics*, **32**, 448–465.

Orchard, T. and Woodbury, M.A. (1972) A missing information principle: theory and applications. *Proceedings of the 6th Berkeley Symposium on Mathematical Statistics*, **1**, 697–715.

Park, T. and Brown, M.B. (1994) Models for categorical data with nonignorable nonresponse. *Journal of the American Statistical Association*, **89**, 44–52.

Press, S.J. (1982) *Applied Multivariate Analysis: Using Bayesian and Frequentist Methods of Inference* (Second edition). R.E. Krieger Publishing Co., Malabar, FL.

Raymond, M.R. (1987) An interactive approach to analyzing incomplete multivariate data. Presented at the annual meeting of the American Educational Research Association, April 20–24, 1987, Washington, DC.

Raftery, A.E. and Lewis, S.M. (1992a) Comment on the Gibbs sampler and Markov chain Monte Carlo. *Statistical Science*, **7**, 493–497.

Raftery, A.E. and Lewis, S.M. (1992b) How many iterations in the Gibbs sampler? *Bayesian Statistics* (eds J.M. Bernardo, J.O. Bergen, A.P. Dawid and A.F.M. Smith), 765–776. Oxford University Press.

Raymond, M.R. and Roberts, D.M. (1983) Development and validation of a foreign language attitude scale. *Educational and Psychological*

Measurement, **43**, 1239–1246.

Richardson, S. (1996) Measurement error. *Markov Chain Monte Carlo in Practice* (eds W.R. Gilks, S. Richardson and D.J. Spiegelhalter), 401–417. Chapman & Hall, London.

Ripley, B.D. (1987) *Stochastic Simulation*. J. Wiley & Sons, New York.

Ritter, C. and Tanner, M.A. (1992) The Gibbs stopper and the griddy Gibbs sampler. *Journal of the American Statistical Association*, **87**, 861–868.

Roberts, G.O. (1992) Convergence diagnostics of the Gibbs sampler. *Bayesian Statistics* (eds J.M. Bernardo, J.O. Bergen, A.P. Dawid and A.F.M. Smith), 775–782. Oxford University Press.

Roberts, G.O. (1996) Markov chain concepts related to sampling algorithms. *Markov Chain Monte Carlo in Practice* (eds W.R. Gilks, S. Richardson and D.J. Spiegelhalter), 45–57. Chapman & Hall, London.

Rubin, D.B. (1974) Characterizing the estimation of parameters in incomplete data problems. *Journal of the American Statistical Association*, **69**, 467–474.

Rubin, D.B. (1976) Inference and missing data. *Biometrika*, **63**, 581–592.

Rubin, D.B. (1984) Bayesianly justifiable and relevant frequency calculations for the applied statistician. *Annals of Statistics*, **12**, 1151–1172.

Rubin, D.B. (1987) *Multiple Imputation for Nonresponse in Surveys*. J. Wiley & Sons, New York.

Rubin, D.B. (1994) Comment on "Missing data, imputation, and the bootstrap" by B. Efron. *Journal of the American Statistical Association*, **89**, 475–478.

Rubin, D.B. (1996) Multiple imputation after 18 years. *Journal of the American Statistical Association*, **91**, 473–489.

Rubin, D.B. and Schenker, N. (1986) Multiple imputation for interval estimation from simple random samples with ignorable nonresponse. *Journal of the American Statistical Association*, **81**, 366–374.

Rubin, D.B. and Thayer, D. (1978) Relating tests given to different samples. *Psychometrika*, **43**, 3–10.

Rubin, D.B. and Thayer, D. (1982) EM algorithms for factor analysis. *Psychometrika*, **47**, 69–76.

Rubin, D.B. and Thayer, D. (1983) More on EM for ML factor analysis. *Psychometrika*, **48**, 69–76.

Rubin, D.B., Schafer, J.L. and Schenker, N. (1988) Imputation strategies for missing values in post-enumeration surveys. *Survey Methodology*, **14**, 209–221.

Ryan, B.F. and Joiner, B.L. (1994) *Minitab Handbook* (Third edition). Wadsworth, Belmont, CA.

SAS Institute Inc. (1990) *SAS/STAT User's Guide, Version 6* (Fourth edition). SAS Institute Inc., Cary, NC.

Satterthwaite, F.E. (1946) An approximate distribution of estimates of variance components. *Biometrics Bulletin*, **2**, 110–114.

Schafer, J.L. (1992) A comparison of missing-data treatments in the post-enumeration program. *Journal of Official Statistics*, **7**, 475–498.

Schafer, J.L. (1995) Model-based imputation of census short-form items. *Proceedings of the Annual Research Conference*, 267–299, Bureau of the Census, Washington, DC.

Schafer, J.L., Khare, M. and Ezzati-Rice, T.M. (1993) Multiple imputation of missing data in NHANES III. *Proceedings of the Annual Research Conference*, 459–487, Bureau of the Census, Washington, DC.

Schafer, J.L., Ezzati-Rice, T.M., Johnson, W., Khare, M., Little, R.J.A. and Rubin, D.B. (1996) The NHANES III multiple imputation project. *Proceedings of the Survey Research Methods Section of the American Statistical Association*, to appear.

Schenker, N. and Welsh, A.H. (1988) Asymptotic results for multiple imputation. *Annals of Statistics*, **16**, 1550–1566.

Schervish, M.J. and Carlin, B.P. (1992) On the convergence of successive substitution sampling. *Journal of Computational and Graphical Statistics*, **1**, 111–127.

Schluchter, M. (1988) Analysis of incomplete multivariate data using linear models with structured covariance matrices. *Statistics in Medicine*, **7**, 317–324.

Searle, S.R., Casella, G. and McCulloch, C.E. (1992) *Variance Components.* J. Wiley & Sons, New York.

Serfling, R.J. (1980) *Approximation Theorems of Mathematical Statistics.* J. Wiley & Sons, New York.

Shih, W.J. (1987) Maximum likelihood estimation and likelihood ratio test for square tables with missing data. *Statistics in Medicine*, **6**, 91–97.

Silverman, B.W. (1986) *Density Estimation for Statistics and Data Analysis.* Chapman & Hall, London.

Smith, A.F.M. and Roberts, G.O. (1993) Bayesian Computation via the Gibbs sampler and related Markov chain Monte Carlo methods. *Journal of the Royal Statistical Society Series B*, **55**, 3–23.

Smith, C.A.B. (1977) Comment on "Maximum likelihood estimation from incomplete data via the EM algorithm" by A.P. Dempster, N.M. Laird and D.B. Rubin. *Journal of the Royal Statistical Society Series B*, **39**, 24–25.

Snedecor, G.W. and Cochran, W.G. (1989) *Statistical Methods* (Eighth edition). The Iowa State University Press, Ames, Iowa.

Tanner, M.A. (1993) *Tools for Statistical Inference, Methods for the Exploration of Posterior Distributions and Likelihood Functions* (Second edition). Springer-Verlag, New York.

Tanner, M.A. and Wong, W.H. (1987) The calculation of posterior distributions by data augmentation (with discussion). *Journal of the American Statistical Association*, **82**, 528–550.

Thayer, D.T. (1983) Maximum likelihood estimation of the joint covariance matrix for sections of tests given to distinct samples with application to test equating. *Psychometrika*, **48**, 293–297.

Thisted, R.A. (1988) *Elements of Statistical Computing: Numerical Computation*. Chapman & Hall, London.

Tierney, L. (1994) Markov chains for exploring posterior distributions (with discussion). *Annals of Statistics*, **22**, 1701–1762.

Tierney, L. (1996) Introduction to general state-space Markov chain theory. *Markov Chain Monte Carlo in Practice* (eds W.R. Gilks, S. Richardson and D.J. Spiegelhalter), 59–74. Chapman & Hall, London.

Titterington, D.M., Smith, A.F.M. and Makov, U.E. (1985) *Statistical Analysis of Finite Mixture Distributions*. J. Wiley & Sons, New York.

Verdinelli, I. and Wasserman, L. (1991) Bayesian analysis of outlier problems using the Gibbs sampler. *Statistics and Computing*, **1**, 105–117.

Wei, G.C. and Tanner, M.A. (1991) Applications of multiple imputation to the analysis of censored regression data. *Biometrics*, **47**, 1297–1309.

Weil, A.T., Zinberg, N.E. and Nelson, J.M. (1968) Clinical and psychological effects of marihuana in man. *Science*, **162**, 1234–1242.

Whittaker, J. (1990) *Graphical Models in Applied Multivariate Statistics*. J. Wiley & Sons, New York.

Wilks, S.S. (1962) *Mathematical Statistics*. J. Wiley & Sons, New York.

Winship, C. and Mare, R.D. (1989) Loglinear models with missing data: a latent class approach. *Sociological Methodology*, 331–367.

Wolter, K.M. (1985) *Introduction to Variance Estimation*. Springer-Verlag, New York.

Woodruff, R.S. (1952) Confidence intervals for medians and other position measures. *Journal of the American Statistical Association*, **47**, 635–646.

Wu, C.F.J. (1983) On the convergence properties of the EM algorithm. *Annals of Statistics*, **11**, 95–103.

Zeger, S.L. and Karim, M.R. (1991) Generalized linear models with random effects: a Gibbs sampling approach. *Journal of the American Statistical Association*, **86**, 79–86.

Index

Absorbing states 70, 82–3, 312, 315
Acceptance ratio 79–80
Adjusted goodness-of-fit statistics 323–4
Agresti, A. 8, 43, 49, 216, 240–2, 290, 292, 297, 300, 302, 313, 326, 369
Aitken acceleration 66
Aitkin, M.A. 383
All variables missing 163, 269
Amemiya, T. 28
Analysis of variance 34, 133, 147, 333
  multivariate 342–4
  relationship to loglinear models 240–2
Analyst's model 108, 140–4
Anderson, R.L. 123
Anderson, T.W. 15, 24, 150, 335, 372
Anti-lexicographical order 334, 395
Arnold, S.F. 70
Association versus interaction 292, 297
Autocorrelation 120–6, 132, 186, 189–90, 207–8
  test for 123
Autocovariance 100, 102

Baker, S.G. 28
Balanced repeated replication 144
Bartlett decomposition 184, 235

Bartlett, M.S. 123
Bartlett's formula 123, 186
Battese, G.E. 383
Bayesian IPF 289, 307, 397
  absorption onto a boundary 312
  cell-means version 314–15
  convergence proof 312–17
  defined 308–9
  example 318–20
  general location model 346, 358
  missing data, see DABIPF
  relationship to Gibbs sampling 318
  relationship to IPF 310
  starting values 310–11
  structural zeroes 311
Bayesian inference 4, 8
  Bayes's Theorem 17, 81
  cell means 313–14
  covariance matrices 153–4, 346–7
  empirical Bayes 57, 254
  general location model 339–41, 346–8
  loglinear models 305–6
  means 153
  multivariate regression 346–8
  proportions 250–1
  regression coefficients 226, 346–7
  with incomplete data 17, 171–2
Bayesianly proper multiple imputations 105–6

Beale, E.M.L. 16, 163
Beaton, A.E. 159
Becker, R.A. 7, 370, 399
Belin, T.R. 66, 382
Bentler, P.M. 384
Berger, J.O. 157
Berliner, L.M. 93
Besag, J. 50, 70
Beta distribution 76, 247
Between-imputation variance 109,
     113
Bibby, J.M. 151, 159, 347
Binary data 42
    imputing as normal 148, 202–4,
       214
Binder, D.A. 145
Binomial distribution 242
Binomial Theorem 244
Birch, M.W. 297
Bishop, Y.M.M. 8, 50, 242, 247,
    292, 294, 299–300, 303, 305
Bivariate normal model 15,
    18–20, 34–5
    alternative parameterizations
       15, 18
    boundary estimates 53–4
    ignorable missingness 24–6
    likelihood ridges 53
    multiple modes 51–2
    nonignorable missingness 26–7
Blenkner, M. 272
BMDP 3, 370, 380
Bollen, K.A. 384
Bootstrap resampling 128, 194,
     208
Boundary estimates 53–4, 63,
    137, 170, 179, 263, 274, 303,
    308, 324, 327
Box, G.E.P. 8, 18, 29, 73, 96, 122,
    155, 252
Bradlow, E. 386
Bromberg, J. 266
Brown, M.B. 28, 266
Brownstone, D. 112
Bryk, A. 382

Burn-in period 91, 119, 133, 138

CM step
    loglinear models 321–2
    general location model 357
    see also ECM algorithm
Canonical form 40
Carlin, B.P. 70, 83, 380, 382
Carnegie Mellon University 399
Case deletion 1–2, 23–4, 201
Case-influence statistics 386
Casella, G. 66, 69–70, 80
CAT software 399
Categorical data 8, 29, 39, 50, 83,
    239
    applying normal model to
       147–8, 202–4, 214, 239
    higher-order associations in 29
Categorizing continuous data 239
Censored data 385
Census 30, 44, 300, 383–4
Centering and scaling 169, 172
Chambers, J.M. 7, 370, 399
Chen, T.T. 44, 260, 282, 303, 331
Cholesky factorization 181–3,
    233, 355, 358
Cholesterol in heart-attack
    patients 175–8, 185–8, 193–200
Clayton, D.G. 380, 382
Clogg, C.C. 240, 253–4, 303, 308,
    384–5
Clustering 30, 376–7
Coarsened data 385
Cochran, W.J. 20, 31, 33, 107,
    196, 373
Coefficient of variation 196
Collapsed table 244, 256, 277
Complete-case methods 24–8, 201
Complete-data estimator 108–9,
    195–6
Complete-data model 9–10
    departures from 29–31, 140–4,
    211–12
    role of 29
Compound symmetry 191, 379

Conaway, M.R. 28
Conditional versus marginal
    association 274, 329
Confidence region 155
Configurations of loglinear model
    294
Connectedness 70, 87
Constraints on parameters 46–9,
    54–5, 62, 341–3
    loglinear 50, 290, 313, 315,
    341–2
Contaminated normal
    distribution 380
Contingency table 50
    2 × 2 tables 42–4, 46–9
    from matrix of categorical data
    240, 257–9, 334
    storage of 395–7
    see also Loglinear models;
    Multinomial model
Contrasts among means 178,
    189–92
Correlated samples 90–3
Correlation coefficient 54, 109
    inferences about 215
Correlogram 122
Covariance matrix
    Bayesian inference for 153–4,
    346–7
    between-imputation 113
    constraints on 191, 379–80
    from EM 62–4
    ML estimate of 150
    residual 157
    restricted 379–80
    singular 155–6
    within-imputation 113
Cox, D.R. 29, 40, 46, 54, 63, 96,
    108, 380, 385
Cross-product ratio, see Odds
    ratio
Current Population Survey 27
Cyclic ascent 50

DABIPF algorithm

general location model 357–9
    examples 359–77
    loglinear models 324–325
    examples 325–31
Data augmentation 2, 8, 37, 90
    binary data example 76–7
    burn-in period 91
    convergence 80, 83–6
        missing information and
        84–5, 137
        of posterior summaries 131–4
        slow 87, 121, 237
        to stationarity 128–31
    defined 70–1
    general location model, see
        DABIPF algorithm
    inconvenient prior distributions
        79
    loglinear models, see DABIPF
        algorithm
    monotone, see Monotone data
        augmentation
    multinomial model 264–7, 396
        examples 267–79, 284–5
    multiple chains 72, 75, 92,
        126–8, 131–4, 139
    multivariate normal model
        181–5
        examples 185–92, 193–217
    nonconvergence 80–3, 123–4,
        205–6
    Rao-Blackwellized density
        estimates from 99
    relationship to EM 37, 73, 80
    relationship to Gibbs sampling
        71
    starting distribution 86–7
    starting values 85–7, 127–8, 133
    univariate normal examples
        73–6, 84–5, 120–4
David, M. 27
Degrees of freedom in loglinear
    models 292, 303
DeGroot, M.H. 155
Deming, W.E. 299

Dempster, A.P. 3, 8, 16, 37–9, 46,
    54–5, 58, 154, 159–60, 163
Density and distribution functions
    empirical 94
    estimation of 94–5, 99
Dependent samples 90–3
    summarizing 93–8
Design matrix
    general location model 342–4
    loglinear models 290, 299, 306,
        316–17, 341–2
Deviance statistic 302–3, 322–4,
    345–6
    with missing data 322–4
Devroye, L. 95
Design-based inference 31, 105,
    107–8, 144
Design variables 31–2, 35, 143
Determinant 158, 170, 224–5
    from sweep 160
Diagnostics 386
Diffendal, G.J. 66
Diggle, P.J. 28, 379
Dirichlet distribution
    as a prior 250–5, 339, 346
    collapsing and partitioning
        255–7
    constrained 306, 346
    defined 247
    factorization of 257
    properties 248–9
    relationship to gamma 249
Discriminant
    analysis 334
    function, linear 349–52, 354
Distinct parameters 11, 17, 32,
    157–8, 246
Dodge, Y. 35
Dorey, F.J. 385
Double precision 169
Double sampling 20, 226, 237
Draper, N.R. 157, 177, 224
Driver injury and seatbelt use
    282–7, 303–5, 318–20, 328–31

E-step
    defined 39
    general location model 352–4,
        357
    loglinear model 320
    multinomial model 261, 396
    multivariate normal model
        164–8
    regular exponential family 40
    relationship to I-step 73
    see also EM algorithm
ECM algorithm 40
    convergence 67–8
    defined 49–50
    general location model 357
    loglinear models 321–2
    Supplemented 68
EM algorithm 2–3, 5, 8, 37–40
    2×2 table 42–5, 46–9
    accelerated 65–6
    convergence 51, 207
        accelerating 65–6
        detecting 61–2
        prior information and 66–7
        rate, elementwise 64–6, 177,
            179
        rate, overall 42, 55–61
        slow 61–2
    covariance matrix from 62–4
    defined 37–9
    examples 41–5, 46–9, 175–81,
        274
    forced 63
    loglinear models 320–1
    multinomial model 260–4, 274,
        396
    multivariate normal model 16,
        163–75
    posterior modes from 46,
        170–5, 262–3
    regular exponential family
        39–40
    standard errors from 62–4
    starting values 169–70, 262
    trajectory of 130

univariate normal data 41–2, 59–61
Efron, B. 13, 128
Eigenvalue 56, 58–9, 61, 64, 67, 130, 170, 179, 185, 201
Eigenvector 56, 58–9, 61, 64, 130, 185
Elementwise rates of convergence 64–6, 177, 179
Emerson, J.D. 29
Empirical Bayes 157, 254
Empty cells, *see* Random zeroes, Structural zeroes
Equal-tailed intervals 96
Ergodicity 82, 297
Estimability of parameters 28, 52
Exchangeability 30
Expectation-Conditional Maximization, *see* ECM algorithm
Expectation-Maximization, *see* EM algorithm
Experiments
  unbalanced 21–2, 32–5
Exponential family 39–40, 41, 149, 243, 297
Everson, P.J. 30, 382
Ezatti-Rice, T.M. 144, 148
Ezzati, T. 373

Factor analysis 384–5
Fay, R.E. 28, 140–1
Fienberg, S.E. 8, 44, 50, 242, 247, 254, 260, 292, 294, 299–300, 303, 305
Finite-population inference 107–8
Fischer, J. 272
Fisher, R.A. 54, 109, 216, 372
Fisher information 57
Fisher scoring 300
Fisher's z-transformation 54, 109, 216, 372
Fixed-point equations 42
Flattening constant 253

Flattening prior 253–4, 263, 266, 274, 368–9
Followup data
  for nonrespondents 20–3
  for response errors 283–4, 303–5, 318–20, 328–31, 385
Foreign Language Attitude Scale 200–11, 338–9, 344–6, 367–72
Fortran 7, 399
Fraction of missing information 42, 58, 61, 110, 129–30, 177
  from EM 62, 64–5, 204, 207
  from multiple imputation 110, 200
Fractional observations 360
Francisco, C.A. 210
Frequentist perspective 105, 112, 155, 171–2, 374
Fuchs, C. 260, 263, 272, 274, 321, 323
Fuller, W.A. 210, 383

Gamma distribution 249, 256
Gamma function 153
Gelfand, A.E. 4, 68–70, 98–9, 126, 318, 380, 382
Gelman, A. 8, 68, 79, 87, 126–7, 132–4, 138, 308, 318, 382, 386
Geman, D. 4, 70
Geman, S. 4, 70
General ignorable procedure 23–6, 35
General linear mixed model 382
General location model
  Bayesian inference 339–41, 346–8
  complete-data likelihood 336
  conditional distributions 348–51
  DABIPF algorithm 357–9
  data augmentation 355–6
  defined 335
  design matrix 342–4
  ECM algorithm 357
  EM algorithm 352–5, 357

examples 338–9, 344–6, 359–77
factorization of likelihood 336,
    341
ML estimation 336–9, 344
observed-data likelihood 354
predictive distributions 348–51
prior distributions 339–41,
    346–8, 368–9
random zeroes 336–7
restricted models 341–8
semicontinuous variables 382
sparse data 337, 341, 360–2
structural zeroes 336
sufficient statistics 336
sweep 351–2
Generalized linear models 144
    with random effects 382
Gentle, J.E. 4, 249
George, E.I. 69–70, 80
Geweke, J. 132
Geyer, C. 68, 93, 132, 138
Ghosh, M. 383
Gibbs sampling 2–4, 8, 69–70
    convergence 70
    defined 69
    nonconvergence 80
    relationship to data
        augmentation 71
Gilks, W.R. 8, 69, 382, 385
Glynn, R.J. 28
Good, I.J. 305–6
Goodman, L.A. 295, 384–5
Graham, J.W. 23
Grand mean 291
Graphical models 380
Greenlees, J.S. 27

Haberman, S.J. 303
Haenszel, W. 326
Hansen, M.H. 21
Harrell, F. 370
Harter, R.M. 383
Hastings, W.K. 4, 78
Hat matrix 178

Heart rate and marijuana use
    178–81, 189–92
Heavy-tailed distributions 380
Heckman, J. 28
Heitjan, D.F. 385
Hierarchical loglinear model
    293–4
Higher-order associations 239, 286
Highest posterior density (HPD)
    method 96–8, 155, 171
Hill, J.R. 128
Hinkley, D.V. 40, 46, 54, 63, 96,
    108
Histogram 94
Hochberg, Y. 282, 303
Holland, P.W. 8, 50, 242, 247,
    254, 292, 294, 299–300, 303,
    305
Homogeneous association 293
Hurwitz, W.N. 21
Hybrid algorithms 4, 79–80, 325
Hyperparameters
    Dirichlet prior 251–5
    normal inverted-Wishart prior
        154–7
Hypothesis testing 96–7
    loglinear models 302–3, 322–4

I-step
    defined 72–3
    general location model 355–6
    loglinear models 324–5
    monotone data augmentation
        230–1, 280–2
    multinomial model 264–6, 396
    multivariate normal model
        181–3
    see also Data augmentation
IPF algorithm 50, 289
    Bayesian, see Bayesian IPF
    comparison to other methods
        299–300
    convergence 299
    defined 298–9

general location model 344,
   346, 357
history 299–300
loglinear coefficients from 299,
   319
missing data, *see* ECM
   algorithm
posterior modes 307–8, 346
random zeroes 300
standard errors from 300
structural zeroes 300
Identifiability, *see* Estimability of
   parameters
Ignorability assumption 11, 17,
   23, 37, 62, 323
defined 11
examples 20–2, 24–7
and proper imputations 105–6
iid assumption 2, 240
departures from 29–30
Imaginary results 155
Imputation
ad hoc 1–2
consistency checks 204
mass 383
mean imputation 1
model 31, 107, 139–45
regression predictions 24
unit-level categorical data
   266–7, 325
see also Multiple imputation
Income in Current Population
   Survey 27
Inestimable parameters 52–3, 54,
   56, 63, 137, 205, 263
Inference, meaning of 90
Intensity parameter 313
Interaction versus association
   292, 297
Interaction models 367–8, 380–1
Internal Revenue Service 27
Interval estimation
in Bayesian inference 95–6
from multiple chains 133–4

Inverted-chisquare distribution
   19, 102–3, 151
Inverted-Wishart distribution 19,
   150–1, 340–1
Item nonresponse 383
Iterated conditional modes 50
Iterative proportional fitting, *see*
   IPF algorithm

Jackknife 144
Jacobian matrix 19, 55, 158–9,
   224–5
Jeffreys prior 155, 252, 285, 347,
   369
Jenkins, G.M.
Jennrich, R.I.
Jensen's inequality 39
Joiner, B.L. 175
Jöreskog, K.G. 384
Justel, A. 386

Kadane, J.B. 44
Karim, M.R. 30, 382
Kaufman, S. 383
Kennedy, W.J. 4, 249
Kent, J.T. 151, 159, 347
Kenward, M.G. 28
Kernel density estimation 94, 103
Khare, M. 144, 148
Kleijnan, J.P.C. 4
Knuiman, M.K. 306
Kong, A. 70, 83, 98, 227
Kott, P.S. 140
Kronecker product 346–7, 358
Krzanowski, W.J. 10, 341

Laird, N.M. 3, 8, 16, 28, 30, 37–9,
   46, 54–5, 58, 66, 163, 306, 382
Lange, K.L. 380
Lange, N. 66, 380, 382
Lansky, D. 66
Latent variables 384–5
Latin square 179
Lauritzen, S.L. 380

Law of large numbers 91, 119
Leonard, T. 306
Leverage 177, 180
Lewis, S.M. 132, 138
Li, K.H. 70, 72, 77, 114–16, 218, 228
Liang, K. 379
Likelihood function
  curvature of loglikelihood 57, 108
  factorization of 12, 15, 18, 20, 32–3, 219–20, 245–6, 325, 336
  ridges in 52–3, 54, 56, 63, 137, 205, 263
  see also Observed-data likelihood
Likelihood-ratio test 12, 47, 135
  2 × 2 tables 48
  general location model 345–6
  loglinear models 302–3, 308, 322–4
  multiply imputed data 116–18, 210–11
  statistic, posterior distribution of 131, 188, 270
Lindsey, J.K. 379
Linear convergence 55, 66, 299
Linear discriminant function 349
Little, R.J.A. 8, 10–12, 16, 28, 37, 42, 159, 163, 169, 171, 218, 223, 260, 323, 341, 351–2, 357, 359–60, 380, 383, 385
Liu, C. 120, 228, 235, 380, 382
Liu, J. 70, 83, 98, 120, 227
Liu, M. 382
Logistic regression 208, 239, 333
  and loglinear models 295–7, 329–31
  multinomial response 297, 369–71
  multiply imputed data 209–11, 329–31
  proportional-odds model 369–71

sparse data 253
Loglinear models 8, 10, 51, 239, 242, 298
  boundary estimates 303, 308, 324, 327
  coefficients, obtaining 299, 319
  configurations 294
  correspondence to logit models 295–7, 329–31
  defined 289–90
  design matrix 290, 299, 306, 316–17
  examples 303–5, 325–331
  factorization of likelihood 325
  general location model 341–2
  goodness of fit 302–3, 322–4
  grand mean 291
  hierarchical 293–4
  hypothesis testing 302–3, 308, 322–4
  interactions 290–2
  interpretation of 295
  loglikelihood 294
  ML estimation 297–8
  main effects 290–2, 295
  missing data, see ECM algorithm; DABIPF algorithm
  odds ratios 289, 292–5
  posterior mode 307–8
  prior distributions 305–6
  random zeroes 300
  relationship to factorial analysis of variance 290–2
  saturated 286, 289, 323
  sparse data 253, 303, 326
  structural zeroes 300, 311, 322
  three-way tables 290–7
  see also Multinomial model; IPF algorithm; Bayesian IPF
Longford, N.T. 383
Longitudinal data 218, 226, 379–80
Louis, T.A. 57, 66

M-step
  defined 39
  loglinear model 320–1
  multinomial model 261–3
  multivariate normal model 166, 172–3
  regular exponential family 40
  restricted parameter space 47
  see also EM algorithm
ML estimation 12
  asymptotic covariance matrix 56–7
  boundary estimates 53–4, 63, 137, 170, 179, 263, 274, 303, 308, 324, 327
  invariance 162, 224
  general comments on 54–55
  general location model 336–9, 344
  large-sample properties 54–7, 63, 108
  loglinear models 297–8
  multinomial model 243
  multivariate normal model 149–50
  nonuniqueness 52–3, 54, 56, 63, 137, 205, 263, 274, 337
MacEachern, S.N. 93
Madow, W.G. 383
Makov, U.E. 384
Malec, D. 383
Manning, W.G. 381
Mantel, N. 326
Mantel-Haenszel test 326
Mardia, K.V. 151, 159, 347
Mare, R.D. 28
Marginal homogeneity in 2×2 tables 49, 267–9
Marginal versus conditional association 274, 329
Marijuana use 178–81, 189–92
Markov chain Monte Carlo 2–5, 8, 68–87
  assessing convergence
    of posterior summaries 131–4

    to stationarity 118–31
  defined 68
  law of large numbers for 91–2
  meaning of convergence 80, 118–20
  properties 80–7
  see also Data augmentation; Gibbs sampling; Metropolis-Hastings algorithm; Hybrid algorithms
Mass imputation 383
Matrices, storage of 169, 351–2
Matrix inversion and sweep 160
Matrix sampling 21, 237
Maximum likelihood, see ML estimation
McCullagh, P. 144, 208, 210, 369
McNemar, Q. 49
Meng, X.L. 8, 37, 49–50, 57, 59, 63–4, 67–8, 116–7, 140–2, 210, 321–2, 386
Metropolis, N. 4, 78
Metropolis-Hastings algorithm 2–4, 8, 78–9
Middleton, R. 79
Misclassification error 283–4, 303–5, 318–20, 328–31
Missing at random (MAR) 10–13, 17, 23, 24–7, 62, 191–2, 323
  defined 10–11
  examples 13–14, 20–2, 25–7
Missing by design 22, 62, 237
Missing completely at random (MCAR) 11, 13, 23, 25–6, 41
Missing information
  convergence of data augmentation and 84–6, 120–1, 137
  convergence of EM and 58–9, 137, 163, 170, 177, 207
  defined 57
  fraction of, see Fraction of missing information

missing observations and 129,
177–81, 229
model complexity and 286
principle 56–8, 66–7
prior information and 66–7
Rao-Blackwell method and 102
Missingness pattern 16, 163
monotone, *see* Monotone
missingness
MIX software 399
Mixed continuous and categorical
data 10, 29, 51, 333–6
see also General location model
Mixture models 384–5
Modern Language Aptitude Test
201
Moment equations 40, 149, 243,
297–9
Monotone data augmentation
226–9, 236–8, 275–6, 325
defined 227
loglinear models 325
multinomial model 280–2,
285–6
multivariate normal model
229–38
Monotone missingness 218, 228–9
multinomial model 284
multivariate normal model
219–20, 223–6
Monte Carlo error
assessing 92, 134, 138, 190
multiple imputation 106–7
posterior summaries 131–4
Rao-Blackwell method 100
Morris, C.N. 30, 382
Muirhead, R.J. 151, 184
Multiparameter inference 97–8
Multiple chains
convergence of posterior
summaries 132–4
convergence to stationarity
126–8
versus single chains 72, 75, 92,
131–4, 137–9

Multinomial model 10, 42
alternative parameterizations
245–6, 276–8
Bayesian inference 250–1,
279–80
collapsing and partitioning
243–5, 261, 277
complete-data likelihood 42,
242, 277–8
data augmentation 264–7
examples 268–79
defined 240–1
EM algorithm 42–4, 46–9,
260–4
examples 44-5, 47–9, 274
factorization of likelihood
245–6, 275–8
ML estimates 42, 243
moments 242
observed-data likelihood 48,
259–60, 264
parameter space 241–2
prior distributions 247, 250–5
random variate generation
265–6
saturated 239, 242, 286, 289,
323
sufficient statistics 42, 243
see also Loglinear models
Multiple imputation 5, 104–18,
139
Bayesianly proper 105–6
choosing number of
imputations 197–99
complete-data estimators 108–9
complex surveys 144–5, 212–13
defined 90–1, 104–5
examples 193–217, 270–2,
329–31, 367–77
frequency evaluations of 112
generating imputations 138–9
inferences for
correlation coefficients
215–16

logistic regression coefficients 209–11, 329–31
means 196, 215
odds ratios 216, 270–1
partial correlations 371–2
proportions 215, 270–1
quantiles 215
ratios of means 196
nonparametric analyses and 144–5
relationship to Rao-Blackwellization 106–7
rules for combining
likelihood-ratio tests 116–18, 210–11
multiparameter estimates 112–14
p-values 115-16
scalar quantities 109–12
proper 105–6, 145
public-use data files 139, 143
simulation studies 114–20, 145, 211–218, 374–7
validity of 140–4
versus parameter simulation 135–6, 144, 198–200
why only a few imputations are needed 106–7
Multiple modes 51–52, 54, 63, 125, 127, 137, 360, 363, 385
Multivariate normal model 10, 29, 147–8
alternative parameterizations 157–9, 161–2, 220–3
application to categorical data 147–8, 202–4, 214, 239
Bayesian inference 151–4
complete-data likelihood
data augmentation 181–5
examples 185–217
density function 148
EM algorithm 163–175
examples 175–181
ML estimation 149–50
observed-data likelihood 16

prior distributions 150–2, 154–7, 171–2, 224–5, 238
random variate generation 181–2
sufficient statistics 149
see also Bivariate normal model
Multivariate t-distribution 127, 347, 380
Murray, G.D. 51
Muthén, B. 384

National Center for Health Statistics 212, 373
National Crime Survey 44–5, 47–9, 267–72
National Health and Nutrition Examination Survey 212–14, 236–8, 372–7
Nelder, J.A. 144, 208, 210
Nested iterations 40, 47, 321, 325
Nested models 302
Newton-Raphson algorithm 16, 40, 50, 300, 385
convergence of 55
Nisselson, H. 383
Nominal variables
applying the normal model to 203
Nonignorable nonresponse 26–8, 384
Nonlinear programming 49
Non-multinomial sampling 246–7
Nonnormal data 147, 203, 214, 239–40, 380–2
Nonparametric methods 31, 109
and multiple imputation 145
Nonresponse followup 20–3
NORM software
Normal distribution
univariate 41–2, 59–61, 73–6, 84–5, 120–4
see also Bivariate normal model; Multivariate normal model

Normal inverted-chisquare
    distribution 19, 152, 226
Normal inverted-Wishart
    distribution 19, 151–4, 171,
    175, 347
    limiting form of 154
    random variate generation
    184–5
Numeric overflow 124

Oakes, D. 385
Observed-data likelihood
    2 × 2 table 48
    bivariate data 14–15
    defined 11–13
    design variables and 33
    general ignorable procedures
        and 23
    general location model 354
    monitoring 61, 131, 170
    monotone missingness 219–220
    multinomial model 48, 259–60,
        264, 323
    multivariate normal model 16,
        173–5
    univariate data 13
Observed-data posterior 17–20, 23
    defined 17
    design variables and 23
    oddly shaped 87, 125, 127, 130,
        137, 360–2
Observed information 57
Odds ratio 45, 48, 268, 272–5,
    272–5, 283, 326, 364–5
    effect of flattening prior on 253,
        274
    loglinear models 289, 292–5,
        326
    multiply-imputed data 216,
        329–31
    pooling 326–31
Olkin, I. 335, 383
Orchard, T. 54, 163
Ordinal data 148, 240, 369–70

applying the normal model to
    202–203, 240
Outlier detection 385–6
Output analysis 119
Overparametrized models 54, 181,
    191, 360–2
Oversmoothing 253–4, 368–9, 371

P-step
    defined 72–3
    general location model 356,
        358–9
    loglinear models 324–5
    monotone data augmentation
        231–4, 281–2
    multinomial model 264–6
    multivariate normal model
        264–6
    see also Data augmentation
p-values 96–7, 112–13
    Bayesian 97
    rule for combining 115-16
Packed storage 169, 185
Parallel chains, see Multiple
    chains
Parameter simulation 6, 89–104,
    137–8
    defined 89–90
    robustness of 136, 144
    versus multiple imputation
        135–6, 144, 198–200
Parameter space
    restrictions on 46–9, 50, 55, 62,
        290, 313, 315, 341–3
Park, T. 28
Partial correlation 371–2
Partitioned table 244, 256–7, 277
Pearson's X^2 statistic 272, 302–3
    with missing data 322–4
Pedlow, S. 8, 37
Peña, D. 386
Pennsylvania State University 201
Periodicity 70, 315
Poisson-gamma model 313–4
Posterior distribution and density

estimation of 94–5, 99
large-sample normality of 96,
    98 *see also* Observed-data
    posterior
Posterior mean 93, 108
    estimation of 91, 93, 98–9, 138
    non-invariance of 252
Posterior mode
    EM algorithm for 46, 170–3,
        175, 262–3, 274
Posterior predictive checks 386
Posterior predictive distribution
    of missing data 105
Posterior quantiles 95
Posterior regions and intervals 95
Posterior tail areas 97
Posterior variance 91–3, 108
Predictive distribution 38, 348–51
Press, S.J. 153, 346, 348, 382
Primary sampling units 374,
    376–7
Prior distributions 6, 55
    bivariate normal model 18
    conjugate 18, 150, 306
    factorization of 11, 17, 244–5,
        257, 278–279
    flattening 253–4, 263, 266, 274,
        368–9
    general location model 339–41,
        346–8, 368–9
    improper 18, 73, 75, 81, 143,
        154, 251, 266, 347
    informative 155–7, 207, 235,
        252–5, 274, 340–1, 347–8
    Jeffreys 155, 252, 285, 347, 369
    loglinear models 305–6
    multinomial model 247, 250–5
    multivariate normal model
        150–7, 171–2, 224, 235
    noninformative 81, 143, 154,
        171, 224, 235, 251–2, 339,
        347
    ridge 155–7, 170, 172, 207, 235
    uniform 252
    univariate normal model 73, 75

Prior information 67, 85
    contingency tables 253–4,
        251–2, 274, 303, 324
    multivariate normal model 155
Product-multinomial distribution
    44, 245–6, 261, 276, 281
Proper multiple imputations
    105–6, 145
Proportional-odds model 369–70
Protective Services Project 272–5,
    325–8
Pseudocode 168–9, 174, 182,
    221–2, 233, 261–2, 264–5, 268,
    301, 310–11
    defined 168

Quadratic convergence 55, 300
Quantile estimation 95
    with multiply-imputed data
        215
Quasilikelihood 144

Raftery, A.E. 132, 138
Raghunathan, T.E 114
Raking 299–300
Random-effects models 30, 377,
    382–3
Random zeroes 263, 266, 300,
    303, 336
Rao, J.N.K. 383
Rao-Blackwell method 75–6,
    98–104, 126, 132, 136, 187–8
    efficiency of 100–4
    relationship to multiple
        imputation 106–7
Ratio of means 196
Rats, weight gain 33–4
Raudenbush, S. 382
Raymond, M.R. 200–1
Regression 32
    linear 15, 24, 34, 147, 157, 220,
        223–6, 371
    logistic, *see* Logistic regression
    missing predictors 33

multivariate 157, 164, 335–6, 342–4, 347–9, 382
ridge 157
Regular exponential family 39–41, 149, 243, 297
Relative increase in variance due to nonresponse 110, 114, 117
Repeated measures 3, 218, 379–80
Replication in Markov chain Monte Carlo 92, 134, 138
Response errors 283–4, 303–5, 318–20, 328–31, 385–6
Richardson, S. 8, 69, 382, 385–6
Ridge prior 155–7, 170, 172, 207, 235
Ripley, B.D. 132
Ritter, C. 120
Roberts, D.M. 201
Roberts, G.O. 69–70, 79, 83, 120, 138
Robustness 30–1, 136, 144, 147, 211–12
Rounding errors 170
Rubin, D.B. 3, 5, 8, 10–13, 16, 28, 37–9, 42, 46, 49–50, 53–5, 58, 63–4, 67–8, 87, 90, 104–10, 112, 114, 116–7, 126–7, 132–4, 138, 140–1, 145, 159, 163, 169, 210, 212, 218, 223–4, 260, 271, 321–3, 372, 380, 382–3, 385–6
Ryan, B.F. 175

S language 7, 399
SAS 370
SECM algorithm 68
SEM algorithm 63–4, 127
Saddlepoint 52, 54, 56
Satterthwaite, F.E. 134
Saturated model 239, 242, 286, 289, 323
Schafer, J.L. 26, 28, 30, 144, 148, 212, 373, 376–7, 384
Schenker, N. 28, 112, 212, 385
Schervish, M.J. 70, 83
Scheuren, F. 383

Schluchter, M.D. 10, 341, 351–2, 357, 359–60, 379
Searle, S.R. 30
Seatbelt use and driver injury 282–7, 303–5, 318–20, 328–31
Sedransk, J. 383
Seemingly unrelated regressions 382
Semicontinuous variables 381–2
Sensitivity analysis 252
Serfling, R.J. 215
Serial correlation 120–6
Shih, W.J. 49
Shihadeh, E.S. 240
Silverman, B.W. 95
Simple random samples 30
Simplex 241–2, 246–7
Simulation
    comparison of complete-case versus ML estimates 24–7
    inference by 4–5, 64
    parameter, see Parameter simulation
    studies of multiple imputation 114–20, 145, 211–218, 374–7
Single chains
    convergence of posterior summaries 131–2
    convergence to stationarity 119–126
    versus multiple chains 72, 75, 92, 131–4, 137–9
Small-area estimation 383
Smith, A.F.M. 4, 68–70, 79, 83, 98–9, 120, 138, 318, 384
Smith, C.A.B. 62
Smith, H. 157, 177, 224
Smoothing
    contingency tables 253–5, 303, 327, 368–9
    covariance matrices 156, 172, 207
Snedecor, G.W. 33
Software for missing data 3, 7
Sörbom, D. 384

Space-filling conditions 321–2
Sparse data 55, 125
    contingency tables 252, 274–5,
        303, 326
    general location model 337, 341
    multivariate normal model
        155–6, 170, 172
Speed, T.P. 306
Spiegelhalter, D.J. 8, 69, 382, 385
St. Louis Risk Research Project
    359–66
Standard multivariate regression
    336
Starting values
    data augmentation 85–7, 119,
        138–9
        multiple 126, 138–9
        overdispersed 86–87, 127–8,
            133, 139
    EM algorithm 169–70, 262
Stationary distribution 3, 68, 72,
    79, 119
StatLib 399
Stephan, F.F. 299
Stram, D. 66, 382
Stratification 30–3, 246–7
Structural equations models
    384–5
Structural zeroes 241, 263–4, 266,
    300, 311, 322, 336
Subsampling a chain 92–3, 106,
    132
Sufficient configurations 294–5
Sufficient statistics
    general location model 336
    loglinear models 294–5
    multinomial model 42, 243
    multivariate normal model 149,
        164–8, 231–4, 172–3
    regular exponential family 40
Sun, W. 145
Superefficiency 141–2
Supplemented ECM, see SECM
    algorithm

Supplemented EM, see SEM
    algorithm
Surveys
    complex designs 29–30, 212,
        373, 383
    Current Population Survey 27
    imputation 31, 107–8, 372–7,
        383–4
    National Crime Survey 44–5,
        47–9, 267–72
    National Health and Nutrition
        Examination Survey 212–14,
        236–8, 372–7
    nonresponse in 20–3, 383
    raking 299–300
    strata and poststrata 31–3, 246
    variance estimation 144, 383
Sweep operator 159–62, 165–8,
    172–3, 181–3, 220–3, 232–3,
    351–2
    defined 159
    general location model 351–2
    reverse sweep 160
    submatrices 220–2
Symmetry in 2×2 tables 49,
    267–269

t-distribution 103, 134, 153
    in multiple-imputation
        inference 109–11
    multivariate 127, 347, 380
Table sampling 265, 267
Tanner, M.A. 8, 69–72, 99, 120,
    126, 385
Target distribution 68
Tate, R.F. 335
Taylor, J.M.G. 380, 382
Taylor series expansions
    EM algorithm 55
    ratio of means 196
Thayer, D. 21, 53, 385
Thisted, R.A. 159, 182
Three-way tables
    loglinear models for 290–7
Tiao, G.C. 8, 18, 73, 96, 155, 252

Tibshirani, R.J. 128
Tierney, L. 68, 70, 79, 83, 91
Time series 120–6
    erratic behavior in 124, 362
    multiple 137
    stationary series 121–2
Titterington, D.M. 384
Total variance 109, 114
Transformations
    of data 29, 147, 169, 217
    of parameters 63, 118, 157–9,
        162, 216, 220–3, 245–6, 279
Two-way associations 239, 293,
    367–8

Unix environment 399

Variance estimation
    complex surveys 144, 383
    from a single chain 132
    from multiple chains 132–4
Verdinelli, I. 386

Wald test 113, 115, 117–8
Ware, J.H. 30, 382
Wasserman, L. 386
Wei, G.C. 385

Weil, A.T. 178, 189
Welsh, A.H. 112
Wermuth, N. 380
Whittaker, J. 380
Wilks, A.R. 7, 370, 399
Wilks, S.S. 248, 255
Winship, C. 28
Wishart distribution 150
    inverted
        see inverted-Wishart
            distribution
    random variate generation 184
Within-imputation variance 109,
    113
Worst linear function of
    parameters 129–31, 185
Wolter, K.M. 144, 373
Wong, W.H. 70–2, 83, 98–9, 126,
    227
Woodbury, M.A. 54, 163
World Wide Web 399
Wu, C.F.J. 39

Zaslavsky, A.M. 386
Zeger, S.L. 30, 379, 382

Printed and bound by CPI Group (UK) Ltd, Croydon, CR0 4YY

17/10/2024

01775680-0006